THE **BODY REPAIR** AND
MAINTENANCE
MANUAL

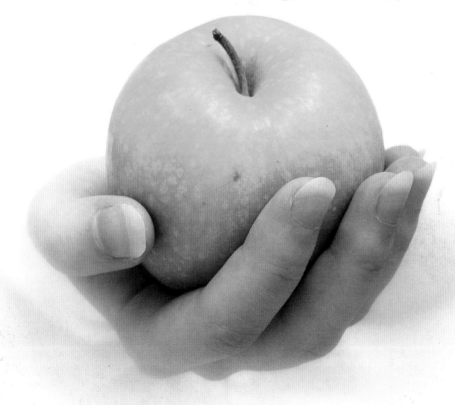

THE BODY REPAIR

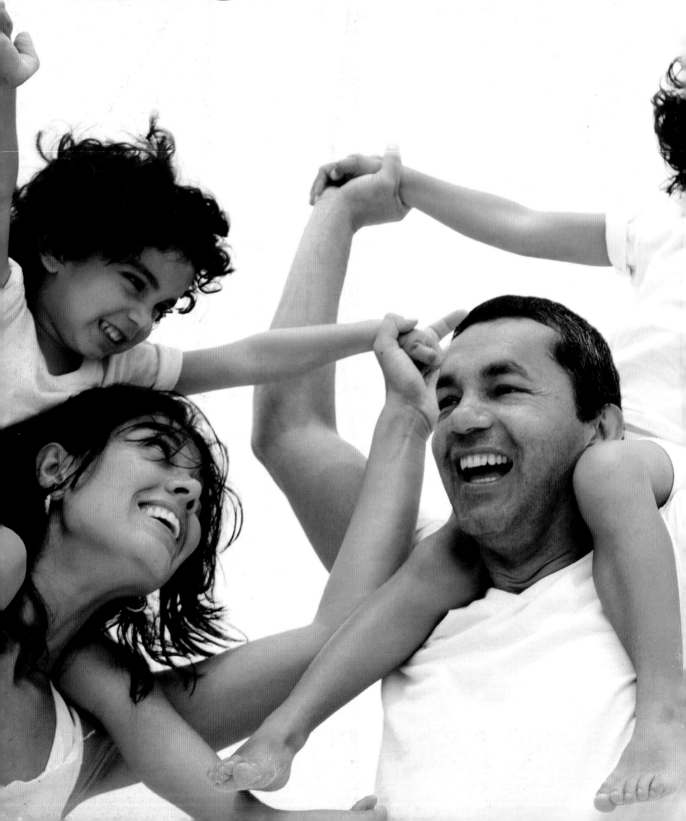

AND MAINTENANCE MANUAL

Published by Reader's Digest Association Ltd

London • New York • Sydney • Montreal

KEY TRUTHS
OF FULL HEALTH

Illness is *not* inevitable

Damage *can* be undone

Good health is a *choice* you make,
not a pill you take

Good health includes *happiness*

Good health *feels* great

To be healthy years from now,
be healthy *today*

1
NEW KEYS TO HEALTH

2
REPAIRING THE PAST

The full-life promise 10

The truth about ageing 14

Seven keys to ageing well 20

Assessing the damage done 38

Body repair: one, two, three ... four 40

Ranking the habits: a doctors' poll 44

Erasing the damage 48

3
LIVING
HEALTHY TODAY

4
PROTECTING FUTURE
HEALTH

Am I leading a
healthy life?   96

Ready, set ... slow!   106

Eat to feel good   110

Move to feel good   174

Live to feel good   238

Take charge of
everyday health   262

Preventing the
diseases of ageing   314

Get the most from
your health care   372

Resources   382

Index   384

NEW KEYS

1

The full-life promise

The truth about ageing

Seven keys to ageing well

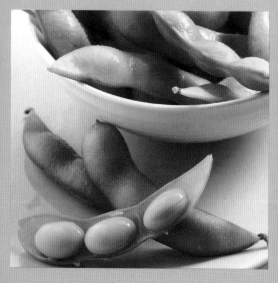

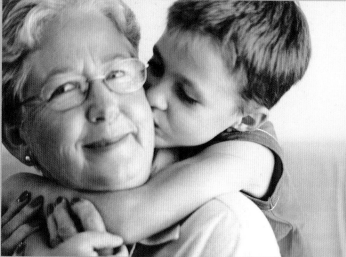

TO HEALTH

Throw out all your old notions about ageing. We are entering a golden era of health in which we can live longer, healthier and **more** energised than before

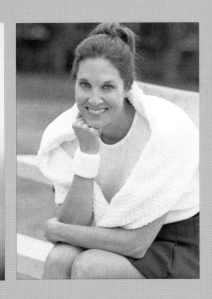

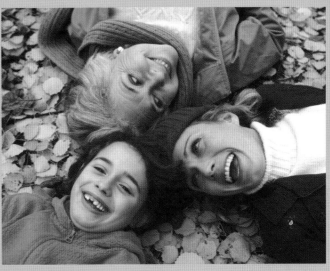

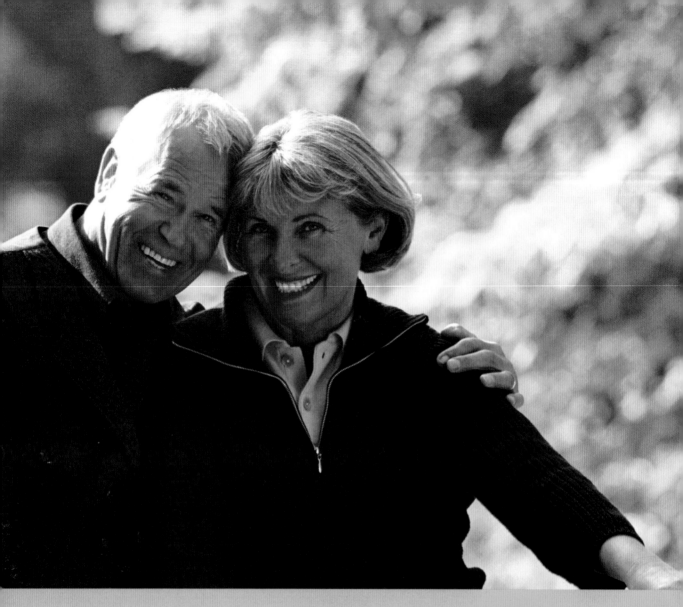

The full-life promise

You may not realise it, but fate has given you an extraordinary gift. You have been born at a point where people live longer than at any time in human history. Compared with the vast majority of people who have passed through this planet, you have been given on average 30 years' more life to enjoy than they had. Do you realise how wonderful this is?

Until a century ago, the average person died in his or her 40s. Before the 20th century, the cycle of life was much more compressed for most people. Your work life might have begun at the age of eight or ten; by 15 you were a parent; by 30, a grandparent; and by 40, your body was more than likely broken, pain-filled and in final decline.

Today, most people who turn 40 believe they have yet to get to the halfway point of their lives. Some are just becoming parents; others are finally launching their 'real' careers. In biological and psychological terms, old age now begins at 80, according to Ian Robertson, dean of research at Trinity College Institute of Neuroscience in Dublin. 'This leaves 30 years – roughly age 50 to 80, a period much longer than youth – for which we have to invent a whole new way of living.'

After all, today's life expectancy in the UK is nearly 77 for men and 81 for women. People aged 85 and older make up the fastest-growing segment of the population in most countries. By 40, we really are just at the middle of our lives – and our wisdom, capabilities and contributions are often just beginning.

Pete Townshend of the famed rock group The Who was only 20 years old in 1965 when he penned the words, 'I hope I die before I get old', a phrase that became the rallying cry for an entire generation. More than 40 years later, Townshend and The Who are still releasing creative, high-intensity rock albums and touring the world. Their appearance might be older, but their energy and attitude aren't. The message: being old no longer has much to do with the number of years you've lived.

So what is 'old'? Old may be your great-grandmother, who was bent, shaky and mentally faded well before her time. Old are the people whose vitality long ago slipped away, leaving them in wheelchairs in nursing homes. Old is the lonely, tired older person who stays in the house and talks to the cats all day in between television shows.

As for the rest of us – we're just getting started.

THE GOAL: LONG HEALTH

Popular phrases such as 'anti-ageing' and 'long life' are deceptive. They imply that the goal of healthy living is to add more years to your life. And, in fact, you *can* add even more years to your life by having a healthy, optimistic outlook. Some scientists hypothesise that the human body, when perfectly maintained, can comfortably last 120 years before naturally giving out.

But as mentioned, modern health care and lifestyles have already given you the opportunity to live to a ripe old age far beyond that of our ancestors. The goal today isn't merely extra years. It is *long health*.

'Long health' means that you are vibrant, creative and energised at any age – be it 44, 58, 72, 85 or 94. It's understanding that although we all have to die one day, an infirm, sedentary life is not the inevitable final chapter of our lives. It means that you do not accept that the diseases of ageing – heart disease, arthritis, insomnia, Alzheimer's, diabetes and so on – are your destiny. Long health is living an active, healthy, happy, purposeful life – now and right up until your very final days.

Sounds ideal, doesn't it?

Better still, long health (as you will discover throughout this book) isn't achieved by swallowing pills, visiting doctors or launching yet another formal exercise routine. Ageing is neither a disease to be treated with medicine nor a process to be reversed through denial, sacrifice or hard work. Instead, achieving long health is a process to be respected and enjoyed. As you'll read over and over, active, happy living every day is the path to long health.

In other words: the best path to being happy, energised and healthy in the future is living happily, energetically and healthily in the present.

So what is the first step to achieving long health? It is recalibrating how you think about ageing. Throw out any notions that ageing is a slow, sad decline towards death, and that your goal is merely to get to some artificial age threshold, like a high-stakes marathon race in which all that matters is reaching the finish line, no matter what torture it causes you.

The truth is that how long you live isn't the issue; it's how well you live. Nothing is more heartbreaking than seeing someone you love confined to a nursing home aged 72. Instead, wouldn't you rather see someone of 72 still playing tennis? Or 75 and running for public office for the first time? Or 81 and completing a 4 mile hike through a forest on a beautiful day? These are not hypothetical examples; these are all activities that real people, real 'old' people, are still doing and enjoying. There is even known to be one centenarian who plays 18 holes of golf three times a week and consistently shoots 15 strokes under his age!

The thing is, these people didn't wait until their 80s to start golfing or hiking. Rather, at some point earlier on, they chose to live more actively and healthfully – perhaps in their youth, perhaps in retirement. That's the beauty of long-health living – the benefits and pleasures it delivers are both immediate and long term.

You are part of a generation that is redefining ageing. It's already happening; when approximately 3,500 people with an average age of 80 were asked their ideas about ageing, more than 60 per cent said their opinions had changed in the past 20 years. Nearly all had thought about how they could age successfully instead of viewing ageing in a negative way. To them, freedom from disease, being able to function independently and remaining actively engaged with life were critical components in successful ageing.

In addition, more than 90 per cent of this group listed 'remaining in good health until close to death' as the most important component of successful ageing. After that followed:

- Being able to take care of myself until close to the time of my death
- Remaining free of chronic disease
- Having friends and family who are there for me
- Being able to make choices about factors that affect how I age, such as my diet, exercise and smoking
- Being able to cope with the challenges of my later years
- Being able to meet all of my needs and some of my wants
- Feeling satisfied with my life the majority of the time
- Being able to act according to my own inner standards and values.

Notice anything missing? Less than a third chose 'living a very long time' as a component of successful ageing. In fact, that statement was last on the list of 20 choices.

THE NEW WORLD OF AGEING

Obviously, we're heading into a new world of ageing. There are no road maps or rules for this new world. But never fear: you won't be alone. Worldwide, the number of people aged 65 and above is increasing faster than any other demographic group, particularly in developed countries. By 2030, 12 in every 100 people will be 65 or older, nearly double the percentage in 2000. In Europe and North America, that figure will be one in five people. And throughout the developed world, those aged 85 and above are now the fastest-growing age group.

In this new world, retiring to the golf course is being replaced with working part-time, with flexible hours; active volunteering; and pursuing new interests and new friendships. Sedentary holidays such as bus tours and cruising the islands are giving way to bike trips through wine countries, volunteer missions to build houses in developing countries, and art courses in Provence.

In this new world, you're less likely than your parents and grandparents to find yourself living with a disability or in poverty, and you are more likely to have completed further education – all markers for successful ageing.

This is a world in which you accept the cosmetic changes time has wrought on your body, as long as your spirit remains robust. A world in which you have finally realised that there's more to good health than not being in bad health. And a world in which our old perceptions of ageing – that cognitive decline and frailty are inevitable, for instance – have been turned on their head.

It is also a world in which the past can be changed, at least when it comes to harmful habits and activities. Even if you got frequent sunburns in your youth, drank a lot or (gasp!) smoked marijuana, the damage can be managed and minimised, as you'll learn in these pages. So, yes, perhaps you wish you'd eaten less junk food, quit smoking earlier, done more to protect your bones and joints and worried less, but it's never too late to change and to see the benefits of those changes. That's what this book is all about. ■

Secrets of the long-lived

In the year 2000, the United Nations estimated that there were more than 180,000 people above the age of 100 throughout the world, a figure that will jump to 3.2 million by the year 2050. Centenarians are the fastest-growing section of the UK population. According to the Office for National Statistics (ONS), between 1911 and 2006 the number of people aged over 100 increased 90-fold, from about 100 to around 9,000 – and by 2031 it's predicted that there will be 40,000.

If you're a man of 40 reading this, you have an 8 per cent chance of reaching the magic 100, and if you're female you have almost a 12 per cent chance. For babies born today the odds are even better – 18.1 per cent for boys and 23.5 per cent for girls.

So, what's the secret?

If only we knew. Despite dozens of studies on centenarians, there doesn't seem to be a typical life pattern or history shared by these long-lived folks. Still, researchers say that they have found some similarities.

People who live to 100 and beyond tend to:
- Complain less about pain and discomfort than younger people with fewer disabilities, suggesting that centenarians are better at adapting to what life hands them
- Remain intellectually stimulated
- Maintain satisfying social relationships
- Keep their interests in creative activities
- Have few sleep problems
- Become anxious or depressed only rarely
- Find great solace in their religious faith
- Be financially secure
- Believe that they can be happy
- Be extroverted

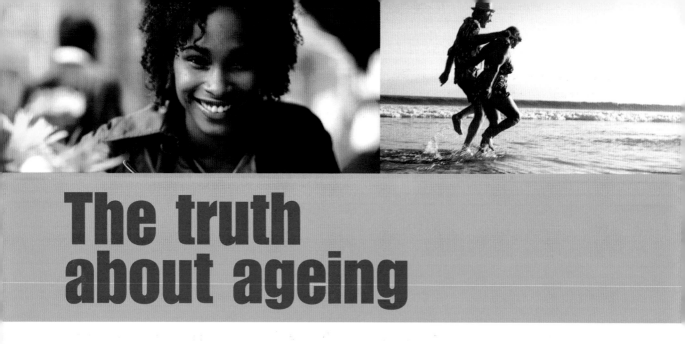

The truth about ageing

I f you rely on what you see on TV, in films or in magazines, old age means frailty, infirmity and dementia. But if you talk to the people actually doing research on ageing, they'll tell you that popular culture has it all wrong. They're questioning every assumption about the effects of ageing on our physical and mental health and finding some pretty surprising results.

Forget everything you ever thought you knew about ageing and memory, says Sonia J. Lupien, PhD, who directs the Center for Studies on Human Stress at McGill University in Canada. She has a rather surprising argument for why we falsely believe older people have worse memories and declining learning abilities. To her, it's because the studies on which we base this opinion are deeply flawed.

You have to consider how the studies are conducted, she says. People have to come to a university setting, typically in the afternoon, where they're tested by a young graduate student. The 'young' participants are typically university students who know where they're going on campus, feel comfortable being tested by someone close to their own age and prefer afternoon testing since they like to sleep late.

Testing for older people Now consider this from the perspective of one of the older participants. You have to drive to the university and find a parking space, or take public transport, then navigate the campus until you find the right room. You're confronted with someone young enough to be your grandchild who asks extremely personal questions then puts you through the tests. You've probably been up since 6am, so afternoons may simply not be your best time. You probably prefer to take a nap around 2pm rather than a test (in fact, studies find memory is strongest in older people in the morning and in younger people in the afternoon).

The stress factor So if you're an older person, Dr Lupien says, the whole experience is really stressful. This is bad in two ways: first, the older you are, the more intensely your body reacts to stress; and second, stress and memory, as she and others have shown in dozens of studies, are like oil and water. The more acute stress you experience, the worse your memory.

Then there's the test itself. If you give older people words to memorise and tell them that you're evaluating their memory, they'll do poorly. If you give them the same words to memorise and tell them that you're evaluating the learning capacity of older adults, they'll do much better. Why? Because everyone – including that older participant – is conditioned to believe that memory gets worse with age. And you know the drill: if you think something *is* a certain way, then it will be. It's a self-fulfilling prophecy.

Here's the important point: when researchers look more closely at the people taking the memory tests, they find that those who are in good physical health, educated, employed and with a good income have memorisation skills just as strong as those of people who are 30 years younger.

'Don't talk to me about any age-related impairment in memory until you take stress into account,' Dr Lupien says. In fact, she's doing just that. In a major study funded by the Canadian Institutes of Health Research, her 70-year-old research assistant asks the questions and conducts the memory tests in the morning in an off-campus location that the older people (but not the younger participants) have already visited for a pre-study cocktail party. 'The young participants hate it,' Dr Lupien says with a grin.

AGEING TRUTHS, AGEING MYTHS

What other myths about the physical and mental effects of ageing exist? Here are some big ones.

Creaky, achy joints are an inherent part of ageing Hardly. A more accurate statement would be that creaky, achy joints are an inevitable part of not exercising. Researchers from the University of Kuopio in Finland studied 55 men and 226 women aged 55 to 75 undergoing knee operations for osteoarthritis,

and calculated their lifetime of physical exercise, compared with 524 people selected at random from the local population. After taking account of factors such as age, weight, physical work stress and past knee injuries, they found that the higher someone's cumulative hours of exercise, the lower their risk of osteoarthritis of the knee severe enough to require surgery. 'Moderate recreational physical exercise is associated with a decrease in the risk of knee osteoarthritis,' they concluded.

Fragile bones and a bent posture are inevitable with age One thing you'll learn from reading this book: *very little* is inevitable with age except death. While osteoporosis is definitely a condition that's more prevalent in older people, it's also one that's very preventable. For instance, a study of 424 female centenarians found that only 56 per cent had osteoporosis, and their average age at diagnosis was 87. That's not bad, particularly considering that these women grew up long before we understood the benefits of diet and exercise on bone.

Your genes are the most important determinant in how well you'll age Ha! If that were the case, then identical twins would age identically. But they don't. A major study from European and American researchers evaluated the lifestyle habits and medical history of 40 pairs of identical twins aged 3 to 74. As the twins aged, the researchers found, not only had their health taken different paths, but their genome changed from identical to one that showed several differences. Genetically speaking, the oldest pair of twins was the least alike.

How so? It all goes back to the 'nature vs. nurture' argument. You might be born with the healthiest set of genes nature can provide, but how you live your life (the nurture part)

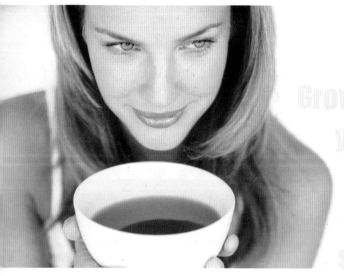

determines how those genes behave over the next 90 years. It turns out that what you eat, how much physical activity you get, even your exposure to chemicals can change your genes through methylation – a process that plays an essential role in maintaining cellular function (changes in methylation patterns may contribute to the development of cancer).

You lose your creative potential as you age Don't tell that to Gene Cohen, MD, PhD, who directs the Center on Aging, Health, and Humanities at George Washington University in Maryland. Dr Cohen, who is in his 60s, started a second career as a game-maker a few years ago. Such creativity offers tremendous benefits for older people, he's found. For the past decade, he and his colleagues have been studying the impact of art and music participation on older adults. In one study of 168 healthy older adults, those who joined a choral group were in better health, used less medication, were less lonely and had fewer falls after a year than a similar group of non-singers.

And according to research by François Matarasso for Comedia, a leading independent research centre in the UK, participation in the arts increases people's confidence, sense of self-worth, self-reliance and involvement in social activity. Another study in Sweden tracking more than 10,000 people found that those who regularly attended cultural events had a lower mortality rate 13 years later than those who did not.

You become less sexual and less able to have sex as you age Not so says Terrie B. Ginsberg, DO, of the New Jersey Institute for Successful Aging. In a major review of sexuality and ageing, she notes that 'contrary to many of our cultural and societal views of the ageing individual, our ageing population continues to enjoy their sexuality'. The key is keeping yourself in shape. Impotence and reduced libido aren't related to age but to medical conditions that can, in most instances, be prevented, such as high blood pressure, heart disease, diabetes and depression. Something as simple as lifting weights a couple of times a week can improve your sex life.

Sexuality in later life has received limited attention from researchers. But according to surveys including more than 1,500 people, published in the *British Medical Journal*, older people are increasingly reporting an active – and fulfilling – sex life. Over 30 years, researchers from Gothenburg University in Sweden questioned groups of 70-year-olds about their sex lives. Between the first sample, in 1971, and the last, in 2000, the proportion saying that they had sexual intercourse increased among all groups: married men from 52 per cent to 68 per cent, married women from 38 to 56 per cent, unmarried men from 30 to 54 per cent, and unmarried women from 0.8 to 12 per cent.

People who reached 70 in the later samples also reported higher satisfaction with their sex lives and fewer sexual dysfunctions, and the number of women reporting having orgasms increased. It is clear, as the researchers say, that 'most elderly people consider sexual activity and associated feelings a natural part of later life'.

A note of caution for any older people re-entering the dating scene, though. A survey for *Saga Magazine* of nearly 8,000 people aged 50 and over found that although most were sexually active, many were risking sexually transmitted infections by not using condoms with new partners. And according to data from the Health Protection Agency, sexually transmitted infections are rising faster among the over-45s than in younger age groups, probably because they have less need to use condoms to guard against pregnancy and are less aware of the need for protection against sexually risky behaviour.

Your brain stops developing after the age of three When this developmental myth was overturned in the 1990s, it created a seismic shift in the way researchers viewed ageing. No longer could they look at the older brain as static. Instead, studies show, your brain continues to send out new connections and to strengthen existing connections throughout your life – as long as you continue to challenge it. It really *is* the ultimate muscle in your body.

Your brain shrinks with age This myth began with studies in 2002 showing that the part of the brain that controls memory, the hippocampus, was significantly smaller in older people than in younger people. Yet ground-breaking research conducted in the 1990s by Dr Lupien showed that chronic stress shrinks the hippocampus. Was it age or stress that was responsible for the shrinking brains of older people?

Probably stress. When she examined brain scans of 177 people aged 18 to 85 she found that 25 per cent of the 18 to 24 year olds had hippocampus volumes as small as those of adults aged 60 to 75. Her point is that perhaps 'the smaller hippocampus in the older person was already there when they were younger, possibly as a result of stress'. In fact, other research she has conducted found that people born *during* the world wars have smaller hippocampuses than those born *between* the two wars; the likely reason is that those born during the wars were exposed to so much stress early in life.

Older people are cranky and unhappy Not quite. When researchers from Heidelberg, Germany, interviewed 40 centenarians, they found that despite significant physical and mental problems, 71 per cent said they were happy and more than half said they were as happy as they'd been at younger ages. Plus, when the researchers compared them to a group of middle-aged people, they found that both groups were just as happy. Most important: nearly 70 per cent of the centenarians said they laughed often.

What does it all mean? That there is no universal definition of ageing. How you'll age is entirely up to you – starting today. ▪

Ageing
through the decades

Here's a quick glimpse at some of the age-related changes that do occur as we move through our decades. It's a surprisingly short list: most other common signs of 'ageing' have little to do with age and everything to do with lifestyle.

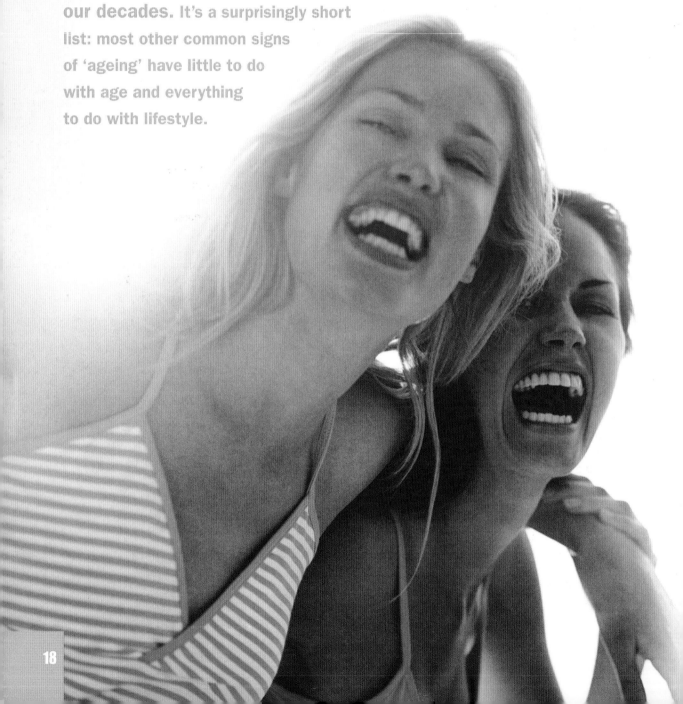

20

● The first signs of age appear in your skin as the collagen fibres that keep your skin taut begin to weaken.

30s

● By the end of the decade, you may find your first grey hair. Men may find their hair colour fading and their hair, well, disappearing.

● You've passed the halfway mark in terms of bone strength. During this decade, bone breaks down faster than it builds up.

● By the time you turn 39, you'll probably find it harder to maintain your weight with the same eating/exercising regimen you followed at the beginning of the decade. Your metabolism is slowing – time to pump up the physical activity.

● This is the time when women's fertility begins waning. It may take longer to get pregnant and you may need to call in the experts for a little boost.

40s

● Gasp! Is that a wrinkle? Yes, this is the time of life when the sun you worshipped as a teen and in your 20s turns on you.

● By the middle of this decade, you're more likely to die of cancer than from accidents.

● By the end of the decade, you may find your days of rock 'n' roll have left sounds slightly muffled. Even if you were a classical-music aficionado, your eardrums have lost elasticity, affecting your hearing.

● Oh, and don't forget the reading glasses. The question is not 'if' you'll develop presbyopia, a type of farsightedness, but 'when'. It occurs because the lens of your eye stiffens with age, making it more difficult to focus.

50s

● One day, you look down at your hands but see your grandmother's hands. Sadly, though, they *are* your hands, and all those brown spots and puffy veins are the result of years of sun exposure and the increasing inability of your skin to rid itself of gunk called lipofuscin – produced when free radicals build up in the skin.

● Early this decade, women will reach menopause. The average age of menopause in most countries is 52.

60s

● Even though you can't see it, you probably have small pockets throughout your intestines called diverticula. They won't bother you unless bits of digested food become caught in them, in which case they get inflamed and infected. To prevent this, make sure you get plenty of fibre.

● Men may find themselves having some urinary problems from an enlarged prostate.

● Your risk of developing cataracts increases. Your optometrist (optician) can detect these during a routine eye check, and they are easily removed with minor surgery.

70s and 80s

● How you'll feel in your 70s and 80s really depends on how you spent the past six decades. If you never exercised, you smoked, drank a lot and considered late-night TV intellectual fare, you may find yourself frail with diabetes and heart disease and fighting chronic pain from arthritis – and you may always be forgetting simple things.

... connect with friends and family

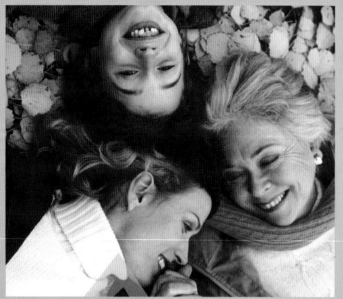

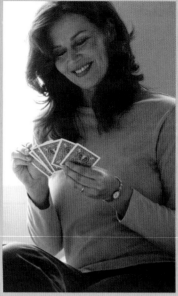

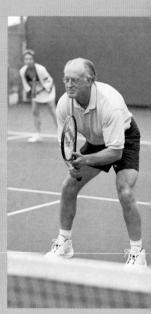

... stress your mind in positive ways

... find something interesting to do

Seven keys to ageing well

A heaped plate of food – and a brimming social calendar. Freedom from diets – and plenty of time for fun and meaningful activities. A peek at the new science of ageing reveals a new view of how to live long and prosper. And we're all for it.

With wisdom gleaned from some of the longest-living, healthiest cultures in the world, as well as new insights made possible by high-tech studies, researchers say that old views of ageing are simply outmoded. Yes, our bodies change. But an inevitable slide in health as we age? Absolutely not! Each of us can live strong, healthy, vibrant, energetic lives for a long time

to come. The key? Actually, there are seven of them. Read on – you may never see your bathroom scales, dinner plate or friends in the same way again.

Be prepared for surprises. Only three of the seven keys involve nutrition and fitness. The other four are related to your attitude, optimism and social interactions. As this book notes over and over, how you choose to live your life has far more impact on your health than any vitamin or pill. The philosopher René Descartes famously wrote, 'I think; therefore, I am', but the new science of ageing suggests that the important truth is really 'how I think is how I am'.

But first, the runners-up

The seven keys in the pages ahead represent the best advice for living a healthy, happy, vibrant, long life. But our experts also pointed to these five actions as being particularly beneficial for long life and long health. So we proudly present this 'silver-medal' advice first.

Drink lots of water After 60, your sense of thirst diminishes, so you may not even realise you're thirsty. The benefits of water are vast – topping up your tank with five to eight glasses a day can cut your risk of a deadly heart attack by up to 54 per cent and at the same time ease constipation, boost flagging energy and even lower your risk of cancers of the breast, prostate and large intestine, research suggests. And drinking three or more cups of tea a day may be as beneficial as drinking plenty of water, according to nutritionists from King's College, London. Tea rehydrates the body just as well as water, they say, and may also protect against heart disease and some cancers due to its high flavonoid (antioxidant) content.

Eat more frequently Three small meals and two or three snacks a day are a great way to get all the nutrition you need – and more. You'll keep your blood sugar lower and steadier to guard against diabetes and heart conditions associated with blood sugar problems. You'll avoid a starve-and-binge pattern that can lead to extra weight. And you'll have more chances to eat with friends and family – as nutritious for the mind and spirit as food is for the body. Let moderation replace deprivation, and you'll be happier and healthier.

Keep junk out of your body It's great to eat organic food when you can. But it's even more important to avoid the common food additives and ingredients that are potent health wreckers: excess sodium, trans fats, saturated fat, sugar and refined carbs. These have little nutritional value, and a diet high in such 'junk' food ingredients can increase your risk of obesity, high blood pressure and heart disease, put your blood sugar on a roller coaster and even fire up body-wide chronic inflammation – a powerful risk factor in everything from heart disease and stroke to cancer and more.

Get the rest you truly need Insomnia – exhausting and mysterious – becomes common as we age. Sleep patterns change radically after 55, when your body clock resets itself and levels of melatonin and growth hormone drop. Medical conditions, prescription or over-the-counter drugs, eating patterns, exercise habits, time outdoors and bedtime routine all play important roles in your sleep as well. And because we often don't know how to adjust, an estimated 41 per cent of women aged 80+ experience insomnia, as do 23 per cent men aged 70+. Feeling sleepy all the time can be annoying and dangerous. But it doesn't have to happen: experts say it's possible to be well rested if you work with, not against, changing sleep cycles.

Learn to relax In a study that followed 202 women and men for more than 18 years, researchers found that those who practised meditation had a 23 per cent lower risk of dying from any cause during the study and a 30 per cent lower risk of death from heart disease. Cutting stress can help your body to heal faster, your mind function better and your digestion work better. You'll sleep better, too. The best news: you don't have to sit alone in a room saying 'Om ... '. Spending time with friends, enjoying nature and listening to music promote the deep relaxation we all need. ■

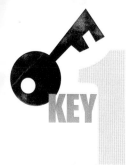

Worry less about losing weight

At some point a few decades ago, it became a widely held belief that you could be healthy – and attractive – only if you were lean. So, for much of our lives, we have gone about our business in a world obsessed with diet plans, mirrors, swimsuits and belly fat.

As it turns out, the 'overweight equals unhealthy' equation isn't quite that simple; even more shaky, particularly for mature adults, is the equation 'losing weight equals better health'.

In fact, new research shows that the drastic calorie-cutting strategies and scale-watching that slimmed jiggly thighs in your 20s, 30s or 40s can set you up for bone fractures, weak muscles and weight *gain* in your 50s, 60s or 70s. Even worse, those popular weight-loss approaches fail to target the belly fat that causes serious weight-related health problems such as diabetes and heart disease. In reality, significant weight loss – either intentional or unintentional – can be life-threatening after the age of 60.

Dieting or trying to return to an 'ideal' weight may not be best for older women, provided they're not obese. It's possible that maintaining body weight may actually keep you more robust and healthy later in life.

In one study of older women, those who maintained their weight for six years had a 13 per cent chance of dying, but those who lost weight increased their risk to 22 per cent.

Women who had up-and-down weight swings also had eye-opening results. Scientists now think that even fairly minor weight swings – from 2 to 4kg (5 to 8lb) for a 1m 65cm (5ft 5in) woman – are associated with a significantly increased risk of death. So unless your waist measurement or BMI is too high (see box opposite), dieting the way you may have done in your 20s *isn't* the healthy option when you're older.

Experts aren't totally sure why weight loss cuts life short in older people. Some lose weight due to an underlying serious illness, but that's not the full story. Dropping pounds on purpose, another study shows, is risky even for the *healthiest* older people. When researchers from the University of California, San Diego, tracked 1,801 women and men over the age of 71 for 12 years, they found that women who lost weight were 38 per cent more likely to die during the study, while men were 76 per cent more likely to die.

Here's what we do know.

Losing weight means losing muscle Older adults naturally have less muscle density than in their 20s, 30s or 40s. So their metabolism slows and thus burns fewer calories during the day. Losing weight accelerates this process. If you lose 5kg (11lb) on an old-fashioned low-cal diet, you'll drop 2.5kg (5½lb) of fat – and 2.5kg (5½lb) of muscle that you can't afford to lose, say experts. Losing that much muscle will lower

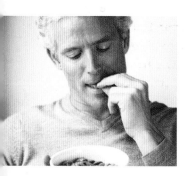

the key Action

Eat for good nutrition and disease prevention. Do that, and your weight will take care of itself your metabolism even further, so you're burning 150 to 250 fewer calories a day.

Less muscle also means you'll be weaker, with less balance and flexibility – raising the odds for a fall. And once your diet ends, you're likely to regain lost weight as fat. If it's around your middle, it will pump out chemicals that fire up chronic, low-level inflammation throughout your body, raising your odds of developing insulin resistance, diabetes, heart disease and even Alzheimer's disease and some cancers.

Dieting threatens bones, too Many studies have shown that among older people, weight loss – whether deliberate or because of illness – leads to loss of bone mineral density. This applies especially to women around the time of menopause and afterwards, and increases their risk of sustaining a fracture during a fall.

You'll never know you've lost bone density or muscle from bathroom scales. And scales won't tell you if you have too much visceral fat – the kind packed inside your abdomen that raises the risk of diabetes and heart disease.

So, rather than eating to lose weight, focus on eating for good nutrition and disease prevention. Then get the exercise you need to build more smooth, dense, strong muscle. Plenty of dramatic studies prove that women and men as old as their late 80s and 90s who stick to a simple, safe, resistance-training programme can build strength and agility, replace puffy fat with sleek muscle, and develop a renewed zest for life.

In one landmark study conducted at the Jean Mayer USDA Human Nutrition Research Center on Aging at Tufts University in Boston, 40 women aged 50 to 70 who swapped their non-exercising routine for a twice-a-week weight-training programme built muscle, lost

Better than the bathroom scales

If you need a number to help you to judge whether your weight is healthy, skip the scales. Instead, try these two. (If your numbers are higher than they should be, make sure you're following a healthy-eating plan and getting regular exercise.)

- **Your waist size** Grab a tape measure. A waist that measures 88cm (34½in) or less for women or 100cm (40in) or less for men is considered healthy. Anything higher could mean you're carrying around the type of visceral belly fat that raises your odds for diabetes and heart disease.

- **BMI (Body Mass Index)** This tells you whether you are the right weight for your height. Divide your weight in kilograms (kg) by your height in metres (m)^2, that is:

$$\frac{\text{weight (kg)}}{\text{height (m)}^2}$$

For example, if you weigh 70kg and you are 1.75m tall, the formula looks like this: BMI = 70/(1.75 x 1.75) = 22.9

Less than 18.4 = underweight
18.5–24.9 = ideal weight
25–29.9 = overweight
30–39.9 = obese
over 40 = very obese

fat, developed stronger bones and became physically stronger than their daughters. They were slimmer, happier, stronger – and healthier. Yet the scales barely budged.

What if you find yourself losing weight without even trying? Do pay attention to the scales in that case – and tell your doctor. Unplanned weight loss may be a sign of nutritional deficiency, hormone imbalance, medication side effects, depression, infection or serious illness. ■

great advice For a comprehensive guide to healthy eating, easy exercise and smart appetite control, turn to the 'Eat to feel good' and 'Move to feel good' chapters.

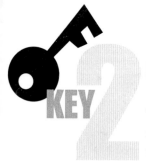

Eat fewer calories, but more food

That's no misprint. When nutrition researchers ate across the globe – from Greece to the Japanese island of Okinawa to Pennsylvania – they found a tummy-satisfying secret to good health: pile your plate high with vegetables and fruits, add respectable portions of beans and whole grains, and downplay high-calorie fare such as burgers and cream sauces.

The result: fewer calories, more health-boosting antioxidants and longer, happier and more active and independent lives. 'Ounce for ounce, people on Okinawa eat *more* food by weight than people who eat a Western-style diet,' says Bradley Willcox, MD, of the Pacific Health Research Institute in Honolulu and lead researcher of the Okinawa Longevity Study. 'They eat a lot of produce and grains and smaller portions of higher-calorie, higher-fat foods. It's the combination of high nutrition and lower calories that gives them a tremendous health advantage: their risk for dementia, heart attacks, strokes and cancer are among the lowest in the world.'

Maintain your body Okinawans aren't starving. They eat about 1,800 calories a day. (In contrast, in many Western cultures, the average adult eats close to 2,500.) 'Slight calorie restriction seems to prime the body for survival,' Dr Willcox says. 'Just cutting back by 10 per cent can have a dramatic effect.

The theory is that this throws genetic "master switches" so that more maintenance work gets done: your cells invest more time and energy in repairing DNA; there's less oxidation (damage from rogue oxygen molecules called free radicals that leads to all sorts of diseases); and insulin, the hormone that tells cells to absorb blood sugar, becomes more effective.'

We're not talking about starvation diets. Yes, eating extremely low-cal diets has extended the lives of earthworms in labs, but the jury's out on whether this impractical and even dangerous practice lengthens human life. Simply refocusing your food priorities by eating smaller portions of calorie-dense foods and copious amounts of plant-based foods is all you need to do.

Lose the belly fat What's more, eating more fruit and vegetables boosts your intake of vitamins and free radical-busting antioxidants.

Researchers at the University of Cambridge have shown in a study of more than 19,000 healthy people aged 45 to 79 that waist to hip ratio is inversely associated with blood levels of vitamin C, independent of body mass index. In other words, no matter how heavy you are, if you have low vitamin C levels you're more at risk of abdominal obesity – the belly fat that's especially hazardous. Meanwhile, in the USA, University at Buffalo researchers have found that a single high-calorie meal boosts the body's production

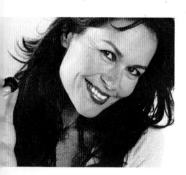

the key Action

Eat as many vegetables, fruits and whole grains as your appetite desires of unhealthy free radical molecules. These rogue oxygen molecules damage cells and cause low-level inflammation throughout the body.

Dump the junk This type of inflammation has been linked with a higher risk of diabetes, heart disease, high blood pressure, stroke and even breast and prostate cancers. The scientists found that a fast-food breakfast sent a rush of free radicals into the bloodstream that stayed at high levels for the next 3 to 4 hours.

'A high-fat, high-calorie meal temporarily floods the bloodstream with inflammatory components, overwhelming the body's natural inflammation-fighting mechanisms,' says Ahmad Aljada, PhD, a researcher at the University at Buffalo School of Medicine and Biomedical Sciences. 'People who experience repeated, short-lived bouts of inflammation resulting from many such unhealthy meals can end up with blood vessels in a chronic state of inflammation, a primary factor in the development of atherosclerosis.'

What's happening? Digesting food requires oxygen. The more calories you eat, the more your body must digest – and the more free radicals are produced as a side effect. Foods loaded with saturated fat, trans fats and refined carbohydrates seem to ratchet up free radical production. In contrast, the antioxidant vitamins and minerals in fruit and vegetables actually mop up damaging free radicals. When Dr Aljada's team tested the blood of volunteers who ate a fruit and fibre-packed meal, there was no increase in inflammatory free radicals.

Scientists now know that free radicals can exacerbate or even cause conditions that become more common in later life, such as cancer, vascular disease, macular degeneration in the

Getting back to natural

Think avoiding fast food, eating brown bread and having muesli for breakfast gives you a more natural human diet? Think again. Remember, we humans were hunter-gatherers for most of our history, and our body systems evolved to process what our ancestors ate – basically what can be felled with a spear or gathered from plants.

So in the Stone Age, the diet consisted mainly of lean meat, fish, eggs, insects, vegetables, fruit, roots, mushrooms and nuts. Then came agriculture and modern mass-production techniques. On a modern Western diet, we get most of our calories from cereal crops, dairy produce, refined sugar, processed vegetable oils and potatoes.

Some experts believe that such a diet underlies many 'diseases of civilisation', such as heart disease, cancer and diabetes, all of them linked to underlying risk factors such as obesity, high blood pressure and high cholesterol.

When scientists at the Karolinska Institute in Sweden put a small group of healthy volunteers on a mock Stone Age diet, they recorded after three weeks an average 36 per cent reduction in calorie intake, with weight loss of 2.3kg (5lb). They had also lowered their body mass index and blood pressure, and levels of a blood clotting factor posing a risk for heart attacks and strokes.

eye and possibly neuro-degenerative diseases such as Parkinson's or Alzheimer's disease. Because the antioxidants in fruit and vegetables help to counteract free radical formation, Help the Aged dubs them the 'anti-ageing remedy'.

What's more, by dumping calorie-dense 'junk' for fruit and vegetables, you can eat much bigger portions while still taking in fewer calories. 'That's a tremendous dietary advantage,' Dr Willcox says. 'You're loading up on the foods that provide you with the most antioxidants, which protect against free radical damage.' ■

great advice For complete details on which foods to eat each day and in what amounts, turn to the 'Eat to feel good' chapter.

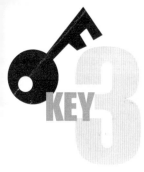

Exercise to slow down ageing

It is no secret that physical activity tones up muscles, protects bones and burns calories. But recently, researchers uncovered a new benefit: exercise acts as a powerful brake on the ageing process.

When University of Florida exercise physiologists put healthy people aged 60 to 85 on weight-training programmes for six months, then tested them for signs of free radical damage, they were surprised by the results. By the end of the study, low-intensity exercisers had a drop in free radical damage, while high-intensity exercisers had a slight *increase* and a control group of non-exercisers had a whopping 13 per cent rise in free radical damage.

In another study, researchers found that an hour of activity a day for just three days raised levels of superoxide dismutase, an important free radical-fighting compound produced by muscle cells throughout the body, including in the heart.

Defend your heart The scientists suspect that aerobic activities such as walking and swimming help heart muscle better defend itself against the cascade of events that leads to a heart attack. The cycle begins when free radicals 'oxidise' LDL cholesterol in the bloodstream. Over time, this damaged cholesterol accumulates on artery walls in the form of gunky, dangerous plaque. When your immune system detects the plaque, it sends in a clean-up crew, which attempts to whisk it away. If a pocket of plaque bursts, it can create blood clots that cause a heart attack. But if your heart muscle pumps out chemicals that disarm free radicals – such as the superoxide dismutase pumped out by the heart muscle cells of exercisers – cholesterol never gets a chance to oxidise, and the process doesn't get started.

Like a flu vaccine that switches on your body's natural defences, exercise works by unleashing a *helpful* amount of free radicals. They're produced naturally by little energy-generating 'machines' in your cells, mitochondria. Your body responds to this surge by pumping out more antioxidants and enzymes to mop up these villains. But if you exercise to exhaustion, the burst of free radicals overwhelms your defences.

Why exercise? Of course, that's not the only reason to take a walk or add extra bursts of activity to your day. Studies show movement can:
- Ease the ache of arthritis
- Lower your Alzheimer's risk
- Keep your bones strong
- Soothe anxiety
- Reduce your chances of developing diabetes
- Lower your odds for colon, breast and prostate cancer
- Help you to sleep better
- Boost your energy levels
- Help you to achieve your healthiest weight

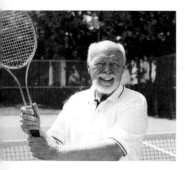

the key Action

Perform simple, natural, strengthening exercises every day, even if just for a few minutes

- Maintain muscle strength
- Improve balance and flexibility.

It is never too late The flip side: not exercising nearly doubles your risk of a heart attack. According to the British Heart Foundation, someone in the UK dies every 15 minutes as a direct result of physical inactivity.

Don't worry if you've never exercised before. People who don't exercise regularly may reap the most benefits from starting, especially if they add some strength-training moves. Muscle strength declines by 15 per cent per decade after age 50 and by 30 per cent per decade after the age of 70, but resistance training can result in 25 to 100 per cent strength gains or more.

Taking regular light exercise can offset the changes to muscle and tendon structure that occur as people grow older and which make them more susceptible to injuries and aching joints. According to research at Manchester Metropolitan University, regular gentle exercise in older people boosts muscle performance, strengthens tendons and increases muscular stability, strength and power – enabling them to remain mobile, independent and active for longer, as well as reducing the risk of falls.

Dr Susan Gilchrist of the Biotechnology and Biological Sciences Research Council in the UK, which sponsored the research, says, 'We aren't suggesting intensive training, but it's worth considering that as we get older a little light exercise can help our muscles to stay strong so they can look after us as we continue to age.'

Break out in a sweat 'Use it or lose it' is the message, according to Dr Iain Lang, of the Peninsula Medical School in Plymouth. Along with US researchers, his team studied data from

Exercise by numbers

Exercising for 20 to 30 minutes most days of the week for a year can offer these amazing rewards. In fact, you'll start to benefit after just six weeks.

3lb	The amount of sleek, energising, calorie-burning muscle you'll build
7%	The resulting boost to your metabolism
25%	The improvement in your body's ability to process blood sugar
1 to 3%	The increase in your bone density
55%	The improvement in your digestion
40%	The drop in your risk of dying in the next eight years
60%	The reduction in your risk of getting Alzheimer's

over 10,000 people aged 50 to 69 and followed them for up to six years in UK and US studies. They found that those who did half an hour's vigorous activity three times a week halved their risk of physical decline and impaired mobility compared with more sedentary study participants.

Vigorous exercise could include mowing the lawn, sweeping leaves or heavy housework, not just sports – indeed, any activity that involves physical labour and makes you breathless or sweaty. What's more, the benefit of exercise occurred across all weight ranges. Irrespective of their initial body mass index, people who maintained a reasonable level of physical activity in middle age were more likely to be able to walk distances, climb stairs and maintain their sense of balance and hand-grip strength as they got older. And fit, obese people fared as well as, or better than, thin, unfit subjects. ■

great advice For a fresh new look at exercise, as well as simple, at-home fitness routines for any age or exertion level, turn to the 'Move to feel good' chapter.

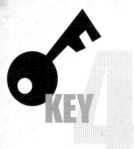

KEY 4

Find something interesting to do

A retired estate agent who helps children to learn how to read. A housewife and mother of five grown-up children – and grandmother of eight – who travels the countryside with her oil paints and easel, capturing nature in all seasons. A retired engineer, always fascinated by the dream of self-sufficient living, who heats his house with wood all winter – and chops every log himself.

Life is perpetually busy no matter what your age, where you live or how well off you are. But the truth is, as careers reach their later stages, as children mature and as home-improvement ambitions are fulfilled, time usually *does* become more available for adults moving through their 50, 60s and beyond.

With this time comes choices. The easy one is merely to relax: to watch more TV, eat out more often, talk on the phone as much as you want. The better choice, not only for your happiness but also for your health, is to discover something more meaningful to devote yourself to and follow it wholeheartedly. Why? Because pursuing your interests – whether it's joining a book group, building hiking trails or doing the things mentioned above – is more than just a pleasant pastime. A growing body of scientific research shows that doing something that interests you offers big mind-body benefits in your 50s, 60s, 70s and beyond.

Do what you love People who maintain hobbies and interests in their later lives suffer less stress and depression, have better moods, improved immune system function and possibly a lower risk of high blood pressure and heart disease. They may even live longer. And this conclusion is coming in from research all around the world.

According to a study at Maastricht University in the Netherlands, men with no hobbies have higher levels of illness and take more sick leave than their more involved counterparts.

It has also been shown that mortality risks are significantly higher in urban men who don't participate in hobbies, club activities or community groups, according to a study of more than 3,000 men by researchers at Gunma University School of Medicine in Maebashi, Japan.

And in Canada, researchers from the University of Manitoba have shown that higher overall activity levels in older people promote happiness, improve functioning and lower mortality rates. What's more, while the social and productive activities tend to produce physical benefits in terms of health and longevity, the more solitary pursuits, such as handiwork hobbies or a love of reading, bring more psychological benefits in providing a sense of engagement with life.

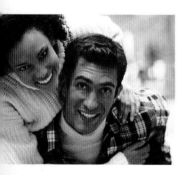

the key Action

Make sure you do something every single day that improves you or the world

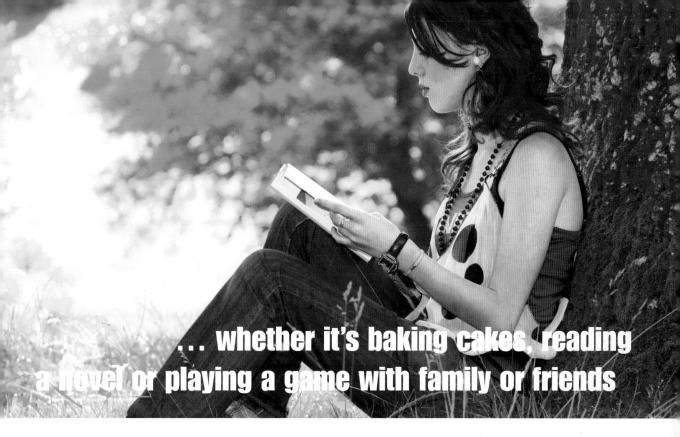

... whether it's baking cakes, reading a novel or playing a game with family or friends

Even in centenarians, and among those with disabilities, 'maintenance of social relationships is of major importance for survival', according to a study from the University of Rome 'La Sapienza'.

Absorb yourself completely The people who think they are ageing well aren't necessarily the healthiest individuals. One factor that emerges from many studies is that older people's sense of what it means to be 'ageing well' does not necessarily match traditional measures of good health and freedom from disability.

In fact, optimism and effective coping styles were found to be *more* important to successful ageing than traditional measures of health and wellness. Self-perception about ageing can be more important than the traditional success markers.

That means getting involved, feeling the sense of flow that comes when you're absorbed in something – whether it's baking cakes, reading a novel or playing a game with family or friends. In many studies, for example, people who found time every day for hobbies, reading and friends ranked their satisfaction with the ageing process higher than those who were isolated and had fewer interests.

The extra benefit of pursuing your interests: by cutting stress, it can lower your blood pressure and tame stress hormones that can wreak havoc with your blood sugar – thereby cutting your odds of having heart disease, high blood pressure, strokes or diabetes. Not bad for an afternoon at the bridge table. ▪

great advice For a complete understanding of the roles active living and personal engagement play in physical health, turn to the 'Live to feel good' chapter.

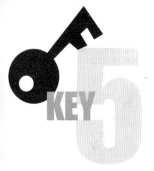

Connect with friends and family

Your spouse. Dear friends. Your children and grand-children. Long-time colleagues. Even Spot and Tabby.

We hope plenty of loved ones – and pets – spring to mind easily when you think about your personal support network. Close connections are a source of joy in the moment and offer a sturdy shield against the stress that can lead to health problems in the long term. Scientific journals are bursting with evidence that having friends around changes the biochemistry of your brain, pumping up feelings of joy and well-being that bolster immunity. The more close friends you have, the greater the odds that you'll be healthy and live longer, while being lonely puts you at risk of an earlier death, high blood pressure, depression and accidents at home and on the road.

Experts are beginning to realise that we're hardwired for friendship. Back in the days when we lived in caves, being alone was perilous – no one was around to help to fend off marauding wolves or forage for roots and berries if you were sick. Fast-forward to today: we're remarkably self-sufficient, yet our ancient responses haven't changed one bit. When you're alone for too long (and the definition of 'too long' is different for each of us), levels of the stress hormone cortisol rise, ratcheting up your odds for heart disease, high blood pressure, depression, muddled thinking and sleep problems. Research even suggests that our brains register social isolation in the same way they register physical pain.

Yet keeping old friends close and building new connections is becoming a lost art. In one study that assessed the social habits of 1,467 women and men in 1985 and again in 2004, they found that the number of people with no close friends at all doubled – to 25 per cent. Overall, the number of companions in whom study volunteers said they could really confide fell by a third.

Stay connected for a healthy heart That's sad news for your heart, according to the scientists who run the Framingham Heart Study. When they checked on 3,267 men, they found that those who were the most socially isolated had the highest levels of interleukin-6 – an inflammatory compound linked to cardio-vascular disease. 'Our analyses suggest that it may be good for the heart to be connected,' says researcher Eric B. Loucks, PhD from the department of society, human development and health at the Harvard School of Public Health. 'In general, it seems to be good for health to have close friends and family, to be connected to community groups or religious organisations, and to have a close partner.'

A spouse or romantic partner may buffer stress best. In one study, brain scans revealed that women had milder reactions to a stressful

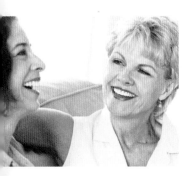

the key Action

To best you can, fill your life with friendship, family, laughter and love event (in this case, a mild electric shock) while holding their husband's hand than when they held a stranger's hand – or no one's hand. And men who made love once or twice a week were 2.8 times less likely to have fatal heart attacks than men who made love less than once a month, report University of Bristol researchers, who tracked the health of 914 Welsh men over the course of five years.

Working on your relationship can make today sweeter and tomorrow healthier, too. Letting hostility and anger take centre stage is a recipe for trouble. In a University of Utah study of 150 couples, those who deployed angry, mean-spirited verbal grenades had more heart-threatening atherosclerosis. The scientists uncovered the connection by videotaping the couples during a 6 minute conversation about a sore marital subject. They also used a CAT scan to check their arteries for calcifications – an early sign of clogging. The surprising link: husbands had a 30 per cent higher risk of severe hardening of the arteries when either spouse was dominant or controlling; wives' risk rose 30 per cent when either partner was hostile.

'People get heart disease for lots of reasons,' says lead researcher Tim Smith, PhD, a professor of psychology at the university. 'If someone said, "What's the most important thing I can do to protect my heart health?" my first answers would be, "Don't smoke", "Get exercise" and "Eat a sensible diet". But somewhere on the list would be "Pay attention to your relationships".'

Pets count, too We're happy to report that four-legged friends are part of the equation for a long, happy, sociable life, too. According to Dr Deborah Wells, a psychologist at Queen's

The *real* health givers

Do you think your doctor and dentist are the sole members of your personal health-care team? Take a second look. The real health protectors in your life may surprise you – and could include any of these people, and more.

- **Your neighbour:** she's offered to start a morning walking club with you – why not say yes? Making a commitment to meet someone for exercise boosts the odds that you'll really do it. And walking with a friend provides soul-satisfying social time, too.

- **Your husband:** every hug, smile and 'I love you' can cut your levels of brain and body-threatening stress hormones.

- **Your dog:** pets soothe stress, many studies show.

- **Your financial adviser:** keeping your money organised and working for you lifts a big burden and eases your anxiety. Studies show that people who think they've got financial woes also have more health problems.

- **Your book group:** discussing new ideas with good friends can cut your risk of Alzheimer's disease, research reveals.

University, Belfast, pet owners tend to be healthier than people who don't own pets. What's more, dog owners do better than cat lovers, with lower blood pressure and cholesterol levels and fewer medical problems, whether minor or more serious conditions. She speculates that 'walking the dog' may promote health through increased physical activity and also by enhancing social contact with other dog owners. Perhaps more important, dogs and other pets also seem to lower their owners' stress levels – thus counteracting one of the major risk factors associated with ill-health. ■

great **advice** For great ideas on how to increase social activity in your life, turn to the 'Live to feel good' chapter.

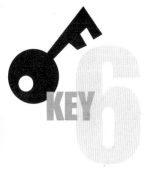

Focus on loving your life

Having an optimistic attitude towards life in your later years can dramatically enhance your chances of living to enjoy more of it. That's the startling conclusion of Dutch research based on nearly 1,000 people aged 65 to 85 at the start of the Arnhem Elderly Study in 1991. Nine years later, those with the highest levels of optimism at the start had almost halved their risk of dying compared with those with the highest levels of pessimism.

Overall mortality among the optimists was only 55 per cent that of the most pessimistic group – and their risk of dying from cardiovascular disease was only 23 per cent in comparison, even taking account of existing disease and major risk factors such as body mass index, hypertension and total cholesterol level. Optimism has a protective effect against mortality in old age, the researchers concluded.

Loving your life, research shows, is a lifesaver. Scientists have found that an optimistic attitude does more than put a smile on your face and make you good company. Studies show that it cuts your risk of getting sick when exposed to the common cold virus; reduces your odds of developing heart disease by 50 per cent; and it increases the likelihood that you'll recover from a heart attack, live longer after a cancer diagnosis and even have fewer everyday health complaints such as upset tummies and breathing problems.

Staying happy and feeling in control in the face of life's challenges builds what experts call 'stress resiliency'. Without this near-magical force field, your mind and body can become steeped in stress hormones, leading to depression, anxiety and a higher risk of everything from colds to Alzheimer's disease and heart disease; it can even make conditions such as glaucoma, rosacea and diabetes worse.

How can you get there? One key element is an ability to enjoy the moment. 'The factors that made later life satisfying included the capacity to enjoy life for its own sake, and finding meaning and purpose,' notes George Valliant, MD, a Harvard Medical School psychiatrist.

Play is not an easy skill for a grown-up to master. 'We're wired from age 20 until age 65 to do things that other people will find valuable – that's how we get paid and how we get our own sense of worth,' says Dr Valliant. He holds up Winston Churchill as a good example of someone who knew how to trade in drive and ambition in favour of fun at retirement. 'Churchill was always looking for other people's esteem. He wrote beautifully and won a Nobel Prize for literature,' he says. 'But as soon as he retired, he stopped writing and took up watercolours. It was simply something he enjoyed for himself.'

Have a laugh It releases endorphins that create a feeling of joy and euphoria, lowers

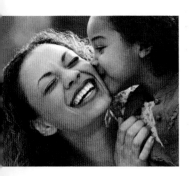

the key Action

Each day, monitor yourself for pessimistic, angry thoughts and replace them with a sense of optimism stress hormones, relaxes muscles and stabilises breathing patterns. Scientists have shown that watching a funny film improves blood flow to a similar extent as exercise – indeed, a really good laughing session can increase calorie burn-off by about 20 per cent. Psychologist Robert Holden, Director of the Happiness Project in Chertsey, Surrey, likens the effect to 'a high-impact internal aerobic work-out'. Regular laughter – some doctors advise 15 minutes a day – has been shown to help people to cope better with pain, fight infection, speed up the healing process and improve general health.

Count your blessings Focusing on what's good in your life really does make everything seem better. Psychologists asked 192 students to make weekly lists for ten weeks of five events they had experienced that week. One group was asked to list things they were grateful for, another group was told to focus on daily hassles, and the third group was given no instructions.

All were also asked to rate their moods, reactions to others, time spent exercising, physical symptoms and general feelings about life. When the results were analysed, people in the 'grateful' group viewed their lives more positively, were more optimistic about the future, responded to help from others with more joy and had fewer physical symptoms than the others.

Create me-time Stress is one of the biggest barriers to happiness, and many studies have shown that long-term stress has detrimental effects on immunity, the nervous system and hormonal balance. It has an adverse influence on other health-related forms of behaviour, such as exercise, eating, smoking and drinking, and can promote depression, memory loss

Happiness is U-shaped

If you're in your middle years and life doesn't seem quite as rosy as it should, don't despair. A major study has found we're most miserable in middle life – but things do perk up later on.

In most countries, measures of average happiness with age form a U-shaped curve – in the UK, the trough is at around age 44, the peak age for depression. The findings are consistent across many groups, irrespective of, for example, socio-economic and marital status or whether or not they have children living at home.

'Only in their 50s do most people emerge from the low period,' says researcher Andrew Oswald from the University of Warwick, one of the study leaders. 'But encouragingly, by the time you are 70, if you are still physically fit then on average you are as happy and mentally healthy as a 20 year old.'

and even some physical diseases, including diabetes mellitus and heart disease – the UK's biggest killer.

A major UK study following the health of civil servants since the 1960s reported in 2008 that consistently high levels of stress damage the heart. The research – part of the Whitehall II study – looked at more than 10,300 civil servants and found a 68 per cent higher risk of heart disease in those with chronic stress.

Dr Tarani Chandola, lead author of the study, says, 'The body is designed to deal with stressful situations, but the important thing is that it returns to baseline levels as soon as possible because of the damage stress hormones can do over a long period of time.'

So make sure that you reserve some time just for you at least once a week and preferably every day. It doesn't matter what you do – jogging, meditation, an art class or gardening – as long as it enables you to forget your troubles. ■

great advice For more on the extraordinary power of optimism and belief in helping you to recover from and even prevent disease, see the 'Live to feel good' chapter.

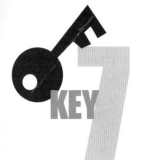

KEY 7

Stress your mind in positive ways

If you think that mental fatigue, forgetfulness, fuzzy thinking and even dementia and Alzheimer's disease are unavoidable in the years ahead, the new science of ageing has news for you: by stressing your mind in productive ways, you can lower your risk of mental decline. And you don't need fancy computer programs or complicated 'brain games' to do it – simple 'brain calisthenics' (one neuroscientist calls them neurobics – aerobics for your brain cells) that involve new ways of doing everyday things are all it takes.

The idea behind neurobics comes from a remarkable discovery: during autopsies of 137 nursing home residents whose mental status had been evaluated during life, ten people were found to have the classic brain changes of Alzheimer's disease despite having had few signs of the disease while alive – indeed, their mental performance had been as good as that of residents whose brains showed no such changes after death. When the scientists looked further, they found a possible explanation: the patients' brains weighed more and had more neurons than residents of the same age without Alzheimer's brain changes. One possible reason: these people had greater 'cognitive reserve' – a savings account of extra pathways that allowed them to offset the changes and function more normally for far longer. Studies since have suggested that up to 20 per cent of people who had no signs of Alzheimer's in their daily lives still have brain changes characteristic of the disease at post-mortem.

Even more exciting: neuroscientists have since found that people who use their brains more often seem to possess these brain-saving reserves. And they believe that stressing the brain in ways similar to how we stress muscles during exercise can produce similar benefits – a stronger, fitter, more flexible brain.

Seek out good stress In one study of 1,772 older people with normal brain function, the odds of developing dementia dropped 12 per cent for each leisure-time activity they took up. Those with the most activities were 38 per cent less likely to develop thinking problems during the seven-year study. Exercise, spending time with friends and intellectual pursuits all helped, but activities that required the most concentrated brain power, such as reading, doing crossword puzzles and playing games that call for strategising, were the most protective.

While 'bad stress' leads to depression and cognitive problems (and even physical ailments), this 'good stress' seems to help the brain by stimulating nerve cells, increasing blood

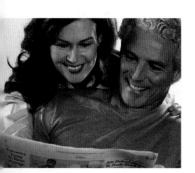

the key Action

Challenge your brain every day through puzzles, reading, thinking and problem-solving flow, and boosting production of neurotrophins – chemicals that protect brain cells. While you're at it, give your body a dose of good stress, too: exercise increases levels of a chemical called brain-derived neurotrophic factor (BDNF), which acts like brain fertiliser. This chemical increases the number of connections between neurons, helps to spur the growth of new blood vessels in the brain, may aid in the growth of new neurons and protects existing nerve cells in the brain from free radical damage.

Add in 'neurobics' Adding 'neurobics' to your mix of brain-healthy pursuits could make an even bigger difference, believes Lawrence Katz, PhD, a brain researcher at Duke University Medical Center in North Carolina. 'Your brain is activated by your senses and you encounter new stimuli all the time,' Dr Katz notes. 'Activities that involve one or more of your senses in a new way, such as getting dressed with your eyes closed, or that combine two or more senses in unexpected ways, such as listening to a piece of music while smelling an aroma, can strengthen synapses between nerve cells and make brain cells produce more brain-growth molecules.

Get connected and stay connected

Continued learning and mental stimulation 'literally grow your brain,' says Professor Ian Robertson, dean of research at Trinity College Institute of Neuroscience in Dublin. More active brains develop a richer and more densely connected network of brain cells, and this brain strengthening may be one reason why dementia is less common among people who have spent more time learning. Reduced mental sharpness is not inevitable in old age,

When left is right

Become left-handed for the day – or, if you're normally a lefty, write and eat with your right hand. Brain scientists say that switching hands activates a big network of brain cell connections, circuits and even regions that normally don't get used.

There are many other instant ways to stimulate new brain connections in fresh, beneficial ways.

- Figure out in your head how to say the name of everyone in your family backwards (Thomas becomes Samoht, for example).
- Similarly, read a whole sentence from the newspaper or a book backwards.
- Multiply numbers in your head. Start with two-digit numbers multiplied by a single digit (for example, 82 x 7) and work up to multiplying by two digits.
- Try counting challenges. For example, count by 13s up to 390.

This isn't as silly as it sounds. Challenging and even frustrating changes in thinking patterns can help to strengthen brain wiring and build new networks that preserve sharp thinking for longer.

he stresses – any decline can usually be stopped or even reversed by mental exercise.

And you don't need to stretch your brain for long to benefit. In a study of nearly 3,000 people aged 65 to 94, just ten hours' training over several weeks in memory, problem-solving and decision-making resulted in significant and prolonged increases in cognitive ability. Booster training sessions a year later yielded further gains in mental function that persisted for more than a year. According to Professor Robertson, 'the training on average took about a decade off the cognitive age of these volunteers'. So the message again is 'use it or lose it'. ■

great advice For more on keeping your memory and other brain skills sharp, see the 'Preventing the diseases of ageing' chapter.

REPAIRING

2

Assessing the damage done

**Body repair:
one, two, three ... four**

**Ranking the habits:
a doctors' poll**

Erasing the damage

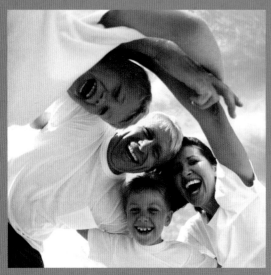
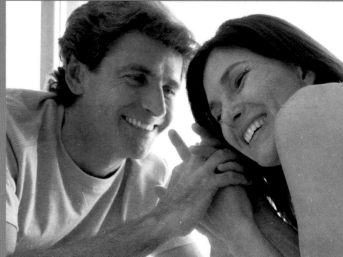

THE ·PAST

The human body has an astounding capacity for healing and regenerating. That includes the ability to undo many of the wrongs of your youth. Here's how

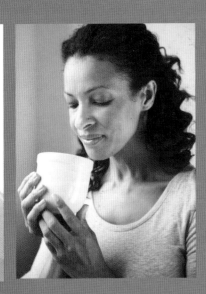

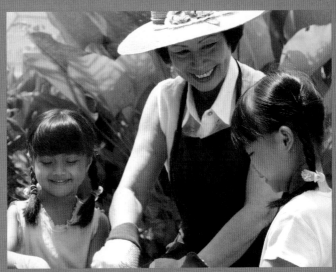

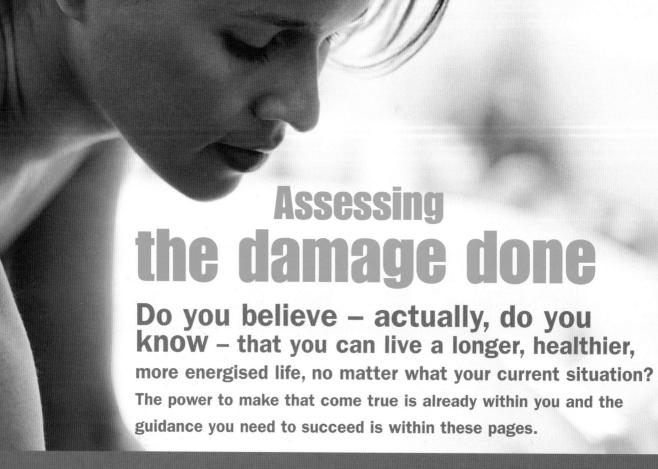

Assessing
the damage done

Do you believe – actually, do you know – that you can live a longer, healthier, more energised life, no matter what your current situation? The power to make that come true is already within you and the guidance you need to succeed is within these pages.

But it's time for some honesty. Decades of abuse to your health is not always easily fixed. For you to take charge of your health, it means coming to terms with your past.

Over the next 56 pages, this book does something that few health books do: it looks backwards. First, you'll discover the fascinating science of how your body repairs and rejuvenates itself. Then you'll explore the habits and lifestyle choices that might have damaged your health along the course of your life. Finally, you'll find out which of these can most influence your future health and what exactly you need to do to minimise the risk.

Be prepared for a few surprises. Some are good: for example, many vices from your younger, wilder days have less of a lingering effect than you might think. But there are challenging facts to learn as well – some lifestyle choices, such as a disregard for summer sun protection in your youth, can have lingering health effects decades after the damage occurred.

To start on this journey into your health's past, there are some tough questions for you to answer. On the facing page is a checklist that probes the unhealthy habits and choices you may have made during three periods of your life: youth, young adulthood and the past few decades. Check off all the statements that are mostly or entirely true.

This isn't a quiz – there are no right or wrong answers, and no one else needs to see this. Instead, use the list as a personal catalyst. If you've checked off a lot of items, your need to correct past health sins is more urgent. If you've checked off just a few, congratulations! You have little holding you back from achieving the longer, healthier life you desire. ■

Q Hard questions about my past

My Youth

- ☐ I frequently got sunburnt
- ☐ I had one or more serious injuries
- ☐ My home life was not happy or supportive
- ☐ I snacked a lot on junk food
- ☐ I regularly ate fast food or frozen dinners
- ☐ I was frequently sick with colds or flu
- ☐ I lived with smokers
- ☐ I lived in a polluted neighbourhood
- ☐ I had a major debilitating disease
- ☐ I watched television every night
- ☐ I was frequently angry or hostile

My Teens and Twenties

- ☐ I smoked cigarettes
- ☐ I smoked marijuana
- ☐ I regularly got drunk
- ☐ I had sex with many partners
- ☐ I snacked a lot on junk food
- ☐ I regularly ate fast food or frozen dinners
- ☐ I gained lots of weight
- ☐ I regularly stayed up much of the night
- ☐ I rarely exercised
- ☐ I lived an isolated existence
- ☐ I was frequently depressed

The Past 20–30 Years

- ☐ I smoked cigarettes
- ☐ I smoked cigars
- ☐ I regularly got drunk
- ☐ I had sex with many partners
- ☐ I had poor romantic relationships
- ☐ I got divorced
- ☐ I had a very stressful job
- ☐ I had workaholic tendencies
- ☐ I spent myself deeply into debt
- ☐ I rarely took holidays
- ☐ I was frequently frustrated, cynical or angry
- ☐ I rarely exercised
- ☐ I lived an isolated existence
- ☐ I gained lots of weight
- ☐ I watched lots of television most days
- ☐ I was a frequent user of painkillers or sedatives
- ☐ I ate fatty or sugary foods most days
- ☐ I lost touch with most of my old friends
- ☐ I rarely saw a doctor

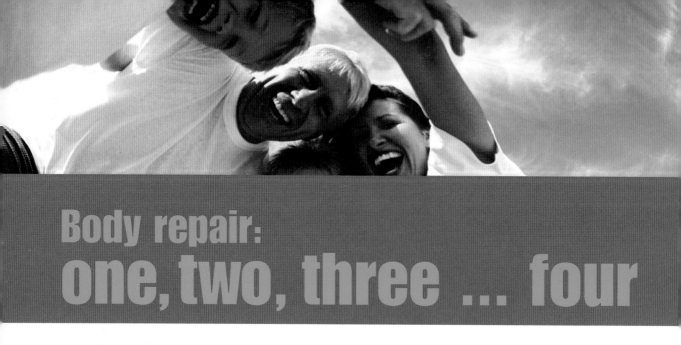

Body repair:
one, two, three … four

Your birth certificate says that you're 53 … or 67 … or 81. But thanks to your body's amazing ability to regenerate continuously, many of your body parts are far younger.

You see, a natural function of your body is to create new cells to replace those that have worn out. Your body generates new blood cells, new skin cells, new hair and new cells for your digestive organs. In fact, most parts of your body are being replaced, to some extent, every day.

Did you know that the muscles in your legs and the tissue within your gastrointestinal system are only about 15 years old? That the red blood cells that deliver oxygen to every cell in your body are only four months old, on average? That the cells on the surface of your skin have a lifespan of just two weeks?

Get motivated If our bodies are constantly rebuilding ourselves, then we all have the chance to improve our bodies greatly and, by extension, our health – starting now.

How well will your body's regeneration system do the job? That's where you come in. While cell turnover naturally slows with age, giving your internal 'mechanic' the right parts for the job

(healthy food) and staying away from the things that slow regeneration (such as too much fat and sugar, smoking, too much alcohol and excess stress) will make all the difference.

TEACH YOUR BODY TO REPAIR

So how can you help? As it turns out, your body has different regeneration modes. We'll call the less helpful one the 'slow mechanic' and the optimal one the 'young mechanic'. You can choose which body-repair mechanic will do the work, experts now believe. The key? Exercise.

Without physical activity, experts now suspect, your body surmises that it is winter – literally. Remember that your genetic coding isn't based on life as its lived today, but as it was lived many thousands of years ago. And if you were sitting around day after day back then, it usually meant it was the cold-weather season, with you and your family huddled together inside for warmth, long past the season for gathering and hunting. And that meant that your body needed to shift into hibernation mode; in fact, your top priority would be to burn as few calories as possible. So the slow mechanic took over, doing minimal work and allowing your bones to thin, your muscles to weaken and more.

But if you get up and move around every day, your genetic coding says, 'Aha! I need stronger bones and muscles, more brain cells to figure out how to hunt that wild boar and a stronger cardiovascular system to keep it all supplied with oxygen and nutrients while I forage for nuts and berries in the woods.' Then, the young mechanic gets to work, bolstering key body systems and creating strong new cells.

Find time to exercise It's up to you whether you allow your body to run down or do all you can to maintain its strength and vitality. The good news is that later in life you have more chances to work on keeping active. A study by the Imperial Cancer Research Fund came to the startling conclusion that older British women are more likely to exercise regularly than younger women. Researchers found that almost half of women over 65 exercised daily, compared with only a quarter of women aged 25 to 34. Overall, the older age group exercised twice as often as the younger ones, who had trouble finding time.

Professor Ian Robertson says that as we get older, aerobic exercise also plays a vital part in maintaining brain function. In one study, people over 60 who exercised regularly showed none of the usual mental decline over the following three years. In another, improved mental performance was seen after four months of moderate aerobic exercise.

Fitness of body and mind are linked, Professor Robertson explains. Exercise promotes the growth of blood vessels in the brain and boosts production of key brain chemicals that encourage cell growth and help to make new neural links. 'For the over-50s, exercise is a sort of wonder-drug that makes you more mentally agile, less forgetful and delays the loss of sharpness that would otherwise happen,' he says.

Make space for friends Another important factor is to stay happy and socially connected. Those who do so live longer and stay healthier, even after major health problems such as a heart attack or cancer. In contrast, anxiety and isolation raise the odds for developing complications and perhaps even dying earlier.

A NEW BODY EVERY DAY

Inside a research lab at Stockholm's Karolinska Institute, researcher Jonas Frisen, PhD, has borrowed a technique normally used to date ancient archaeological treasures and focused it on the human body. Dr Frisen checks levels of radioactive carbon-14 in cells using this high-tech system to determine the age of various cells and tissues. He announced recently that while some tissues in the human body date from before birth, others arrived on the scene less than a month ago.

Cells that face lots of wear and tear, such as skin cells, red blood cells and those that line the stomach and intestinal tract, turn over quickly. The liver, which detoxifies every piece of food, every beverage and every drug you ingest, replaces all its cells in less than 18 months.

The oldest tissues in your body? The muscle cells of your heart; the inner lens of the eye, which forms before birth; and the nerve cells of your brain's cerebral cortex. Dr Frisen estimates that the average age of your cells is seven to ten years old – making you a youngster at any age.

The power to regenerate Scientists at the Juvenile Diabetes Research Foundation Centre at Vrije Universiteit Brussel in Belgium have discovered a progenitor cell in the pancreas of mice that can generate new insulin-producing cells – exciting news that could one day help people with type 1 and even type 2 diabetes to regrow a natural insulin supply instead of relying on medication.

Meanwhile, researchers at the British Heart Foundation are investigating the limited ability of human hearts to regenerate cells, in the hope of developing methods to grow new heart muscle – an advance that scientists hope one day to exploit to help survivors of heart attacks and congestive heart failure to develop stronger, better-functioning tickers.

The biggest news came a decade ago, when neuroscientists turned the conventional wisdom about brain cells upside down. Once, experts agreed that the human brain didn't grow new nerve cells, believing we received a lifetime's supply at birth (or grew the rest soon after, as the brain developed in early childhood). With age, these cells grew weak and began to die … and that was that. But now, we know that, at least in some areas, your brain can develop stronger connections and even brand-new cells.

The bottom line: your body has a vast capacity for repair – and you don't have to be a scientist in a lab to experience the benefits.

MAXIMISING REGENERATION

There are four strategies that have proven to be the best for nurturing your body's repair system – and ensure that the young mechanic is doing the work. These are strategies that keep coming up in this book – in one case, for maximum body rejuvenation; in other cases, for maximum disease prevention, healing, energy, mood and beyond. Hopefully, with each new mention, you will become increasingly convinced of their powers to give you long life and long health.

strategy 1 Exercise

The new Fountain of Youth: a daily walk plus three strength-training sessions each week. As mentioned, exciting research is proving that physical activity flips the youth switch, signalling

to your body to grow younger as it repairs, maintains and regenerates itself. Among the key body systems that benefit:

Muscles In one research study, 70 year olds who performed regular strength-training exercise were as strong as 28 year olds who didn't work out. Skip exercise and you'll lose muscle strength with every passing year.

Brain Once, experts believed that age-related drops in memory and cognitive skills were the inevitable result of dying brain cells. Now, scientists know that the brain can strengthen old cells and generate new ones. Exercise releases a fertiliser-like substance called BDNF.

Heart A heart-threatening lifestyle – replete with high-fat foods, too many calories, little exercise and smoking – can leave you with stiff, clogged arteries 40 years older than your biological age. Ageing also weakens the heart's ability to contract and pump blood. Exercise makes heart muscle contract more forcefully, makes arteries more supple and slows atherosclerosis.

Bones Your skeleton grows lighter with time. But research shows that strength-training pumps up the body's natural bone-building system so that bone density increases. Without it, you can lose 2 per cent of density per year, raising your risk of fractures.

strategy 2 Shed stress, make connections

People's brains are hardwired to live in groups. After all, in a group was the safest place to be in prehistoric times. So when we're isolated, our stress levels rise; to our subconscious minds, prolonged periods of isolation aren't safe or natural, so our brains respond by producing stress chemicals to goad us into action.

Some proof of the powerful influence that stress reduction and social connections can have on your body's repair system:

● Men who survive a heart attack are four times less likely to die from a second heart attack if they come home to family members than if they come home to an empty home.
● Women with more friends and relatives in their lives are more likely to survive heart disease and cancer than those with few.
● People with heart disease who had been anxious, but then lowered their stress levels, significantly cut their risk of a heart attack, according to one Harvard Medical School study.

strategy 3 Supply the correct 'parts'

A Volvo won't run with replacement engine parts pulled from a beaten-up car. And your body won't be able to repair itself with the wrong parts, either. Every time you eat junk food, refined sugars or grain products such as white bread, trans fats and highly processed foods, you're doing just that. Nature's top-of-the-line parts list for the human body are all the nutrients you'll find in lean protein, oily fish, nuts, berries and – especially – antioxidant-rich fruit and vegetables.

The proof that it works:
● Every daily serving of veggies you add to your diet cuts your heart disease risk by 4 per cent (or more) and your stroke risk by 3 to 5 per cent.
● Just five servings of fruits and veggies a day lower diabetes risk by 39 per cent.
● Subjects aged 70 and older who ate the most fresh produce, in one Australian study, had the fewest wrinkles.
● Eating one extra apple a day could reduce your risk of an early death by 20 per cent concludes a University of Cambridge study that measured blood levels of vitamin C (a marker of fruit consumption) in almost 20,000 people. Adding two or more daily portions of fruit and vegetables could roughly halve your risk, regardless of age, blood pressure or smoking habits.

How old are you, really?

Here are the average ages of the cells in your body, based on new studies.

Stomach lining	**5 days**
Tastebuds	**10 days**
Skin surface	**2 weeks**
Eyelashes	**2 months**
Red blood cells	**4 months**
Liver	**300–500 days**
Bones	**10 years**
Rib muscle	**15.1 years**
Stomach	**15.9 years** (excluding the lining)
Cerebellum	**2.9 years** younger than you are
Inner eye lens	**Older** than you are

strategy 4 Ditch the stuff that interferes with repair

Smoking. Exposure to secondhand smoke. Drinking to excess. This bad stuff thwarts your body's regeneration efforts. The up side: study after study proves that your body's repair system goes back to work the moment you give them up:
● Within minutes of stopping smoking, your lungs and cardiovascular system begin repairing themselves. Blood pressure falls closer to a healthier level within 8 hours. Within 24 hours, your heart attack risk begins to fall. Within a month, lungs work better. (There's more on the benefits of quitting smoking in the pages ahead.)
● Your brain can repair itself even after damage inflicted by heavy drinking. In a study from the University of California, San Francisco, researchers found that alcoholics who stayed sober for nearly seven years performed as well as non-alcoholics in brain-function tests.
● Heart attack rates among non-smokers plummeted when a smoking ban was instituted in restaurants and bars in one mid-sized American town – something researchers attribute to a drop in exposure to second-hand smoke. ■

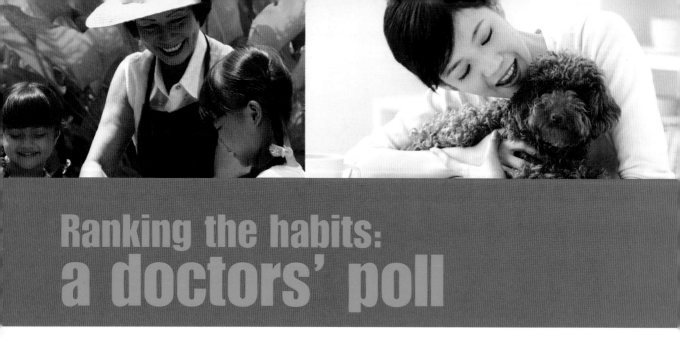

Ranking the habits:
a doctors' poll

ake control. Don't put off healthy changes. But above all, stop worrying and start enjoying life.

When the health editors at Reader's Digest asked nine doctors who specialise in anti-ageing to rank the impact of dozens of lifestyle habits – both past and present – on future health, their answers were both intriguing and amazing.

As expected, the informal expert panel took a serious stance on notorious health wreckers such as tobacco smoking, drinking to excess and being too sedentary. But these doctors and psychologists were equally concerned about *hidden* health threats – issues such as worry, unhappy relationships and debt.

Plenty of research suggests that these extra-strength stresses can lower immunity and raise the risk of everything from diabetes to heart disease to migraine headaches and more. The result? The panel in some instances ranked these seemingly unrelated-to-health issues ahead of better-known health risks such as not exercising, breathing second-hand smoke and ignoring troublesome medical symptoms as the most dangerous to your future.

Their fixes surprised us, too, going beyond the conventional wisdom of 'eat more vegetables' and 'get more exercise' to emphasise the pleasurable. Good company, relaxation, holidays and fun, they told us, are as important for a healthy future as that whole-grain bread you had at breakfast this morning or the solitary walk you plan to take this afternoon.

THE DEADLIEST HEALTH SINS

Among current bad health habits, eight out of nine doctors rate these three as having the potential to cause significant harm:

- Smoking
- Chronic anger, stress or worry
- Feeling out of control at home or in your relationships.

'Certainly smoking is the biggest killer,' notes geriatrician Robert Stall, MD, of Buffalo, one of the panellists. 'My feeling is the tobacco companies are the biggest drug cartel in the world, killing more people than all illicit drugs combined.'

Tobacco smoke makes the risk of lung cancer and heart attack soar, but that's only the beginning. 'Smoking is the most destructive habit when it comes to lung health,' Dr Stall notes. 'It triggers conditions like emphysema and chronic obstructive pulmonary disease [COPD], where you're literally suffocating. It's as if you're holding your nostrils shut so that you can barely get any air through, and breathing that way every moment of every day. It's torturous.'

What was the next tier of unhealthy habits? More than half the doctors identified the following as having the greatest chances of causing significant future harm to your health:

● Not having a regular exercise routine
● Drinking to excess on a weekly basis
● Breathing secondhand smoke regularly
● Taking sleeping pills to fall asleep most nights
● Gulping large quantities of sugary drinks every day.

Being stuck in an unhappy relationship – with your spouse or with your own body – got top rankings, too. Experts said that ignoring warning signs and symptoms of potential health problems could be as damaging as living with a spouse or partner with whom you fight or maintain an icy silence.

Poor food habits set off alarms, too. All of the experts agreed that regularly indulging in high-calorie, high-fat, high-salt fast-food meals could cause moderate to significant health effects. And eight out of nine saw similar risks for those who skimped on veggies or rarely drank plain old water – as well as those who filled up on meat, pastries, sweets or ice cream.

Dieters, beware: gaining and losing the same 5 to 10kg (10 to 20lb) repeatedly was deemed dangerous by most. So was skipping breakfast.

What happens after meals mattered, too. Do you brush and floss? Eight out of nine said that neglecting dental health could be the cause of moderate to significant harm – an opinion

Hurting your health

The panel of surveyed doctors rated the following ongoing habits, eating patterns and attitudes as most harmful to present and future health.

Habits

1 Smoking cigarettes
2 Spending yourself deeply into debt
3 Needing sleeping pills to get a good night's sleep
4 Drinking too much at least once a week
5 Taking painkillers every day

Eating patterns

1 Drinking a lot of sugary drinks
2 Eating four or more meals a week at fast-food restaurants
3 Eating sugary or fatty foods every day
4 Rarely eating vegetables
5 (tie) Skipping breakfast most mornings

    Losing and regaining the same 5 to 10kg (10 to 20lb), over and over again

Lifestyle choices

1 Being angry, worried or stressed more than happy
2 Feeling a loss of control over home, career or family
3 Living in an unhappy relationship for some time
4 Ignoring most health problems and symptoms
5 Not exercising beyond everyday living

corroborated by research linking gum disease with more chronic inflammation and a higher risk for diabetes, heart disease and even stroke.

Why did the experts come down harder on current bad habits than on health sins from your past? Is a current fizzy drink habit really worse than getting drunk in your 20s? It turns out that the answer is usually yes. 'We all have a health reservoir called functional reserve – it's the extra capacity that helps to protect us against illness, helps us to recover when we get sick and maintains body functions,' Dr Stall notes. 'As we get older, this reserve naturally lowers. And if you add insults such as smoking, drinking too much, overeating or avoiding exercise, the threshold is lowered even further. You can maintain a bigger safety cushion between health and disease, even in your 80s and 90s, if you eat well, exercise and relax.'

The experts also weighed in on 21st-century vices. Eight out of nine thought too much debt, too much coffee and too much intense, stressful driving could have moderate to significant health effects. Six warned that skipping holidays isn't a good thing, and seven were concerned that being a workaholic could damage health.

RATING YOUR PAST

What could be the riskiest health mistake you made in your youth? Perhaps surprisingly, it might not prove to be drinking too much, using marijuana or even having had lots of sexual encounters with different partners. Yes, most of the experts rated these as having moderate to significant power to harm your present or future health, but there is an innocent and often-unavoidable practice that might have subjected you to the greatest risk: frequent sunburn in childhood or adolescence. Research confirms that early sunburns – a consequence of days spent in the open air and sunshine, without the benefit of sunblock – are an important risk factor for skin cancer later in life.

Meanwhile, more than half of the panel thought that several other unavoidable childhood health experiences – a major illness, an accident or exposure to pollution – could also play important roles in shaping your future health. Research confirms that all three can influence your well-being decades later, yet studies show that most survivors of childhood illnesses and accidents don't receive the follow-up care they need (and long-term effects of environmental toxins are still not well known in many cases).

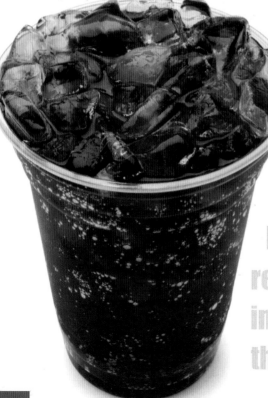

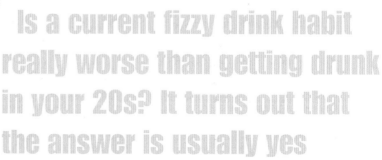

Is a current fizzy drink habit really worse than getting drunk in your 20s? It turns out that the answer is usually yes

HEALTH AND EMOTIONS

It is impressive that 'worrying less and having more fun' earned the number five spot when the experts listed their favourite ways for adding more healthy years to your life. On the flip side, it was also surprising that eight of the nine ranked feeling out of control and feeling worried, stressed or angry most of the time as sources of significant harm.

But the results didn't surprise psychologist and researcher Michael J. Salamon, PhD, director of the Adult Developmental Center in Hewlett, New York. Dr Salamon, one of the doctors who took the Reader's Digest survey, says his own research illuminates the power of feelings and attitudes to extend life. 'In a study, we surveyed older people about their life satisfaction, then went back ten years later to see how they were,' he says. 'What we found was that those with the highest life-satisfaction scores were much more likely still to be alive a decade later than those who had had the lowest scores. Something was going on with the way they approached life.'

A growing stack of research confirms the connection. Stress, unhappiness, loneliness and hostility have been linked with higher levels of stress hormones, higher blood sugar levels and clogged arteries. 'The people who were still alive had an accepting attitude. One person told me, "You bless the bad as well as the good",' Dr Salamon notes.

If you think the satisfied people were simply richer or more popular or maybe started the study in better health, Dr Salamon has news for you. 'We found no correlation between health or wealth or popularity and satisfaction,' he says. 'It's purely attitude. So if you don't have a happy personality naturally, you can cultivate satisfaction by acknowledging your innate grumpiness and making an effort to appreciate the good things in your life.'

The top six fixes

When asked which activities would be most likely to add healthy years to a person's life, the doctors had numerous responses, but these six came out on top:

1 Exercising more

2 Quitting smoking

3 Eating more fruit and vegetables

4 Eating less junk food and fatty food

5 Worrying less and having more fun

6 Getting enough sleep

THE FIX: TAKE CHARGE TODAY

More good news: the experts thought most current lifestyle mistakes are moderately easy or even simple to fix. Among the easiest in their estimation were: taking more holidays, cutting back on TV, eating more veggies, drinking more water, having breakfast, cutting back on fizzy drinks and sweets and having less coffee. Slightly more challenging were: getting more exercise, cutting back on junk food, calling a halt to yoyo dieting and reducing meat consumption (to make room for healthy main dishes with fish, beans and grains).

The toughest to change: smoking, a dependence on sleeping pills and an ingrained fast-food habit.

Their best advice: just do it.

'It's never too early to start taking good care of yourself, but it's never too late, either,' one survey-taker wrote. 'There will always be some benefit.' Added another, 'This is not unique advice, but … today is the first day of the rest of your life. [You] are in charge of caring for yourself and enjoying each day.' ∎

... from smoking cigarettes

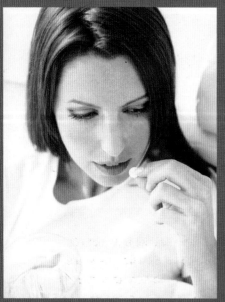
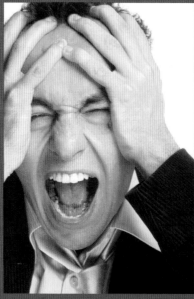
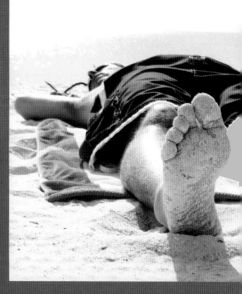

... from a youth spent in the sun

... from many sexual partners when I was young

Erasing the damage

When it comes to health, some sins of our past are not so easily forgiven. As it turns out, several youthful indiscretions have a potentially long-lasting effect on our bodies. That was our discovery on reviewing a mountain of medical research and interviewing doctors about such excesses as binge drinking, marijuana smoking and having multiple sexual partners.

But there is a very positive side to the story. By halting bad habits and embracing healthier ones, you can *almost always* minimise the risks, to the point where statistically they can have almost negligible influence on your health today. In fact, five straight days of eating ice cream or cakes in the past week probably has more bearing on a person's health than any escapades of 30 years earlier, experts made clear.

So it's time to put most of your concerns about your past to rest. In the pages that follow, we examine 34 habits and lifestyle choices of your distant and recent past, and explain how they might affect your health today and tomorrow. More important, we reveal the best ways to mitigate any damage the habit or lifestyle caused, to make sure that what's done is finally done. Because when it comes to health, you want your best to begin today, and to increase with age. ■

I'm a former smoker, but I quit a year or more ago

PAST HABIT

Damage done

If you've kicked the habit, you are to be congratulated and admired. Breaking a nicotine addiction isn't easy. With each smoke-free year that passes, you lower your odds for heart disease, serious breathing problems and cancers of the lungs, mouth, throat, oesophagus, bladder and possibly the pancreas, too.

But you may not be in the clear yet. Your heart and lungs remain at higher risk of disease than those of a non-smoker for up to 20 years after you quit.

Can I undo it? Absolutely

You'll see immediate health improvements shortly after quitting, but the full benefits of quitting take years to reap. Your heart disease risk drops by 50 per cent within a year after you kick the habit, but it's not until 15 years later that your risk of heart disease and stroke fall to the level of someone who's never smoked. As for lung cancer: after ten smoke-free years, your risk is about a third to half that of continuing smokers; it falls almost to that of someone who's never smoked within 20 years.

Good news: if you take additional steps to improve your health beyond staying smoke-free, you can accelerate the recovery and end up with even more immunity to the diseases most linked to smoking.

Plus benefits

Your skin will look younger and less wrinkled than someone who continues to smoke. You're saving money (cigarettes are expensive) and life's little pleasures – the taste of good food, the smell of spring flowers, the sensation of taking in a big lungful of fresh, rain-washed air – are yours to enjoy again. And then there's the big one: lowered risk of most of the life-threatening diseases.

Repair plan

● **Be vigilant** Habits and addictions do not die easily. Even if you've been smoke-free for years, it might take just one weak moment to restart your habit. Always be mindful of the benefits of not smoking and the self-respect you've earned in kicking the habit, and do not allow yourself to be tempted.

● **Stay away from second-hand smoke** Passive smoking nearly doubles your odds for a heart attack – and may be even more risky for former smokers whose lungs and cardiovascular systems are still recovering from past insults. Avoiding smoke at home, at work and when you're out socialising may be the biggest preventive step a former smoker can take.

● **Eat lots of fruits, veggies and whole grains** These natural foods are packed with cell-shielding antioxidants that further protect against heart disease, stroke and several forms of cancer. Bonus: you get extra vitamins and cholesterol-lowering fibre.

● **Get checked out** Stay up to date with blood pressure and cholesterol checks. Make regular appointments with your doctor in advance so you don't forget.

● **Monitor lung health** Stay alert for signs of lung problems, such as persistent coughing, shortness of breath and chest pain. Tell your doctor right away if you have these. ■

● FOR MORE ON OVERCOMING BREATHING PROBLEMS, SEE PAGE 368.

My skin is freckled and worn from a youth spent in the sun

PAST HABIT

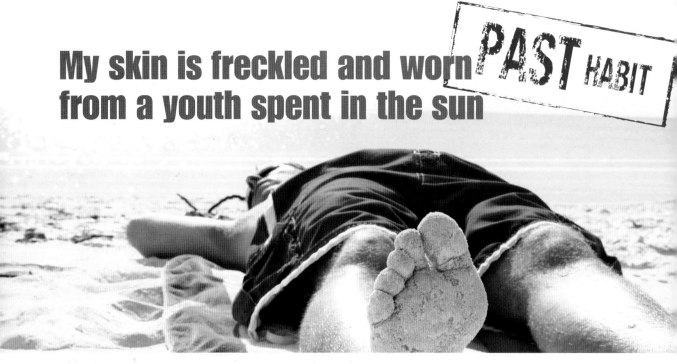

Damage done

Experts believe that most skin cancers are caused by excessive sun exposure before the age of 18. And an estimated 80 per cent of signs of skin ageing as you get older are related to cumulative sun exposure over your lifetime. So the more sun exposure you had, the more likely you are to face wrinkles, splotches, freckles and skin discoloration after the age of 50.

Your odds of developing skin cancer are higher if you have pale skin, blonde or red hair and/or blue eyes: all signs that your skin has low levels of protective melanin. If you endured three or more blistering sunburns before the age of 15, you're at higher risk of melanoma, the most deadly form of skin cancer. Five early sunburns doubles it. Not surprisingly, people who work outdoors and athletes – who spend a lot of time outside – are at higher risk of all forms of skin cancer.

Oddly, a history of being careful may also be a risk. Sunburn is more common among people who use sunscreens, which do not reduce the risk of melanoma and may even increase it, according to Cancer Research UK. Why? Perhaps because those most likely to use sunscreen have a greater natural sun sensitivity. It has been suggested that chemicals in certain sunscreens could actually promote cancers, though most experts deny this. Or it could be because people who use sunscreens stay in the sun from 13 to 39 per cent longer than those who don't, so say scientists at the International Agency for Research on Cancer in Lyon, France. And the stronger the stated protection, the longer they toast.

Can I undo it? Maybe

Various cosmetic treatments can undo some signs of sun-related ageing on the skin (see page 83). There is also now hope that it may even be possible to reverse sunburn damage.

Scientists from the universities of Bath and Nottingham are working on a new type of sunscreen that could repair sunburnt skin and perhaps help to prevent skin cancer. And a study of people with skin cancer at the Queensland Institute of Medical Research in Australia found that those who ate at least three weekly servings of green leafy vegetables, such as spinach, more than halved their risk of a recurrence over the following 11 years.

Plus benefits

Taking steps now will help you to prevent further damage to your skin and help to ensure early detection of skin cancers. You'll also experience reduced skin inflammation, meaning less strain on your immune system.

Repair plan

● **Take your sun in small doses** Scientists have recently been debating whether all sun exposure is harmful. That's because vitamin D, vital for healthy teeth and bones and protection against certain cancers and other diseases, is made in the skin on exposure to sunlight. A short burst of sunshine – no more than 10 to 15 minutes – on unprotected skin at noon can maximise vitamin D production, according to University of Manchester researchers. Although you can also get vitamin D from foods, many people in Britain are deficient, especially over the winter months.

● **Eat more tomatoes** Evidence has also emerged recently that lycopene, a powerful antioxidant found in tomatoes, especially when cooked, could be a more effective skin-protector than sunscreens, according to a University of Manchester study. Just five tablespoons (55g) of tomato paste daily significantly reduced both sunburn and signs of sun-induced skin ageing.

● **Don't rely on sunscreens** Limit intentional sunbathing, especially in the middle of the day. Wear a hat to protect your face, neck and ears, and use lipbalm containing sunblock. Wear sunglasses when outdoors in strong sunshine between 10am and 4pm, and choose wrap-arounds that protect against 99 per cent of both UVA and UVB rays, the two types of ultraviolet radiation in sunlight that can do most damage.

● **Choose sunscreens with care** If you must sunbathe, pick a 'broad spectrum' sunscreen effective against both UVA and UVB, and with an SPF of 15 or greater. Apply 30 minutes beforehand and increase your sun exposure in small stages. A 'waterproof' sunblock gives protection for twice as long as a 'water resistant' one. Most important: don't overdo your time in the sun even if you are wearing sunscreen.

● **Don't smoke** Smoking also increases your risk of skin cancer.

● **Check your own skin regularly** After a shower or bath, take a hand mirror into a well-lit room and examine your entire body, including between your toes. Becoming familiar with your own birthmarks, moles and blemishes will allow you to spot changes and potentially dangerous newcomers at your next check. Remember that 95 per cent of skin cancers are treatable if they are detected early.

● **Watch for danger signs** Follow the British Association of Dermatologists' ABCD-Easy guide to check for signs of melanoma – the deadliest type of skin cancer. Look out for:

● Asymmetry – the two halves of the area may differ in shape
● Border – the edges of the area may be irregular or blurred, and sometimes show notches
● Colour – this may be uneven. Different shades of black, brown and pink may be seen
● Diameter – most melanomas are at least 6mm in diameter. Report any change in size, shape or diameter to your doctor
● Expert – if in doubt, check it out! If your GP is concerned about your skin, see a consultant dermatologist, the person with the most expertise in diagnosing skin cancer. Your GP can refer you.

● **Be extra-careful in the sun if you take medication** Several drugs can make your skin more sensitive to sun damage. If you're off abroad or likely to be out in the sun for long periods, check with your doctor for any medications that could increase your vulnerability. ■

● FOR MORE ON MANAGING SKIN PROBLEMS, SEE PAGE 297.

I used to smoke marijuana

PAST HABIT

Damage done

More than you realise. Marijuana smoke contains 50 to 70 per cent more carcinogenic hydrocarbons than tobacco smoke, plus high levels of an enzyme that converts certain smoke components into their most potent, cancer-causing forms. 'Cannabis poses a serious health risk to the lungs, and smoking a joint can be more harmful to the lungs than smoking a cigarette,' says Dr Keith Prowse, Chairman of the British Lung Foundation. This, combined with the fact that marijuana smokers inhale more deeply and hold smoke in their lungs for longer than cigarette smokers, means that regular pot smokers may have an even higher risk of lung cancer than former cigarette smokers.

Cannabis may also double or even triple your risk of head or neck cancers, according to a study that compared the health histories of 173 cancer patients and 176 cancer-free people.

But that's not all. According to a study from Sheffield Hallam University published in 2008, cannabis users have deficits in verbal fluency, visual recognition, delayed visual recall and short and long-term prospective memory compared with groups of tobacco smokers and non-smokers. And increasing evidence implicates cannabis use in the development of psychotic illnesses such as schizophrenia.

Can I undo it? Unknown

There are no studies that show the long-term health effects of a short-lived marijuana habit. But healthy living is likely to reduce any lingering damage your youthful indiscretion caused.

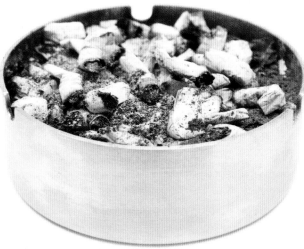

Plus benefits

You can work towards having a much lower chance of stroke and cancer.

Repair plan

- **Don't smoke cigarettes** Just because tobacco is legal and marijuana isn't doesn't make it healthier. As noted, nothing is worse for your health than a smoking habit of any kind.
- **Eat well** A diet packed with fruit, vegetables and whole grains can help to cut your risk of stroke – and may help to lower your risk of lung and other cancers.
- **Avoid second-hand smoke** Passive smoking is risky for the lungs of former cigarette smokers. The same goes for former marijuana smokers, too.
- **Get checked** Make regular appointments with your doctor so you stay up to date with blood pressure and cholesterol checks.
- **Stay alert for signs of lung problems** Tell your doctor right away if you have persistent coughing, shortness of breath or chest pain. ■

● FOR MORE ON PREVENTING CANCER, SEE PAGE 330.

I used to get drunk a lot

PAST HABIT

Damage done

Possibly less than you think. The key words here are 'used to'. Many people drink fairly heavily in their late teens and early 20s, but few carry on doing so into their 30s and 40s, when the average drinking pattern settles to more moderate – and healthy – levels. Although you may vividly remember the dire morning-after effects of acute alcohol intoxication, generally there is little lasting harm to health from those early extravagances – as long they weren't too frequent and didn't last too long.

In fact, the main long-term danger from youthful bouts of excessive drinking is from the aftereffects of the vastly increased risk of accidents, involvement in violent altercations and risky sexual behaviour. Progress to a pattern of either heavy regular consumption or sporadic 'binges' for decades, though, and the catalogue of alcohol-related damage increases sharply (see also pages 66-67).

Can I undo it? Yes

There's plenty you can do to help your body repair damage caused by alcohol and to offset added risks. Experts are just beginning to look at how much of the physical and mental effects of drinking can be reversed. Proof that the body can heal: in one study of nearly 1,600 people, former drinkers' risk of cancer of the oesophagus dropped to normal after a decade.

Plus benefits

Choose to replace your overindulgent past with a healthy present and future, and the benefits are widespread. You'll protect yourself from heart disease and several forms of cancer. You'll feel more energised and upbeat. And you'll give your self-esteem a huge boost as well, knowing you have the will-power to know when to stop.

Repair plan

● **Quit smoking** People who drink alcohol are more likely to smoke, which is one of the worst things you can do if you want to stay healthy. Smoking and drinking together increase your risks of cancer even more. If you're still hooked follow the advice on pages 62 and 63 to help you to kick the habit.

● **Drink sensibly now** Enjoying a drink in moderation, especially red wine, can have positive health benefits as you get older. But these evaporate quickly if you overdo it. Follow recommended drinking limits, don't (ever) binge drink, and have some alcohol-free days, to give your system time to recover.

● **Eat plenty of fruits and vegetables** Eating well and exercising regularly both help to offset your added risk of heart attack, stroke, diabetes and even some cancers. ■

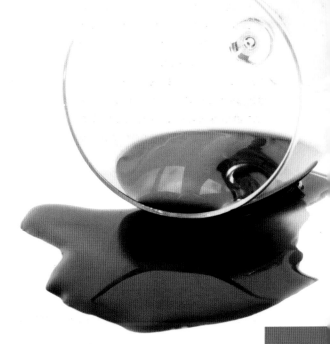

I had many sexual partners when I was young

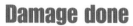

PAST HABIT

Damage done

If your wild days are well behind you, so are most of the immediate risks of sexually transmitted diseases. There is one important exception: the more sexual partners a woman has had, the higher her odds of developing cervical cancer at any age. Most cases of cervical cancer are caused by specific strains of the human papilloma virus (HPV). A persistent, silent infection could linger for years before the cancer is discovered: slightly more than 20 per cent of women with cervical cancer are diagnosed when they are over 65 years old.

Your odds of developing cervical cancer after an HPV infection double if you're also a smoker, if you ever used oral contraceptives for five years or longer (your risk may rise four times above normal if you were ever on the Pill for longer than ten years), if you've given birth to several children, if your mother or sisters have had cervical cancer or if you've had any illness that lowers your immunity.

If you've resumed an active sex life with new partners, or had more than one partner in the past few years, here's something else to ponder: your knowledge of sexually transmitted diseases (STDs) may be out of date. Some doctors are beginning to see an increase of STD infections in older patients, as more single or even newly married older people enjoy new intimacies. The rules for safe sex have changed radically in the past 15 years – you may need to catch up.

Can I undo it? No

You can't 'undo' an HPV infection, but you can get tested and treated (with surgery or other procedures). If you've become sexually active again, you can learn new preventive rules to protect yourself.

Plus benefits

You can have a greater sense of control and safety in your intimate relationships. Plus, being proactive will greatly lower your risk of STDs and help to catch signs of cervical cancer earlier.

Repair plan

● **Get double-tested if you are a woman** Both a cervical smear and an HPV check are necessary to be sure of your cervical health. Cervical smears test for early warning signs of cervical cancer, but can miss precancerous cells 25 to 50 per cent of the time. In contrast, an HPV test looks for the actual cause of cervical cancer: the 13 potential strains of this nasty, carcinogenic virus. If you test positive, you can have infected cells removed early, before damage is done. HPV testing is not yet being performed alongside routine cervical screening in the UK, though this is being considered. Some women with mildly or borderline abnormal smear test results may be offered an HPV test (the test is available privately if you're unable to get it on the NHS).

● **Get tested every three years** Even if you are not currently sexually active or you have negative

The rules for safe sex have changed radically in the past 15 years – you may need to catch up

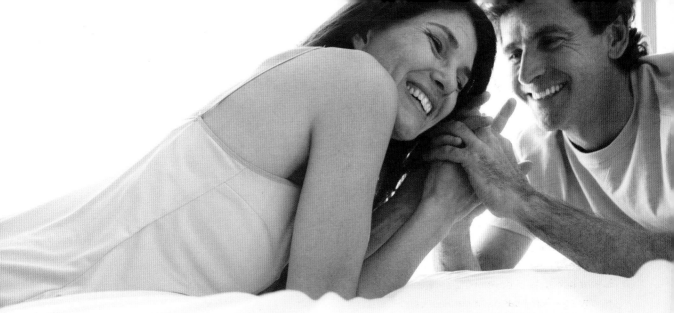

cervical smear and HPV results, get tested. It takes at least three years for a new HPV infection to begin causing cells to change in precancerous ways. Cutting-edge cervical cancer-screening guidelines suggest that rechecks every three years, with another smear and another HPV test, are sufficient to catch problems.

● **Talk to your doctor about the HPV vaccine** Although the highest rates of HPV infection are in women under 25, and rates decline from age 30, there is a second, smaller peak among women over 45, according to researchers at the University of Western Australia in Perth. The current UK vaccination programme is aimed at teenage girls, but vaccination has been shown to be effective in older women. Now that it is licensed in the UK, doctors should be able to offer it privately.

● **Ask if you can stop testing** If you are over 70 and have had three or more normal cervical smear tests in a row in the past ten years plus at least one negative HPV test – and no new sexual partners in at least three years – it may be safe to stop cervical cancer screening. If you've had a total hysterectomy, you may also be able to skip cervical checks. If you still have your cervix or if the surgery was done to treat cervical cancer or precancer, continue to have checks done regularly. Ask your doctor.

● **Have a fruit salad and a yellow, orange or red vegetable every day** Studies suggest that getting plenty of the antioxidant beta-carotene – from food, not supplements – may cut cervical cancer risk.

● **Play by the new rules** Sexually active again? Don't be fooled by the proverbial wisdom of your age: your odds for contracting an STD are not much different from those of a teen or 20 year old who's just becoming sexually active. You'll need condoms (even if the risk of pregnancy is nil). It's also a good idea to ask your partner a few tough questions: are you HIV-negative? Do you have herpes or other STDs? Have you had other sexual partners recently? While such questions once seemed out of line, today's sexual landscape is much more open and honest. Use your maturity to ask them in a sensitive, appropriate way. And if you don't like the answers – or trust them – it's still okay to say 'no'.

● **Watch for signs of STDs** Call your doctor if you develop rashes, blisters, sores, itching, pain, fever, discomfort during sex or an unusual discharge.

● **Be honest with your doctor** Your doctor may not realise that you're active, or may be reluctant to ask. Say if you've had new sexual partners or are in a new relationship so your doctor knows to be concerned about sexual health issues. ■

I had a major illness when I was young

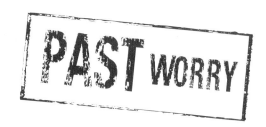
PAST WORRY

Damage done

It is human nature to believe in full recoveries and happy-ever-after endings, particularly when it comes to children. But in reality, major diseases can sometimes cause lasting damage to children's bodies, even if their recovery seems complete.

The reasons are varied. For example, survivors of childhood cancers may face more risks from the treatments they had than from recurrences of the cancer itself. Harsh chemotherapy drugs and radiation can damage healthy cells throughout the body. The result: you're three times more likely to have a chronic health problem than someone who's never had cancer, and eight times more likely to have a severe condition.

According to one Dutch study, reduced bone density means you're more likely to develop osteoporosis and have an increased risk of fractures in later life. The same is true for people who had systemic lupus erythematosus (SLE) as children and were treated with steroids, according to rheumatologists in Norway. And even using inhaled steroids for asthma can, in the long term, increase your risk of brittle bones and fractures later in life. Survivors of childhood polio (cases of polio peaked in the early 1950s) often experience progressive muscle weakness with age.

Can I undo it?
Unfortunately no

You can't erase the lingering damage of a major childhood disease. But you can live healthily now and, by doing so, reduce the risk of new disease. You can nip any emerging problems in the bud if you work with your doctor to stay current with any health screenings.

Plus benefits

Healthy living has many benefits, but for those who had major challenges as a youth, the mental rewards of a healthy, active adulthood are particularly sweet. Plus, by being mindful of the long-term effects of your past challenges, you'll catch related health problems earlier, when they're most treatable.

Repair plan

● **Tell your doctor about your medical history** Ask what screenings you need now. Knowing about your childhood diseases helps a doctor to know what to watch for and how to help you to achieve better health.

● **Lead a healthy life** Good food, ample exercise, a healthy attitude and life-affirming habits such as getting plenty of sleep, water and relaxation are the ticket to long life and good health for everyone, but particularly those whose bodies have been challenged. Make the mental commitment to health, and you will find that your past might become increasingly irrelevant to your future.

● **Take up offers of follow-up appointments** People who have survived childhood cancer have a more than six-fold risk of developing a second tumour, according to a study at Birmingham Children's Hospital. Although the risk declines the more years that pass since successful treatment, it may never go away entirely, so if you're offered a long-term follow-up, take the opportunity.

● **Be smart about bone health** Get enough calcium, vitamin D and weight-bearing exercise to protect your bones. ■

I had some major injuries when I was young

PAST WORRY

Damage done

Most childhood injuries – from a skinned knee when you fell off your bike to a bumped head when you took a tumble out of the neighbourhood tree house – heal swiftly, causing no further problems. But more serious injuries – the result of car accidents, bad falls or major sports injuries, for example – can have consequences that show up or grow worse later in your life.

Childhood fractures can change the way the bones finish growing. About 15 per cent of injuries to a child's or teen's growth plate – the vulnerable area of growing tissue at the ends of the long bones – can slow future growth of the arm or leg bones. While a slight difference in the length of your arms won't cause problems, even a tiny discrepancy in leg length could. Foot pain, knee pain, hip pain and lower back pain have all been linked to small leg-length differences that can be difficult to detect on your own.

Knees are especially vulnerable. Growth-plate injuries at the knee can lead to crooked legs and knee pain. And if you ever tore your anterior cruciate ligament – the key ligament that keeps the knee joint stable – you may be at higher risk of arthritis later in life.

If you were a serious athlete at school or university you may well have been concussed at some point. If you experienced more than two such concussions, you may now be at higher risk of headaches, depression and memory problems as well as sleep problems, mood swings, ringing in the ears and poor concentration.

Can I undo it? No

But you can take important steps to compensate for some problems and to prevent future damage.

Plus benefits

You'll have less joint pain and, perhaps most important, less chance of a recurring injury.

Repair plan

● **Seek help for limb or back pain** If you have foot, knee, hip or lower back pain, see your GP promptly. A difference in the length of your legs could be the cause – and could perhaps be corrected with something as simple as an orthopaedic lift in your shoe.

● **Tell your doctor if you had multiple concussions earlier in your life** This can help your GP to make decisions about how to treat memory, sleep and mood problems.

● **Protect your head** If you had several concussions earlier in your life, skip sports and activities that could cause more damage if you fall, such as roller-skating or ice-skating. Be sure to wear a helmet if you cycle or ski.

● **Exercise regularly, but not too intensely** Stronger muscles can relieve some of the strain on joints that have previously been injured, and properly exercised joints get lots of nourishment and care from your bloodstream and immune system. Exercise also helps to prevent the risk of arthritis and other aches and pains of ageing. Avoid high-impact exercise, however, as it can actually hurt or aggravate existing joint conditions. ■

● FOR MORE ON MANAGING JOINT PAIN, SEE PAGE 286.

I grew up in a heavily polluted area

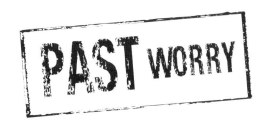

Damage done

Children's lungs are more vulnerable to damage from air pollution and excess ozone than adults' lungs, since they are still developing and growing. The result is a high propensity for lung-related disease in those with constant exposure to smoke and pollution. This was vividly revealed in a study that compared healthy children in a heavily polluted area of Mexico City against similar children raised in rural Mexico. X-rays of the children's lungs revealed that more than half of the city children already had lung damage that may be predictive of future problems.

Another study shows that exposure to pollution for many years can raise your lung cancer risk by as much as 24 per cent and can be as destructive as breathing second-hand tobacco smoke. In a different study that tracked 500,000 people from 100 cities for 16 years, researchers found that dirty air also increased the risk of dying from heart disease by 6 per cent or more. The more polluted the air, the higher the death rates.

Can I undo it? No

Damage done to young lungs doesn't get repaired by your body. But there's plenty you can do to keep your lungs healthy and to protect against future damage.

Plus benefits

Achieving better lung health means improved, deeper breathing. Delivering better-quality air to your lungs results in greater stamina and overall energy, too.

Repair plan

- **Avoid smoke and dirty air** The only way to avoid polluted air consistently is to live far from heavy traffic, factories with large chimneys and highly crowded neighbourhoods. If you live in an urban area, though, there are still many things you can do. Pay attention to the pollution forecast for the day, especially on hot summer days when there may be higher levels of ozone in the air. Take frequent trips out of town. Stay indoors during peak traffic times.
- **Don't smoke** Tobacco smoke irritates fragile, already-vulnerable lung tissue.
- **Pay attention to your lung health** Call your doctor right away if you have chest pain or aches when you inhale or exhale or if you are coughing up blood. These, along with unexplained weight loss, can be symptoms of lung cancer, as can shortness of breath, a hoarse voice, difficulty swallowing, pain under your ribs and/or swelling of your face or neck.
- **Watch for COPD** See your doctor if you're coughing frequently, wheezing, have frequent lung infections or have a lot of mucus. These symptoms can be a sign of a complex breathing problem that doctors call chronic obstructive pulmonary disorder, or COPD.
- **Exercise** It strengthens the muscles that help you to breathe.
- **Eat lots of fruits and vegetables** The antioxidants can help to protect lungs from future damage.
- **Learn to control your breathing** If you have COPD, your doctor or a respiratory therapist can teach you how to relax when you're feeling short of breath. ∎

● FOR MORE ON BETTER BREATHING, SEE PAGE 368.

I watch a lot of television

Damage done

The more TV you watch, the higher your odds of being overweight and developing type 2 diabetes. In one study of more than 9,000 women and men, normal-weight people watched about 2.3 hours of TV a day, while overweight people watched 2.6 hours and obese people watched 3 hours or more. The connection? More screen time means less activity and increased eating.

In the same study, people who watched more than 2 hours of TV a day ate 150 more calories a day, downing more pizza, more sugary soft drinks and more high-fat, high-calorie, low-fibre processed snack foods than those who watched less TV. Small wonder, then, that other studies have linked television viewing with the risk of diabetes in both sexes. In one, those who watched for 40 hours or more a week were three times more likely to develop diabetes than those who watched for less than 10 hours a week. Watching 21 to 40 hours doubled the risk.

If you watch TV instead of keeping up with an old hobby, visiting friends or stretching your mind, you may also hasten memory loss, research shows.

Can I undo it? Completely

By turning TV time into active time, and by committing to a healthy TV/activity balance, you can burn more calories, become fitter and reduce your odds of related health problems quickly.

Plus benefits

You'll have a fitter body and more time for sleep plus more energy, better moods, a sharper mind and more social connection, which may even help you to gain more self-confidence.

Repair plan

● **Follow the 2/30 rule** Experts suggest watching no more than 2 hours of TV a day – and doing at least 30 minutes of exercise every day.

● **Set a no-repeat rule** That is, never watch something you've watched before. If you find yourself watching that same old sitcom or film late at night, instantly turn it off.

● **Set a 'no channel surfing' rule** Turn on the TV only when there is something you truly want to watch. If you are turning on the TV without any particular show in mind, take that as a sign that you need to be more active.

● **No snacking in front of the TV** It's far too easy to eat hundreds of calories' worth of crisps and barely realise it. In fact, many weight-loss programmes smartly advise you never to allow food to go beyond your kitchen table. That also means no snacking in bed and no chocolate bars while paying the bills.

● **Exercise while you watch** Walk on the spot, do sit-ups or try the 'Easy Does It!' strengthening and stretching programme, beginning on page 200, while your show is on. Or drag your treadmill into the TV room and use it while you watch.

● **Clean during commercials** Empty wastepaper baskets, vacuum a room, put in a load of washing … it can add up to 20 minutes' worth of calorie-burning chore time every hour. When you're finished, your home will shine – and you will have saved hundreds of calories by moving instead of snacking. Added bonus: you won't have to watch all the food commercials designed to make you want to overeat.

● **Resolve to leave home more often** See more friends, do more interesting things and stimulate your mind every day. ■

● FOR MORE ON GETTING FIT THE EASY WAY, SEE PAGE 174.

I take painkillers and sedatives as a matter of course

CURRENT HABIT

Damage done

While these drugs can be beneficial when taken for legitimate health problems, long-term habitual use can cause more problems than it solves. Taking non-steroidal anti-inflammatory drugs (NSAIDs) such as ibuprofen or diclofenac for arthritis or muscle pain can, over time, raise your risk of ulcers, gastrointestinal (GI) bleeding, high blood pressure and heart attack. It is estimated that every year in the UK, NSAID use causes about 65,000 upper GI emergencies, resulting in 12,000 hospitalisations with stomach ulcers and GI bleeds and approximately 2,600 deaths.

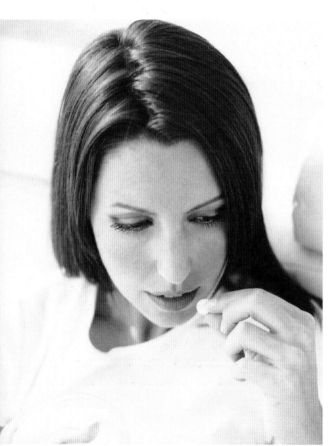

The annual NSAID-related death rate is higher than that of asthma, cervical cancer or malignant melanoma.

If you take an NSAID regularly, even for less than two weeks, you have a 3.6 per cent chance of developing a stomach ulcer and a 3 per cent risk of a duodenal ulcer, according to one study. Take the drug for more than four weeks, and the ulceration rates rise to 6.8 per cent and 4 per cent respectively. The risk increases with age and is higher in women than in men.

NSAID users also have a doubled risk of kidney failure. And an estimated 300 deaths and 30,000 hospital admissions annually from congestive heart failure may be linked to NSAID use. In one Oxford University study, the risk of heart attack or stroke increased by 51 per cent among people taking high doses of ibuprofen (800mg three times a day) and by 63 per cent for high-dose diclofenac (75mg twice a day).

Because the same drugs tend to pop up in many different remedies, if you use over-the-counter medications regularly it's easy to take too much inadvertently. For example, you may pop one pill for a headache then later take a cold remedy containing similar ingredients, then your usual tablet to ease joint pains. Automatically reaching for pills for minor aches and pains can easily become a habit. About one in five people who take painkillers for frequent headaches develop so-called 'rebound headaches' when the drug wears off – and so may be tempted to take yet another pill.

Over-the-counter or prescription sedatives can also cause serious problems – and may also be habit-forming. You can become dependent on sleeping pills in just two weeks, then, when you try to stop, wham, you get rebound insomnia – and need another prescription.

Suppose that, like one in three older people in the UK, you're taking a sleeping pill from your GP. You add an over-the-counter antihistamine for hay fever, then a codeine-containing painkiller for backache. They're all sedating. So you're putting yourself at high risk of side effects like dizziness, impaired balance, confusion and disorientation – which can lead to serious consequences such as falls, accidents and car crashes.

According to a major analysis reported in the *British Medical Journal* of 24 studies carried out over 37 years and involving nearly 2,500 people aged over 60, the risk of side effects from sleeping pills alone considerably outweighed the benefits of such drugs.

Can I undo it? Yes

New pain-relief strategies can ease muscle, joint and head pain with fewer pills – and fewer side effects. And kicking the sedative and prescription pain pill habit is possible with commitment and support. Once the pill taking has ceased, your body will quickly recover from the effects.

Plus benefits

You may cut your risk of heart and high blood pressure problems as well as gastrointestinal ulcers and bleeding. You'll be more alert, less at risk of falls and other accidents, and you won't be increasingly dependent on pills that do less and less good over time.

Repair plan

● **Watch for warning signs of GI trouble** If you take prescription or over-the-counter NSAIDs or other painkillers regularly, tell your doctor about any unusual symptoms right away. These might include abdominal pain, bleeding or black, tarry stools (a possible sign of upper GI bleeding).

● **Talk to your GP about NSAID side effects** If you need these drugs on a long-term basis, whether you're using over-the-counter tablets or prescribed drugs, check whether there are alternative drugs that might work – especially if you have risk factors such as being over 75, obesity, high blood pressure or a history of GI ulcers.

● **If you must take ibuprofen on a regular basis, protect your stomach** Make sure that your GP is prescribing a proton-pump inhibitor, a drug that blocks the production of irritating stomach acid, reducing your risk of stomach ulcers and bleeding.

● **For frequent headaches, see your doctor about a migraine-stopping drug** Many headache-prone people have migraines, which can be stopped quickly with the right medication.

● **Check out alternate pain-relief strategies** For arthritis pain, strategies could include weight loss, gentle exercise, acupressure and adding more omega-3 fatty acids to your diet. And topical NSAIDs – creams and gels – applied directly over the site of the pain may work just as well as tablets with fewer side effects, according to a 2008 study of almost 600 patients aged over 50 with chronic knee pain at Queen Mary University of London. For back pain, exercise and stress relief are tops. For headaches, avoid triggers such as certain foods, drinks and situations (stress, sleeplessness, getting too hungry).

● **Adopt 'sleep hygiene' strategies instead of sleeping pills** Avoid late-evening caffeine and too much activity or excitement (no late-night horror films). Have a small snack containing the sleep-promoting amino acid tryptophan, such as a banana or a small piece of chicken or turkey, about an hour before bedtime. Or make yourself a soothing chamomile tea or some warm milk and honey. And make sure your bedroom is dark and quiet. ■

● FOR MORE ON AVOIDING CHRONIC PAIN, SEE PAGE 335.

I am a cigarette smoker

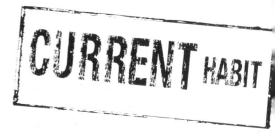

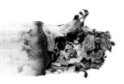

Damage done

As far as health goes, no popular habit on this planet is as harmful as smoking. Cigarettes directly cause 30 per cent of deaths from heart disease, 30 per cent of cancer deaths and a whopping 80 to 90 per cent of all lung cancers. They also increase people's risk of developing mouth, throat, oesophageal, bladder and possibly pancreatic cancer. No wonder smoking is officially the number one cause of preventable deaths in the developed world.

As few as eight cigarettes a month – just 100 a year – raises your smoking-related lung-cancer risk, especially if you've kept it up for years. In fact, any smoking raises your risk. In a study of British doctors, smoking just 1 to 14 cigarettes a day raised the risk to eight times higher than normal; smoking 15 to 25 cigarettes raised the risk 13 times; and smoking more than 25 a day pushed the risk up 25 times.

The 4,000 chemicals in tobacco smoke are lethal for your cardiovascular system – raising your odds enormously of heart attacks, strokes and high blood pressure. Chemicals in tobacco smoke increase cardiovascular risk by strangling the body's oxygen supply, making artery walls stiff, slashing levels of 'good' HDL cholesterol and making blood platelets stickier and more likely to form heart-threatening clots. Smoking also promotes premature skin ageing.

Then there's lung damage. Smoking can trigger or exacerbate short-term breathing problems including bronchitis and asthma attacks. Smoking is also closely linked to chronic obstructive pulmonary disorder, or COPD – a cluster of incapacitating airway problems. These disorders, which include chronic bronchitis and emphysema, are some of the fastest-growing and most debilitating lung issues among older people. In fact, COPD is the fifth leading cause of death in the UK – and 80 to 90 per cent of cases are linked to smoking.

Scientists don't yet understand why some smokers develop COPD while others don't, but an intriguing study by doctors at the Royal Devon and Exeter Hospital revealed that middle-aged smokers with heavily lined faces are five times more likely to develop COPD than smokers with fewer wrinkles, suggesting some kind of genetic susceptibility to both.

Can I undo it?
Yes, if you stop in time

No matter how long or how much you've smoked, you can reverse much of the damage – if you stop smoking once and for all. According to a major study by British and Danish researchers that tracked more than 8,000 people aged 30 to 60 for 25 years, at least a quarter of long-term smokers will eventually develop COPD if they carry on smoking. The longer people smoked, the higher the risk. The good news though is that no one who gave up smoking early in the study developed severe COPD.

Your lungs and cardiovascular system begin repairing themselves within minutes of your last cigarette. Within 8 hours, your blood pressure begins falling to a healthier range and high levels of toxic carbon monoxide gas in your bloodstream drop. In a day, your heart attack risk begins to fall. Within two days your sense of taste and smell sharpen. Within a month, your lungs will work better and you should be coughing less, feel more energetic and have less congestion and shortness of breath.

Plus benefits

Quitting smoking has countless health benefits. Significantly reduced threat of cancer or heart disease, an improved sense of taste and smell, better endurance and fewer colds and infections are just a few. You will also reap confidence-boosting rewards such as fresher breath, younger-looking skin and no more tobacco smell on your clothes.

Repair plan

● **Treat it like an addiction, not a habit** Non-smokers – and oddly, many smokers themselves – often fail to understand how thoroughly addictive smoking can be. Ending a long-running smoking habit cannot be done casually. You need to prepare yourself mentally and physically, and to have a strategy, a support team and a Plan B in case some methods fail.

● **Get help and support** You can get nicotine-replacement therapy – patches, gum, nasal spray, inhalators, lozenges or microtabs – over the counter or, for a certain period, on prescription from your GP or NHS stop-smoking facilities. Some prescription drugs can also help you to quit and counteract cravings. Using these treatments, doubles your chance of success – with treatment and the support of stop-smoking services, you are up to four times more likely to succeed.

● **Take care of yourself** Get plenty of sleep, exercise every day, drink plenty of water and stay busy; this will give rewards that help to replace whatever benefits smokers feel they get from the habit.

● **Time it right** Plan to start your life as a non-smoker during a calm period.

● **Eat lots of fruits and veggies** Studies show that smokers and former smokers who eat plenty of produce, in a variety of brilliant colours, have lower rates of lung cancer. The reason? Probably the protective antioxidants in fresh fruits and veggies.

● **Try 'nicotine fading'** If nicotine cravings have kept you from quitting in the past, this longer-term, slower-quitting technique could help. Use a nicotine patch or gum to help you to become accustomed to life without cigarettes as you gradually step down your nicotine exposure. Keep using the patch or gum for as long as you need to, being sure to follow the package directions.

● **Remember, a lapse isn't a failure** Most successful quitters have lapsed many times. Use the lapse to discover your personal obstacles to quitting, and create a plan for dealing with your needs. If you use cigarettes to relax, try a walk, a phone call or a piece of fruit instead. If it was part of your after-meal routine, replace it with a cup of tea. ■

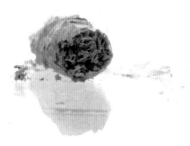

● FOR MORE ON BETTER BREATHING, SEE PAGE 368.

I enjoy a good cigar every now and then

Damage done

Even if you don't inhale, smoking the occasional cigar raises your odds of heart disease and a wide variety of cancers. While no one's figured out the precise risk, consider this: because cigars are bigger than cigarettes, take longer to smoke, use tobacco that's aged and fermented, and are rolled in slower-burning wrappers, a single large cigar emits up to 20 times more ammonia, 5 to 10 times more cadmium (a carcinogenic metal) and up to 80 to 90 times more highly carcinogenic nitrosamines.

'All smokers, whether or not they inhale, directly expose the lips, mouth, throat, larynx and tongue to smoke,' says a definitive US National Cancer Institute report on cigar smoking. 'In addition, smoke constituents in the saliva are swallowed into the oesophagus.'

If you smoke one or more cigars every day, you've raised your odds of heart disease, serious lung problems and a wide variety of cancers on virtually every part of your body that is exposed to tobacco smoke, from your lips, tongue, mouth and throat to your oesophagus, larynx and lungs. The more you smoke, the higher the risk: while one or two cigars a day doubles your risk of cancers of the mouth, puffing three or four raises your risk to more than eight times above normal; smoking five or more cigars a day boosts it to 16 times higher than that of non-smokers.

Can I undo it?
For the most part

If you've smoked an occasional cigar, quitting will probably wipe out most cigar-related risks within a few years. But for long-term heavy cigar smokers, the heart disease and lung cancer risks may not fall to that of a non-smoker's for decades.

Plus benefits

Stop smoking cigars and you'll not only lower your risk of mouth and lung cancers but also save money, banish cigar breath, and leave your clothes, car and house smelling much better.

Repair plan

● **Commit to never buying cigars again** When you run out of your current stock, switch to a healthier pastime, such as sipping a good glass of wine. Unlike cigarette smoking, smoking cigars is usually an occasional vice, not a dependency, making quitting a little easier.

● **Don't buy into the cigar culture** While it might seem that the occasional cigar with the fellows is bold, classic, even elegant, it isn't. There are many better ways of showing solidarity with your friends and associates that won't do such harsh damage to your body.

● **Downsize** Can't give up the occasional cigar? Smoke the smallest size possible.

● **Monitor for the effects of past smoking** Get regular blood pressure and cholesterol checks to catch heart disease risks early. Tell your doctor about your smoking history and watch for lung cancer warning signs, such as constant chest pain, shortness of breath or coughing up blood.

● **Be sure your dentist checks for oral cancers** Stay alert for oral cancer warning signs such as a sore on your lips, gums or inside your mouth that won't heal; a thick spot in your cheek; numbness; difficulty swallowing; or a feeling that something's caught in your throat. ■

I snack all the time, whether or not I'm hungry

CURRENT HABIT

Damage done

Losing touch with your body's natural hunger and satisfaction signals can lead to chronic overeating – and unhealthy extra pounds that can lead to diabetes, heart disease and other serious conditions. When Swedish researchers compared the eating habits and weights of 4,359 people, they found a consistent pattern: overweight people ate more snacks than normal-weight people. And if you snack on junk foods, you're also flooding your body with trans fats and saturated fats, excess sodium and sugars and refined carbohydrates.

Can I undo it? Yes

With determination, anyone can fix bad eating habits and get to a healthier, more natural weight. By acknowledging the psychological issues behind your snacking, you'll find that there are other choices besides eating that provide what you need. And by paying attention to your hunger signals and switching to healthy snacks, you can boost nutrition, control cravings, lose weight and avoid energy slumps.

Plus benefits

Your weight will fall to a healthier level. You'll replace unhealthy trans fats, saturated fat, sugar, refined carbohydrates and extra sodium with nutritious, high-fibre fare.

Repair plan

● **Reacquaint yourself with hunger** If you've lost touch with feelings of hunger and satisfaction, try postponing eating until your stomach is truly hungry and your body is craving fuel.

● **Before you eat, rate your hunger on a 1-to-10 scale** On the hunger scale, 1 is 'starving, feeling light-headed'; 5 is 'comfortable'; and 10 is 'so full I feel sick'. Your goal: eat only when you reach a 3.

● **Stop eating well before you're stuffed** Finish when you reach a 6 on the hunger scale – just a little bit full. You'll eat less – and be truly hungry again in time for your next meal or snack.

● **Satisfy emotional hunger the right way** Much of snacking is related to stress, boredom, even sadness or depression. If you need a psychological boost, don't turn to chocolate. Treat yourself to relaxation or fun: take a walk, call a friend or make plans to socialise. Express anger, sadness and other emotions to a confidant, a diary or the one who's triggering your feelings.

● **Put a stop to mindless eating** If snacking is simply a long-held bad habit that helps you to get through the day, it's time to ban crisps, biscuits and all other snacks from every room except the kitchen or dining room. If you can't take a break, and chewing and drinking are a comfort, turn to sugarless chewing gum and tea or ice-cold water.

● **Replace junk food with real food** Throw away crisps, crackers, biscuits and sweets. Instead, stock fruit, veggies, whole-grain crackers, nuts and low-fat or fat-free dairy products. Make your snacks beneficial to your health.

● **Plan snacks like real meals** Try healthy, high-fibre fruit and fresh vegetables such as baby carrots or cherry tomatoes, and for a more substantial snack, perhaps some whole-grain crackers with a dab of peanut butter. Put your snack on a plate, pour a glass of water or a cup of tea, and sit at the table to enjoy it. ◾

● FOR MORE ON HEALTHY-EATING HABITS, SEE PAGE 110.

I drink to excess at least once a week

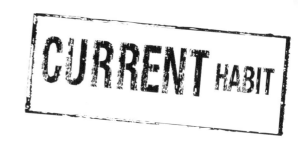

CURRENT HABIT

Damage done

Alcohol can be a tonic – or toxic. If you've enjoyed a glass of wine with dinner throughout the years or the occasional cocktail at a party or beer after work with friends, you're a moderate drinker. For you, alcohol delivers benefits: in more than 100 studies, moderate drinkers enjoyed a 25 to 40 per cent reduction in heart attacks, ischaemic (clot-caused) strokes, peripheral vascular disease, sudden cardiac death and death from all cardiovascular causes. Why? Alcohol in moderate amounts raises levels of 'good' HDL cholesterol and discourages the formation of small blood clots that can lead to heart attacks and strokes. It may even help to protect against type 2 diabetes and gallstones.

But if you drink to excess regularly, alcohol can be a poison. Women who regularly consume two or more drinks a day and men who regularly down three or more are at higher risk of liver damage, pancreatitis (inflammation of the pancreas), various cancers including those of the liver, mouth, throat, larynx and oesophagus, high blood pressure and depression. Women, who are more sensitive to alcohol's inebriating effects and its long-term health effects, may develop heart disease, brittle bones and even memory loss.

Each extra daily drink raises a woman's risk of breast cancer by 6 per cent, according to a study by Cancer Research UK of drinking patterns among 150,000 women around the world. Although the overall impact is small, especially in young women who are at low risk, it may become more important with age. The average lifetime risk of breast cancer is about 8.8 per 100 by the time a woman reaches the age of 80. One alcoholic drink a day increases the figure to 9.4 cases per 100, and six daily drinks raises it 13.3 per 100. However, in older women the effect on breast cancer may be offset by the beneficial effect of alcohol in reducing heart disease. Several studies have found a higher risk of prostate cancer among men who drink a lot or who have been long-time drinkers. Too much alcohol can pack your liver with fat, and can lead to a reversible liver problem – alcoholic hepatitis – or to irreversible scarring – cirrhosis.

The list continues: if you've been drinking to excess for years, you may need screening and treatment for thinning bones or an enlarged heart. Alcohol can also age your brain, making memory and thinking problems worse.

Can I undo it?
For the most part

Soon after you cut back or stop, your digestion will improve: your stomach won't have to cope with the irritation caused by the alcohol and the excess stomach acids it triggers. You'll sleep more soundly. Your blood sugar will be lower and steadier. Your blood pressure may fall towards a healthier range. Even your brain will bounce back. Alcoholics who stayed sober for nearly seven years performed as well as non-alcoholics in brain function tests in one study. Even if you have liver damage, cutting back on alcohol and eating a healthier diet could help your liver to regenerate itself to some degree.

Plus benefits

Without a doubt, you'll have a healthier liver and cardiovascular system. You will have a far-reduced risk of car crashes and other accidents. You'll also feel more energetic and you may have better relationships with family and friends if drinking has caused problems before.

Repair plan

● **Stick with healthy limits** That's two or fewer alcoholic drinks a day for men, one for women. Health dangers begin to rise for people who drink more than that.

● **Reserve alcohol for meals** You're more likely to sip a beer or a nice glass of wine slowly if you're enjoying it along with a good meal. At parties or before you eat, stick with iced tea, water or sparkling water with a splash of lemon or lime.

● **Drink for taste, not to get drunk** For a teenager, feeling drunk might seem novel and cool. As a mature adult, there is no sound reason ever to get drunk. If you discover that you are drinking for the effects of the alcohol – be they to escape a bad day, give you courage in new situations or merely to be 'one of the gang' – stop immediately. Work hard to find a healthier coping mechanism.

● **If you can't stop, acknowledge the addiction** If you can't stick with a healthy drink limit, if you drink secretly or if you need more alcohol to get the same 'drunken' effect, it's time to get help. You may have an alcohol-use disorder. Talk with your doctor and contact a support group such as Alcoholics Anonymous for the support you'll need to make a healthy change.

● **Take your health seriously** Report any symptoms to your GP promptly, and follow advice about any health issues such as high blood pressure or brittle bones. Don't smoke – smoking and drinking together multiplies the potentially harmful effects on your body. And make sure you eat a healthy diet – excess alcohol consumption can deplete vital vitamins and minerals. ■

I have spent myself deeply into debt

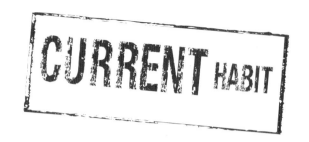

Damage done

Money worries can have serious health consequences. In one telephone survey of 3,121 women and men, half admitted to having stress about money, 23 per cent said their anxiety was severe and 12 per cent called it overwhelming. The damage? Survey-takers said financial stress contributed to high blood pressure, depression, insomnia, headaches, digestive disorders, aches and pains, ulcers, excessive smoking and drinking and gaining or losing weight.

Debt is strongly linked with poor mental health – more so than low income as such, according to a study at the Institute of Psychiatry in London. Among 8,580 people assessed, those with low income were twice as likely to have a mental disorder (psychosis, neurosis, alcohol or drug abuse), but the association with income vanished when debt and other social variables were taken into account. Of those with a mental disorder, 23 per cent were in debt compared with just 8 per cent of those without a mental disorder, and the more debts people had, the more likely they were to have a mental disorder, even taking account of income and other variable factors.

Can I undo it? Yes

But let's be honest: it's not going to be easy. Getting yourself out of debt is analogous to losing large amounts of weight: it takes time, the process can be hard on your ego and your lifestyle, you must be constantly vigilant and it's easy to revert back to old habits. But for those who succeed – and many do – the results are stunning.

Plus benefits

You are going to feel more in control of your life with less stress and fewer worries. You'll be able to sleep better, stop overeating and have fewer headaches. Finding ways to focus on the simple joys in life will help to improve your relationships.

Repair plan

● **Learn about money management** You can't master your money if you don't understand the rules and methods of personal finance. Find a straightforward book, magazine or website and learn all you can about credit cards, mortgages, electronic banking, budgeting and investing.

● **Put your credit cards on ice** Literally. Put them in a cup, add water and place it in the back of the freezer so you can't use them. It will stop you increasing your debt immediately.

● **Create a budget** How much money is coming in each month? How much are you spending on essentials and how much are you spending on frivolous purchases? An hour of honest assessment can go a long way.

● **Pay at least the minimum due each month on bills** Pay more than the minimum on your highest-interest credit card. After you pay that off, move to the one with the next-highest interest.

● **Automate good money habits** Have your wages paid directly into your account and bills paid automatically from it; have small amounts automatically diverted to savings accounts. Use technology to help you to manage your money.

● **Change money priorities** Banish shopping as a form of entertainment. Instead, go for a walk, take up a hobby or meet friends. Identify what you want to spend money on in the future. ■

I'm a workaholic

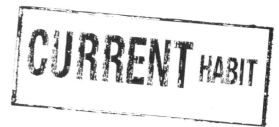

Damage done

Non-stop thinking about your job. Never-ending work emails and phone calls, at all times of the day and night. Repeatedly prioritising work over family, friends and personal pleasures. Workaholics are people who are out of balance with life. And that imbalance is unhealthy – workaholics are at risk of stress-related high blood pressure, heart disease, being overweight and type 2 diabetes.

A workaholic's biggest health threats: stress and self-neglect. In one British study of small-business owners, those who worked the longest hours were the most likely to cancel doctors' appointments or to wait and 'store up' illnesses so that they wouldn't have to take as much time off to see the doctor. And thanks to fatigue and overscheduling, one in five never exercised. If you feel chained to your desk, you're probably not eating well, either.

You're also missing out on the joys of life – and the experiences and relationships that can sustain your health and happiness in the years ahead. In one study of 1,000 women, researchers found that those who were married to workaholic men were more likely to get divorced, and had fewer happy feelings about their relationship.

Can I undo it? Yes

It takes just one thing: convincing yourself to do it. Half the battle is in your mind. As with any habit or addiction, once you truly commit to pull back and regain the balance you once had, changing is a simple, step-by-step process, with measurable benchmarks and outcomes.

Plus benefits

You'll enjoy the novel concept of having time for yourself, your family and your friends. You'll get better, more restful sleep and have less stress. You are likely to lose weight and have a healthier heart. It's all about balance.

Repair plan

● **Set a stopping time – and stick to it** That means telling all the people you work with that between certain hours, you are not going to be available, and enforcing that by not answering the phone or responding to emails.

● **Make healthy eating and exercise a priority** Put them on your calendar and keep these 'health appointments' with yourself as religiously as if they were meetings with an important client.

● **Fill your free time in ways you enjoy** If you cut back on work only to sit in front of the television, you will go back to working. Instead, commit to social activities, family time, cooking or a home project. Fill your time in a way that's more fun than work, and you will help to end your work addiction.

● **De-stress before, during and after work** A few minutes of stretching, deep breathing or yoga helps to release tension and keep priorities straight. Take better care of your mental health, and you'll quickly see the world in a new way.

● **Turn off the electronics** The combination of wireless communications technology and worldwide corporations mean that you can instantly plug into work at any time, at any place. Fight this urge! When you are not working, turn off your mobile phone, your laptop, your electronic organiser and any other devices that link you to your work world. ■

● FOR MORE ON A HEALTHY, HAPPY LIFESTYLE, SEE PAGE 238.

I drink a lot of coffee or caffeinated beverages

Damage done

Minimal. For most of us, years of coffee drinking will have no ill effects – in fact, surprising research suggests that coffee drinkers have a 30 to 60 per cent lower risk of type 2 diabetes, as well as reduced rates of Parkinson's disease and liver disease. However, a high caffeine intake has been reported in some studies to reduce bone mineral density and increase the risk of fractures, although studies are not consistent, and the risk, if any, appears concentrated mainly among women with a low calcium intake.

But if you're extra-sensitive to caffeine, drink several cups a day of supercharged espresso or cappuccino or have cut nutritional corners in your diet, a highly caffeinated lifestyle could pose health problems. Downing more than four cups of regular coffee (or as few as two espressos or other high-caffeine options) can cause anxiety, insomnia and nervousness. Experts say that once your body is used to caffeine, it probably doesn't affect blood pressure. But some research suggests that in the short term, the amount of caffeine in two to three cups of coffee can raise systolic blood pressure (the top number) by 3 to 14 points and diastolic blood pressure (the bottom number) by 4 to 13 points.

Can I undo it? Yes

Since caffeine's effects are relatively short-lived, cutting back will lessen them in a day or two.

Plus benefits

You'll feel calmer, sleep better and know you're protecting your bones from fracture risks.

Repair plan

● **Skip caffeinated drinks after noon** If you drink caffeinated drinks for their energising effects, drink them in the morning. Caffeine lingers in your system for 3 to 7 hours. A cup after lunch could create sleep problems at bedtime.

● **Avoid caffeinated drinks for a few days before your next blood pressure check** If your numbers drop after cutting caffeine, consider switching to decaffeinated versions of your favourite drinks.

● **Get plenty of calcium** If you love coffee but hate dairy products, take enough calcium supplements to get 700 milligrams a day.

● **Switch to decaf slowly** If caffeine is jangling your nerves, but you love the taste, buy a bag of decaffeinated coffee and one of your favourite caffeinated blends. Mix a little decaf into your morning brew. Over the course of a month, add more and more decaf and less and less caffeinated. Your tastebuds will adjust, and you'll feel less anxious without all that caffeine. ■

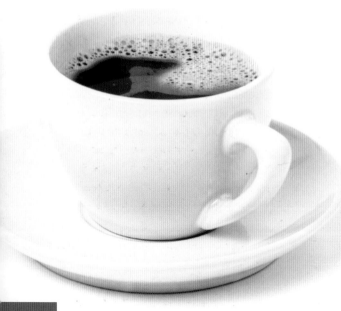

I eat ice cream, cake or other sugary foods every day

Damage done

A lot. In the early 1800s, we ate about 7kg (15lb) of sugar a year. But by the turn of the 21st century, sugar consumption for people with modern diets reached nearly 73kg (160lb) a year – with serious consequences for health and weight. A steady diet of sugar, fat and refined carbohydrates means that you're eating far more empty calories than you should, yet getting less of the high-fibre, high-nutrition foods such as fruit, vegetables and whole grains that your body needs. It also puts your blood sugar on a roller coaster, swinging between dizzying highs and energy-draining lows – and leaving you with intense cravings for even more sugar.

The combination of high calories, low fibre and a dearth of vitamins, minerals and protective antioxidants works together to raise your odds of heart disease, stroke, a pre-diabetic condition called insulin resistance, Alzheimer's disease, some cancers and even sexual problems. In one Dutch study of 16,000 women, those who ate the most sweets and refined carbohydrates had an 80 per cent higher risk of heart disease than those who ate the least.

Can I undo it? Yes

Saying 'no thank you' to cakes, biscuits, chocolate and sweets can reduce sugar cravings and improve energy levels in a matter of days.

Plus benefits

Better moods – no more irritability caused by blood sugar fluctuations. You'll attain a healthier weight and a lower risk of heart disease, diabetes and other blood sugar-related problems.

Repair plan

- **Make healthy substitutions** Rather than turning your back on sweet treats, start by choosing some healthy alternatives. Fruit is a terrific choice, particularly watermelon, peaches and berries. All are sweet and satisfying. Instead of ice cream, have no-fat frozen yoghurt or fruit ices. Instead of cake, have a biscuit and fruit.

- **Splurge weekly, rather than daily** Allow yourself a moderately sinful dessert once a week. That way, you don't have to feel deprived.

- **Ask yourself why you're treating yourself so often** So much of snacking is out of habit, boredom or stress. The best rule of all is to find healthier ways to fulfil your emotional needs than through food. Take a walk, call a friend, do a stretch, read a book. Limit your food intake to satisfying your hunger.

- **Start a new after-meal routine** Go for a walk instead of having dessert. Or, if you still want a family dessert ritual, schedule it for 60 minutes after the main meal, when the kitchen has been cleaned up and everyone has done something active. Then choose something healthy, such as watermelon or cantaloupe slices.

- **Make your kitchen a sugar-free safety zone** Don't keep treats, or even sweet baking ingredients, such as chocolate chips, in the house. Instead, go out for an occasional dessert.

- **Don't rely heavily on artificial sweeteners** It's far better to retrain your tastebuds to appreciate the natural sweetness of fruit than to maintain your unnatural craving for refined sugar. ∎

● FOR MORE ON HEALTHY CARBOHYDRATES, SEE PAGE 110.

I usually skip breakfast

Damage done

More than you realise. Missing breakfast can have serious consequences for your weight, your energy levels and even your blood sugar.

Breakfast-skippers tend to weigh more than people who eat breakfast, studies show. Skipping the first meal of the day leaves your metabolism in 'sleep mode' – a thrifty state intended by nature to get your body through the 12 hours or more between dinner and the break of day. Munching a piece of toast or crunching a bowl of cereal signals to your metabolism that it's time to gear up by burning more calories. Skipping the fuel keeps your metabolism on low, which can make you gain weight and feel sluggish.

You've also created a starve-now-indulge-later eating pattern. Breakfast-skippers tend to overeat later in the day.

Breakfast-avoiders may also have a higher risk of diabetes – perhaps because they tend to eat fewer whole grains, produce and dairy products.

Can I undo it? Yes

Starting a breakfast routine is easy. And the moment you do, you take a major step towards fixing the problems it has caused, including excess weight and unhealthy blood sugar swings.

Plus benefits

Eating breakfast will result in more stable blood sugar. This means fewer food cravings and hunger pangs later. Because you are refuelling your body early, you'll have more energy in the morning, and you may start to control your weight easier, too.

Repair plan

● **Work with your body** Not hungry first thing in the day? Wait an hour or two then have a piece of toast with peanut butter, a bowl of cereal or some fruit, a hard-boiled egg and a glass of milk.

● **Eat foods you like** Breakfast foods are a marketer's creation, nothing more. There's no rule that says you have to start the day with them. Have a sandwich, a bowl of soup or last night's leftovers, if that is your pleasure.

● **No time? Make a portable breakfast sandwich** One great combination is peanut butter and banana on whole-wheat. Any kind of protein between two pieces of bread would also work. Bring along a piece of fruit and you're set. If you like milk, add a cup of skimmed milk, poured into a take-away coffee mug with a lid.

● **Grab an energy bar and pot of yoghurt** Together they contain the perfect amount of nutrients and calories to start your day. And both are instantly ready for eating.

● **Have a smoothie** For the ultimate on-the-go breakfast, whiz low-fat yoghurt, frozen berries, half a banana, a little orange juice and some honey in a blender. (For more volume, add ice cubes before blending.) It tastes like ice cream, but is packed with fibre, calcium, protein and antioxidants.

● **Set things up in advance** Get breakfast ready the night before, so that you can eat it at the kitchen table in 10 minutes or less. Pour cereal into bowls, lay out cutlery and cups, set up the coffeepot and wash, chop and refrigerate fruit. ■

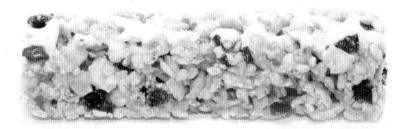

I keep losing then gaining the same 10 to 20lb

Damage done

More than you think. Experts say that this common dieting phenomenon (also known as yoyo dieting or weight cycling), can alter your body composition in frustrating and even dangerous ways. Repeated weight gain and loss lowers the amount of muscle mass you have. This raises your body-fat percentage, lowers your body's ongoing calorie burn and reduces your body's ability to regulate blood sugar. All this is a set-up for more weight gain and related health problems.

Muscle mass declines naturally with age; moving into your later years with a deficit due to weight cycling can leave you even weaker and more prone to balance problems. And if the extra body fat you've gained has settled around your middle, you'll be at higher risk of heart disease and diabetes. Meanwhile, other researchers have found that yoyo dieters have lower levels of 'good' HDL cholesterol.

If you've followed faddy weight-loss plans – from the grapefruit diet to the low-carb or low-fat crazes – you may also have skimped on important nutrients such as calcium or protein or the cornucopia of vitamins and antioxidants in fruit, veggies and whole grains.

Can I undo it? Yes

Switching to a consistently healthy diet will end the yoyo weight effect, and adding strength-training to your routine will rebuild muscle mass and get your metabolism back to where it belongs. All this can be achieved within a few months.

Plus benefits

The obvious benefit is a sleeker, stronger, more-energetic body – thanks to strength-training. Exercising will also improve balance and prevent falls. Better nutrition will aid in lowering your risk of heart disease, diabetes and premature death.

Repair plan

● **Give up faddy diets** It's time to convince yourself once and for all that formal diets don't work. Science shows that short-term regimens or gimmicks to lose weight fast aren't healthy or sustainable. Eat healthy foods in healthy portions, and you'll get to a stable, appropriate weight for your body. Talk to your doctor about what's right for your age and body type.

● **Give up your feast-or-famine eating style** Instead, plan to have three normal-sized meals a day, and three small snacks, too. Never allow yourself to get very hungry.

● **Focus on portion control** Most diets fads are built on demonising certain foods or overstating the importance of others. But at the end of the day, only one thing matters for weight – whether you are eating too many calories. So rather than focusing on what's on your plate, learn first to focus on how much is on your plate. Portion control is the best method of all for losing weight. Learn to eat a little less at your meals and the pounds will slowly but permanently disappear.

● **Rebuild lost muscle mass** Muscle is crucial to long-life living, and if yoyo dieting has weakened you, you have an obligation to yourself to regain strength. To start, try our fitness plans in our 'Move to Feel Good' chapter. Do something to challenge your muscles each and every day. ∎

I drink a lot of fizzy or other sweetened drinks

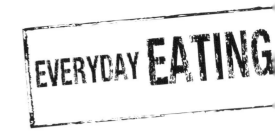

EVERYDAY EATING

Damage done

Surprise! Our panel of doctors rated this as the worst daily food habit of all. But they're right: sipping lots of sugary drinks as well as fruit drinks, sweetened iced teas and other soft drinks is a set-up for weight gain, diabetes, brittle bones and more.

When Harvard School of Public Health researchers looked at the diets and health of tens of thousands of women, they found that those who drank at least one sweetened soft drink a day had twice the risk of type 2 diabetes as women who downed soft drinks less than once a month. The culprit? Extra calories ... and all that sugar. Downing a few hundred excess liquid calories a day seems to be responsible for a hefty weight gain: women who drank soft drinks put on more than 5kg (10lb) in just four years. In contrast, women who quenched their thirst with water, milk and unsweetened (or diet) drinks gained far less weight, the study found. In a study from Finland, people who drank the most sugary beverages had a 68 per cent higher risk of type 2 diabetes.

Think of soft drinks as liquid sweets – a sneaky source of calories that does little to fill you up, but is certain to fill you out. In another study, researchers found that when volunteers drank roughly three cans of fizzy drinks a day – totalling 450 calories – it didn't have any impact on how much they ate at meals. In contrast, when they munched jelly beans, they automatically ate less throughout the day.

Soft drinks can also weaken your bones, possibly because if you consume a lot of sweet drinks, you're less likely to be drinking bone-protecting, calcium-rich milk, or perhaps because the phosphoric acid in carbonated beverages, especially colas, may be particularly damaging to bone health. In one study, women who had more than three cola drinks a day had 4 per cent lower bone mineral density at the hip. Experts suspect that phosphoric acid in colas interferes with natural bone-building in the body, even if you're getting plenty of calcium.

Can I undo it? Yes

You can fix the damage, and you can kick the soft drink habit, but it's harder than you might think. We have programmed our tastebuds to crave sweetness, so weaning ourselves off sugar can be difficult. Like any habit, it takes persistence truly to break it for ever.

Plus benefits

Cutting back on fizzy drinks will result in lower, steadier blood sugar levels, which means a lower risk of diabetes, heart disease and stroke. Eliminating the 150 calories in each fizzy drink from your diet will help you to lose weight or maintain your weight. And since these drinks can etch the surface of the teeth, you'll have stronger tooth enamel.

Repair plan

● **Quench thirst with water** Treat fizzy and sweetened fruit drinks strictly as snacks. For thirst, drink water.

● **Carry water with you** Start the day with a large bottle of cold water, and constantly refill it as the day goes by. You'll find that it is a very effective way to cut back on sugary drinks.

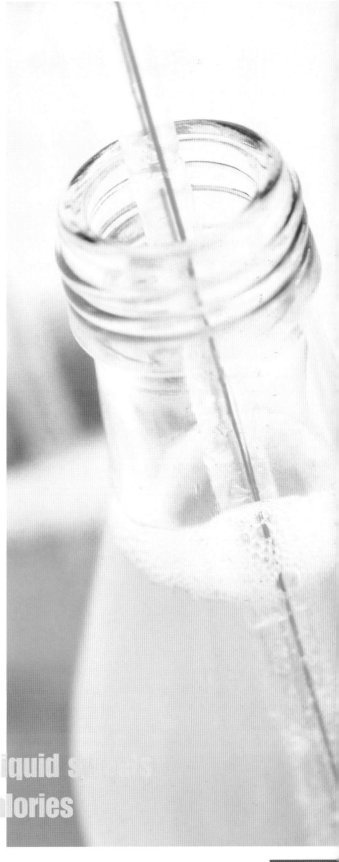

● **Think through your daily beverage intake** After water, daily drinks that are good for your health include coffee, tea, milk, natural unsweetened fruit juices and even wine. Spread those out throughout the day, and you diminish the need for fizzy drinks.

● **Discover the art of iced tea** Brew your own fruity, herbal iced tea the easy way – drop four tea bags into a litre (2 pints) of filtered water and refrigerate overnight. Give it extra zing with a spritz of lemon and enjoy as much as you wish, as an alternative to water.

● **Bypass diet versions of fizzy and sweetened juices** Diet drinks are one way to wean yourself off of a fizzy drink habit, but they should be a temporary solution, not a permanent one. There's new evidence that having more than one a day raises your risk of metabolic syndrome, a pre-diabetic condition that also threatens the heart.

● **Sweeten your milk** Have a cup of cocoa every day: add a tablespoon of pure cocoa and a teaspoon of sugar to skimmed milk, heat and enjoy. One teaspoon of sugar is a fraction of what's in most fizzy drinks.

● **Make a rule: just water at restaurants** Save calories – and money – by skipping fizzy drinks at restaurants. This is particularly true at fast-food restaurants: have a bottle of water instead.

● **Avoid caffeinated cola in particular** Colas containing caffeine were associated with lower bone mineral density than decaf versions in one study. One alternative: home-brewed iced tea (see above), made with black tea for a little caffeinated pick-me-up. ∎

Think of soft drinks as liquid sweets – a sneaky source of calories

I rarely drink water

Damage done

If you barely drink any water, you may be living on the verge of dehydration – or flooding your body with hundreds of extra calories a day if you are drinking mostly juices and soft drinks instead.

Even mild dehydration can make you feel tired. It can also lead to constipation. Over time, dehydration can raise your risk of a heart attack simply because your blood may be slightly thicker and more likely to clot. If you're taking a diuretic to control your blood pressure, or you take laxatives, you may need to drink extra water to maintain a healthy fluid balance in your body. Dehydration can happen faster with age, because your body already contains about 10 per cent less water than it did when you were younger – so there's less of a safety margin.

Can I undo it?
Yes, immediately

Developing a water-drinking habit is easy, and it will quickly improve your health and energy levels.

Plus benefits

Hydrating your body means more energy, less chance of confusion and dizziness, and less risk of falling. Water aids digestion and leads to a lower risk of heart disease.

Repair plan

- **Aim for five to six glasses of pure water, herbal tea or pure juice a day** Sparkling water with a splash of juice or a twist of lemon counts, too.
- **Eat juicy fruit** Enjoy watermelon, oranges, peaches, berries ... the juicier, the better.
- **Check your urine every time you relieve yourself** If it's pale and has almost no odour, you're probably getting plenty of fluids. If it's dark, strong-smelling or you simply don't urinate very much or often, you probably need to drink more water.
- **Always have a glass of water first thing in the morning, and with each meal and snack** Don't wait until you feel thirsty to have a drink – the sense of thirst grows fainter after the age of 60, but your need for fluids remains the same or increases.
- **Drink moderately when you're active** It's vital to stay hydrated when exercising, but don't overdo it. Drinking too much during prolonged physical exertion can reduce blood sodium levels and lead to collapse, confusion or even death from excess water on the brain, according to a study of London Marathon runners. Excessive water intake 'can be extremely dangerous,' warns Dr Dan Tunstall-Pedoe, medical director of the London Marathon. Organisers suggest that while trained, faster runners need a litre (2 pints) of fluid an hour, slower runners should drink no more than half that.
- **Be alert to signs of mild dehydration** These include sudden thirst, fatigue, headache, dry mouth, muscle weakness, dizziness and light-headedness. ■

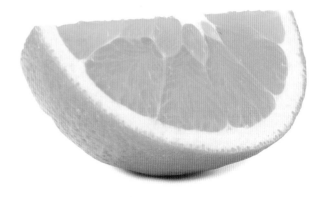

I rarely eat vegetables

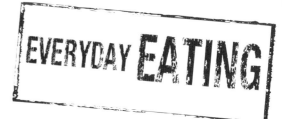

EVERYDAY EATING

Damage done

Significant. If you routinely shun salads, pass up the peas and banish broccoli from your plate, you've denied your body fibre, folic acid and antioxidants that help to guard against heart disease, diabetes, cancer, memory loss and stroke. Chances are high that you've filled your plate with extra potatoes, bread or rice and, as a result, may have put on extra pounds and elevated your risk of a pre-diabetic condition called insulin resistance, too.

Repair plan

- **Start with 'nibble' vegetables** The easiest way to reintroduce yourself to vegetables is to munch on crunchy raw choices such as cucumber and carrots. Getting into that habit will make it easier to move on to eating cooked vegetables as well.
- **Have a salad at every lunch and dinner** It's hard not to like crunchy lettuce with a tasty dressing. Start each meal with a salad and you'll not only greatly increase your vegetable intake but also lower your appetite for the rest of the meal.

The benefits of adding vegetables to your diet are immeasurable

Can I undo it? Absolutely

Finding veggies you like – or new ways to prepare and serve the ones you've been avoiding – can lower your blood pressure, decrease levels of 'bad' LDL cholesterol, smooth out your blood sugar, improve your digestion and perhaps even lower your risk of lung cancer. Several well-designed studies show benefits in as little as four weeks. Every serving of veggies you add to your day cuts your heart disease risk by 4 per cent (or more) and your stroke risk by 3 to 5 per cent.

Plus benefits

The benefits of adding vegetables to your diet are immeasurable, but some of the biggest ones include better digestion, stronger bones and a lower risk of heart attack, high blood pressure, stroke and some cancers. But that's not all: you may end up with fewer wrinkles!

- **Put more vegetables into your stews, soups and casseroles** There's no reason that your chilli can't be bolstered with diced carrots, celery, peppers, onions and even green beans.
- **Add a little fat** A dab of olive oil, a teaspoon of margarine or a sprinkle of Parmesan heightens the flavour of cooked broccoli, spinach, green beans, squash and other veggies. Fat boosts the absorption of nutrients, too.
- **Sip your veggies** Low-sodium tomato juice or vegetable juice counts as a vegetable serving.
- **Double the amount of lettuce and tomato on your sandwich** And use a dark green lettuce, such as romaine, or switch to baby spinach for an extra-nutritious kick.
- **Buy pre-sliced** No time to chop? Pre-cut carrots, broccoli, cauliflower, green beans and more are waiting for you in the produce section of your supermarket. So is shredded cabbage. Take advantage – let someone else be your sous chef. Just microwave, steam or sauté. ■

● FOR MORE ON GETTING MORE PRODUCE INTO YOUR DIET, SEE PAGE 110.

I eat many of my meals from fast-food restaurants

Damage done

Significant. A diet of double cheeseburgers and fries washed down with an oversized fizzy drink or milkshake often leads to a bigger waistline and other related health problems. When University of Minnesota researchers tracked 3,031 women and men for 15 years, they found that those who ate fast food twice a week compared to less than once a week gained 5 extra kilograms (10lb) and were twice as likely to have a pre-diabetic condition called insulin resistance. What's more, people in the UK are even more attached to fast food than those in the USA, according to a BBC survey of 9,000 people in 13 countries, in which Brits topped the table for their junk food addiction.

Because fast food is extremely calorie-dense, it fools people into consuming more calories than their body needs, according to a study by the UK's Medical Research Council. The average fast food meal has 1.5 times as many calories as a typical British home-cooked meal, and 2.5 times as many as a traditional African meal. But our bodies are not geared to recognising the excess energy and fat content, and smaller portions are rarely available. It's all too easy to consume extra calories, creating weight gain and, ultimately, obesity from regular fast-food consumption.

Another risk is from the content of harmful 'trans' fats that until recently predominated in most of the oils used in fast-food frying. Trans fats raise levels of the 'bad' blood fats – LDL cholesterol and triglycerides – that contribute to hardening of the arteries and fire up inflammation, an immune-system response that's involved in the build-up of fatty plaque

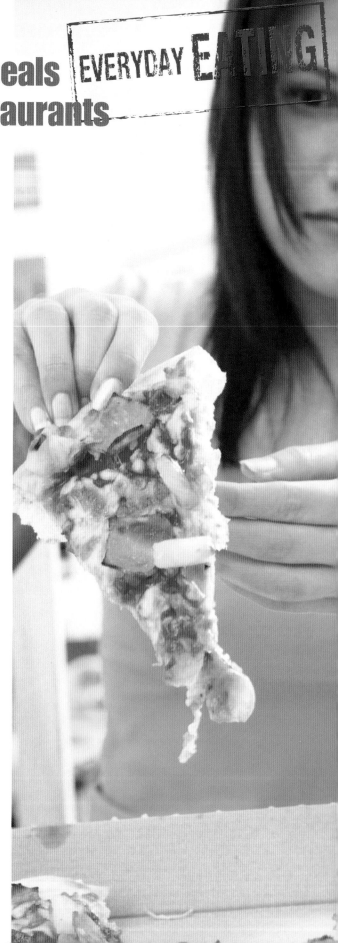

in artery walls. They also lower the 'good' HDL cholesterol that could mop it all up, and add to the abdominal fat that is most associated with diabetes and heart disease. Consuming just 5g of trans fat a day may raise your risk of heart attack by 25 per cent.

Can I undo it?
Yes, with commitment

It will take permanent lifestyle changes that won't be easy at first. Fast food is super-convenient, surprisingly inexpensive and, thanks to all its fat, salt and sugar, undeniably tasty. Healthy eating takes more time and thought and, in some cases, more money. But the health benefits are immediate and substantial.

Plus benefits

In addition to losing extra weight, slimming your waistline and protecting yourself from heart disease and diabetes, you'll save money if you make your own meals instead of buying fast food.

Repair plan

● **Wean yourself off slowly** Most people cannot end a habit cold turkey, and that holds true for fast-food consumption. Cut back a little each week, and each time you go, buy a little less than you used to and start ordering the healthier choices such as fruit slices or yoghurt.

● **Start off by cutting out the fizzy** As discussed earlier, fizzy drink consumption really hurts your health. And fast-food restaurants love to serve up monster-sized cups of it. Switch to milk, coffee or bottled water to save hundreds of calories.

● **Switch from burgers to chicken** In particular, switch to grilled chicken, which is one of the healthiest choices on a fast-food menu. Get dressing on the side and use just a tiny bit.

● **Switch from fries to salad** Those fries are cooked in pure fat and are covered in salt. Fast-food salads may not have the crunch of a French fry, but they are more satisfying than you might realise, and they are considerably more healthy.

● **End the impulse visits** The worst health sin is to spot a takeaway restaurant and impulsively go in for a quick burger, even if you aren't all that hungry or it's not mealtime. Put a firm halt to these kinds of mad meals.

● **Switch to supermarkets** On the road and need a fast meal? Go to a supermarket and get some fruit, a pot of yoghurt, a prepared salad or maybe even some sushi. Every major supermarket chain has responded to the need for fast meals with lots of healthy choices. You are likely to eat a greater volume of food and consume fewer calories.

● **Make your own** You can eat with confidence in your own kitchen. How about leftover roast beef on a crusty roll, a handful of plump cherry tomatoes, crunchy carrots and a juicy orange? Wash it down with unsweetened iced tea.

● **Get your health tested** Eating frequent fast-food restaurant meals is indicative of a generally unhealthy lifestyle. If you want to switch to the healthy side, ask your doctor to check your blood pressure and cholesterol. Finding out the damage that has been done can be a strong motivation for ending your fast-food restaurant visits. ■

It's all too easy to consume extra calories, creating weight gain and, ultimately, obesity from regular fast-food consumption

I have a piece of meat for dinner most days

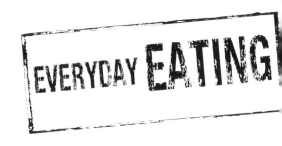

Damage done

A tender steak or juicy chop is one of life's simple pleasures. But increasingly research is linking daily red meat consumption with a higher risk of cancers of the breast, colon, pancreas and prostate – as well as greater odds for arthritis. Eating lots of meat may also raise heart disease risk, especially for people with diabetes.

In a study of 150,000 women and men, those who ate 50 to 90g (2 to 3oz) of red meat a day were 30 per cent more likely to develop colon cancer than those who had less. Overall, when compared to vegetarians, meat-eaters have a 40 per cent higher risk of a range of cancers. Why? It could be that meat lacks the fibre, antioxidants and other nutrients found in fruits, vegetables, beans and whole grains, putting meat-eaters at a nutritional disadvantage. But there seems to be more: the fat in meat boosts human hormone production, which could fuel some breast and prostate cancers. Experts also think that when meat is cooked at high temperatures – grilling, for example – compounds called heterocyclic amines (HCA) and polycyclic aromatic hydrocarbons (PAH) form that seem to raise cancer risk.

Then there is the portion issue. A 'nice piece' of meat too often means a slab three to six times the size of what is considered a healthy serving. Many cuts of meat are inherently high in fat, so lots of meat often means a high-calorie diet that's adding pounds to your frame.

Can I undo it?
For the most part

While you cannot reverse cell damage that may be caused by HCAs and PAHs, there's plenty you can do to lower your future risks. For example, eating fish and poultry (plus plenty of produce and whole grains) rather than red meat, potatoes and refined grains could lower your heart disease risk by nearly 25 per cent.

Plus benefits

You'll broaden your taste in food, save money if you buy beans instead of meats for some meals and, most important, cut your risk of cardiovascular disease and some cancers.

Repair plan

● **Set a goal of eating three or fewer meat-centred dinners a week** Go with chicken, fish/seafood or vegetarian meals the rest of the nights.

● **Skip processed meats such as sausages and cold meats** Filled with salt, chemicals, preservatives and fat, there's evidence that these may raise the risk of diabetes.

● **Order fish when dining out** It's an easy way to get an extra serving of this super-healthy protein.

● **Use meat as an ingredient, not as a meal in itself** That means using meat in salads, stews, soups or stir-fries, rather than served up as a single hunk.

● **Grill smarter** To reduce the creation of unhealthy PAH and HCA chemicals, use low-fat meats, trim the fat and use low-fat marinades to avoid flare-ups from fat drippings.

● **Go for game** If you can't do without red meat, experiment with venison instead of beef – it has a much lower saturated fat content than other meats and contains more iron and higher levels of beneficial omega 3 fatty acids. ∎

● FOR MORE ON EATING MORE LEAN PROTEIN, SEE PAGE 148.

I tend to ignore health problems and symptoms

Damage done

It is one thing to neglect your health when things are going fine, but to ignore symptoms and 'let nature take its course' is highly risky. Your immune system can battle minor infections well enough, but beyond that, 'nature taking its course' often means you get worse, not better. Everyday symptoms such as indigestion, lethargy, dizziness or chronic coughs can often indicate the emergence of more serious diseases – including heart attacks, strokes and cancers.

Yet people ignore symptoms all the time. In a recent survey of 1,100 men, 30 per cent said they wait as long as possible before seeing a doctor about troubling symptoms of any kind. The problem then is you lose the chance to get small health problems treated before they become big problems. Catching many cancers early boosts your chances of survival significantly. Reversing high blood pressure, high cholesterol or high blood sugar as soon as possible lowers your odds of fatal heart attacks, strokes and a wide range of diabetes-related complications such as kidney failure, blindness and amputation due to infections in the feet and legs. Even ignoring a seemingly small problem such as bleeding gums could raise your risk of serious gum infections, which contribute to diabetes and heart disease.

Can I undo it? Possibly

If you have your health, you are lucky – no clear damage has come about as a result of your self-neglect. But treat all symptoms as a wake-up call and have them checked by your doctor. Then adopt a new approach to health, in which you are highly mindful of your body's signals.

Plus benefits

Early diagnosis of chronic problems is worth far more than you can imagine. So is losing the uncertainty related to your undiagnosed symptoms and health problems. These benefits far outweigh any inconvenience or embarrassment from consulting a doctor.

Repair plan

● **Change your attitude** So many men – and plenty of women – have an I-don't-need-a-doctor attitude, as if suffering in silence is a virtue and going to see a doctor a defeat. It's time to change that. Just as success in business almost always relies on a team, so does success in health. Your doctor is essential to your achieving long life and long health. Treat him or her as a welcome participant in your successful future.

● **See your doctor more often** As well as revealing any symptoms, ask for a check on blood pressure and cholesterol and discuss any risk factors such as being overweight or a family history of serious illnesses.

● **Don't forget your eyes and your teeth** Once every two years is the minimum for seeing your optometrist. And don't forget to attend dental check-ups as often as is recommended by your dentist.

● **Resolve to take aches and pains seriously** Pain specialists agree that early pain relief is best. Left alone, chronic pain can create hard-to-break feedback loops in your brain.

● **Set a two-week limit** Do you have an odd-looking mole? An abnormal bulge? Unusual bloating? Take any strange symptom to your doctor if it persists for more than two weeks. ■

I get sunburnt a few times each summer

Damage done

Unquestionably some, potentially a lot. If you love sunbathing or make an effort to maintain a golden-bronze tan, you've unwittingly contributed to the ageing of your skin. Sunbathing destroys the elastic fibres that keep skin looking firm and smooth. That leads to earlier wrinkles, blotches, freckles and discoloration. More important, sunburns contribute significantly to cancers of the skin.

If you've augmented a sun-kissed colour with trips to the tanning salon, beware: using tanning beds doesn't, as advertisements suggest, build up a 'safe' base tan – it raises your risk of skin cancer and wrinkles. In one study, researchers found that tanning-bed aficionados were as much as 2½ times as likely to develop one of the three common forms of skin cancer as people who don't use tanning beds. Some beds put out higher levels of ultraviolet (UV) rays than the UV levels emitted by the midday summer sun.

Also beware of using sunscreen as an excuse to stay in the sun for longer. In two European studies, people who used sunscreens with a Sun Protection Factor (SPF) of 30 had up to 25 per cent more daily sun exposure than those using

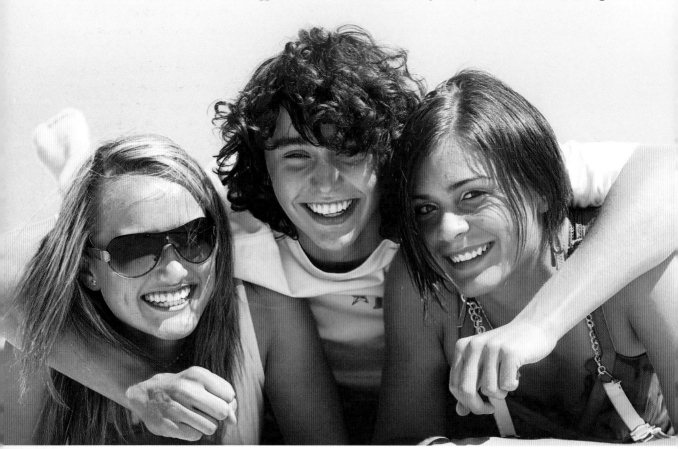

SPF 10 products. Sunscreens also reduce vitamin D formation – vital for strong teeth and bones and an important factor in protection against certain cancers and other diseases – far more effectively than they protect against sunburn.

Can I undo it? Maybe

Sun exposure, especially if your quest for the perfect tan has left you sunburnt, damages skin in ways that it was previously thought couldn't be repaired. However, nowadays various cosmetic treatments such as dermabrasion, chemical peels, laser and pulsed light therapy, and drugs such as retinoic acid, may help to reverse some of the signs of sun-related ageing. Researchers now think it may even be possible to reverse sunburn damage.

Plus benefits

Protecting your skin results in softer, more supple skin with fewer wrinkles and less discoloration. The main advantage, however, is your lowered risk of skin cancer.

Repair plan

● **See your doctor with any skin problems** If you develop any unusual lumps, bumps, colour or shape changes in a mole, see your doctor promptly for a proper evaluation.

● **Know a danger sign when you see it** A melanoma may be blackish/brownish with irregular edges – but it could also be red, pink or waxy, or it could be a sore that just won't heal. Other warning signs include itching, bleeding, sensitivity to touch or obvious growth. Basically, anything that doesn't look right to you on your skin deserves to be checked by a doctor. (See the list of danger signs on page 51.)

● **Always wear sunscreen when outdoors** Keep high SPF (sun protection factor) sunscreens by your back door, in your car, in your bag or anywhere else handy. Get in the habit of taking 30 seconds on your way out the door to rub some on your face, scalp and exposed areas of the arms and legs.

● **Get your glow from a self-tanning product instead of the sun** Tanning creams and gels can give your skin a bronzed look without the cancer risk.

● **Stay safe in the sun** Stay in the shade or wear a broad-brimmed hat, sunglasses, long sleeves and trousers during the peak sunburn hours of 10am to 4pm.

● **At the beach, wear a sun-protection water shirt. Surfers do** They are the equivalent of a high SPF sunblock lotion, and they don't wash off in water.

● **Try the tomato diet** Eat more tomatoes – they're packed with lycopene, a powerful antioxidant, and may help to protect against sun damage even more effectively than sunscreen, according to research by the University of Manchester. Dermatologist Professor Lesley Rhodes says that 'the tomato diet boosted the level of pro-collagen in the skin significantly. These increasing levels suggest potential reversal of the skin ageing process.'

● **Sip green tea** There is some evidence that polyphenols in green tea may protect your cells against cancer-causing sun damage. ■

Eat more tomatoes – they're packed with lycopene and may help to protect against sun damage even more effectively than sunscreen

● FOR MORE ON HEALTHY SKIN, SEE PAGE 297.

I've lived in an unhappy relationship for some time now

Damage done

Surprisingly high. A study of 105 middle-aged British Government employees found that women and men with more marital worries had higher levels of the stress hormone cortisol as well as higher levels of stress and high blood pressure – factors that raise the risk of heart attack and stroke.

In a larger study, researchers at University College London quizzed more than 9,000 civil servants about the quality of their relationships, then followed them for 12 years. Those who had negative aspects in their relationship had a 34 per cent raised risk of subsequent heart disease even after adjustments for age, sex, status and known heart risk factors. Other studies show that an unhappy relationship can raise your odds for weight gain, depression, lowered immunity, stomach ulcers and heart disease risk.

studied 180 older people having flu jabs at general practices in the city, they found that those who were married had better antibody responses to the immunisation than those who were single, divorced or widowed. Those who reported higher marital satisfaction had better responses than married people who didn't. In contrast, people who had recently been bereaved had lower antibody levels.

Can I undo it? Probably

Numerous studies have shown that just being married is associated with a longer lifespan, while never having been married raises the risk of an early demise, especially in men. People who have been divorced also have a higher mortality rate, even during a subsequent stable marriage.

The protective effects of marriage may be due to emotional support or to other health-promoting

A happy relationship may protect your health and enhance recovery from illnesses

In contrast, a happy relationship may protect your health and enhance recovery from illnesses. Researchers from Manchester Royal Infirmary assessed 600 patients in the days following a heart attack. Those who reported having a close relationship with someone in whom they could confide had half the risk of a further heart attack over the next 12 months compared with people without such a supportive relationship.

Being married, especially happily so, may also boost your infection-fighting abilities. When researchers from the University of Birmingham

factors. Research has shown that married people are more likely than single people to take simple health-promoting steps on a daily basis such as eating breakfast, wearing seat belts, getting physical activity, having regular blood pressure checks and not smoking.

Nevertheless, there's no doubt that a happy relationship is better for you than an unhappy one, and if your union has been unhappy or hostile for a long time, pay attention to your mental and heart health. Be realistic – one Swiss study of more than 15,000 couples showed that most went through a 'honeymoon period' of intense happiness, but this generally lasted only about a year. After that, most couples reported less satisfaction with married life and with each other. But be patient: in another study, most unhappy couples who simply stayed together were very happy within five years.

According to Relate, the UK's leading organisation providing advice and support for couple and family relationships, many relationships struggle at common stress points, such as the birth of a first child, the approach of redundancy or retirement or the discovery of an affair. Couples who can adapt and negotiate to accommodate change are more likely to stay together – and if you can't do it between you, get help. Even if you decide to separate, it will help to make the break-up less painful.

Relationship problems affect people physically as well as emotionally – in one study, 40 per cent of Relate clients reported a reduction in visits to their GP after seeking support, and many also cut back on prescription drugs.

However, if you find yourself suffering physical violence within your relationship, contact Women's Aid or your nearest branch of Relate for help (numbers are listed in *The Phone Book*).

Plus benefits

Happy marriages deliver on just about every conceivable health benefit: a lower risk of major diseases, longer life, less stress. Then there are the emotional benefits: happiness, fun, joy, intimacy. A close, loving relationship is among the best things in life for your long-term health.

Repair plan

● **Stop expecting perfection from your mate** Experts say most couples – even those in happy marriages – have 6 to 10 areas of disagreement that may never be resolved. Your marriage may not be broken at all – just normal.

● **Keep your love account in the black** According to experts, it takes 5 to 20 positive statements to outweigh the damage wrought by one negative remark. Do more of the former, less of the latter.

● **Don't try to change your partner** When things aren't going right, change the way you act. Marriage experts say that trying to force your partner to change rarely works and, worse, it creates resentment. If you take good-hearted steps to improve, it'll be noticed – and often, this will cause your spouse to respond in kind.

● **Touch** Human touch triggers the release of feel-good endorphins – for giver and receiver.

● **Study the art of small acts of love** You know how to push Mr or Mrs Right's buttons, and that should include his or her joy buttons, too. That doesn't just mean sex, but it's not a bad place to start. Greet him with a glad-to-see-you hug and kiss when you get home. Surprise her by waking her up with coffee on a rainy Thursday morning.

● **Spend time together every day** You clear your schedule for hair appointments, favourite TV programmes and your book group – how about your spouse? Spend 20 to 30 minutes a day chatting together about your daily lives, your dreams, your plans. And make time for intimacy – even if it means scheduling it in a day planner.

● **Skip the blame game** Setting your partner up as the bad guy ignores the 80 to 90 per cent of him or her that's really wonderful. Criticism, contempt, confrontation and hostility don't help anything. Instead, express concerns by talking calmly and honestly about how you feel.

● **Listen carefully to your spouse** Don't try to defend yourself or argue ... just respect what he or she has to say. This alone can go a long way towards ending the fights and finding a healthier common ground.

● **Raise concerns when you both have time and energy to discuss them** Late at night, when you're rushing out the door, or when you are hungry isn't the right time. ■

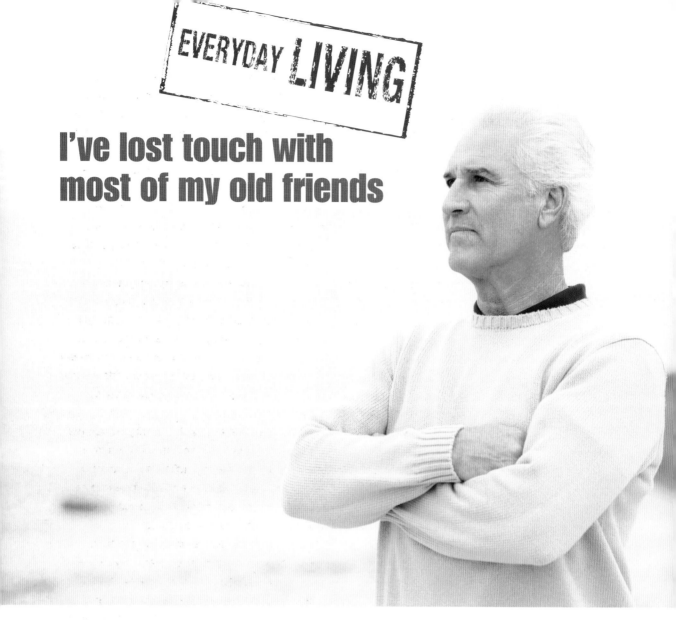

I've lost touch with most of my old friends

Damage done

If you have read the opening chapters of this book, you will know already where the science stands on this question – positive social connections are crucial to your health and well-being. Unless you're the rare type of person who truly thrives on going solo, spending too much time by yourself or having too few friends to confide in and socialise with can, over time, raise your odds of heart disease, high blood pressure, depression, muddled thinking and sleep problems.

Why? Loneliness raises levels of stress hormones in the bloodstream and, as a result, may play a role in firing up chronic inflammation – a risk factor in heart disease, diabetes and even some forms of cancer.

The biggest danger posed by having too few friends: it becomes a habit that could rob you of happiness in the future, when you may need it most. When researchers from Cardiff University analysed data from the 2002 Health Survey for England, they found that good social networks and contacts were strongly linked with better self-reported health, irrespective of health-affecting behaviour such as smoking, alcohol intake and fruit/vegetable consumption.

And according to the Australian Longitudinal Study of Ageing, which involved 1,477 people aged 70 or over, strong social networks lengthen survival among older people. Those who reported having most friends were 22 per cent less likely to die in the ensuing ten years than those with the least – and the protective effect of friendship outweighed even close contact with children and other relatives, which had little impact on survival rates. What's more, the benefit of having lots of friends was still evident even among people who had been through major changes such as the death of a spouse or close family members.

There's no magic number of friends, or number of times a week or a day to reach out by phone, email, old-fashioned letter or in person. But you do need at least one friend other than your spouse – something that 25 per cent of participants in one friendship study didn't have.

Can I undo it? Yes!

All you need to do is get past the mental blocks that have prevented you from reaching out. For some, that isn't easy – shyness, insecurity and low self-confidence can all get in the way of making new friends or reviving old ties. But all these can be overcome, and the benefits of doing so will be immediate.

Plus benefits

More social interactions will have a less-than-subtle positive effect on your mood, making you much more happy, engaged and confident. And with these emotions, every aspect of your health will benefit.

Repair plan

- **Make a list** With whom from your past would you most enjoy being closer? The answer could be friends, former co-workers, family members, even people you have met just once or twice but with whom you were highly impressed. Put them in order, and commit to a plan to contact them in a slow but steady sequence.
- **Use the Internet to get started** Today, email has become a wonderful way of reconnecting with long-lost friends and colleagues. Write a short note saying hello, confirming the address and asking if it's okay if you send a longer note. Who can turn down such an offer?
- **Work on your personal script** As you begin to make social connections new or old, you are going to be asked a lot of questions about you, your recent past and your plans for the future. Anticipate them and work on your answers ahead of time. This will greatly help your confidence and will help you to focus on giving out positive, appealing messages.
- **Turn a hobby into a social activity** Do you play the clarinet? Join the town band. Do you love the theatre? Volunteer to take tickets at local productions ... or dare to audition for a role on stage. Have you a special skill or collection? Find others with the same interests.
- **Do lots of little interactions** For example, if you see a neighbour, walk over and chat for a few minutes. Linger after church services, classes or work and chat with acquaintances. Engage local shop owners in a little conversation. Talk to shoppers at the supermarket who are buying the same products as you are. You'll find that these little conversations are great fun and bolster your confidence.
- **Volunteer with a local organisation that performs good works in your community** With age, each of us should be more willing to donate our wisdom, time and skills to help our communities. The benefit will include great conversations and new-found relationships. ■

I'm angry, worried or stressed more than I'm happy

Damage done

Substantial, and not merely for your mental health. Anger, stress and worry release a cascade of stress hormones that increase your blood pressure and blood sugar, depress your immunity, slow your digestion and just make you feel mean. Nature intended stress to be a short-lived fight-or-flight response to a threat. But modern life can lead to chronic stress – and to far-reaching impacts on your health.

For a start, people who react more strongly to psychological stress have a higher risk of becoming obese. According to a study at University College London (UCL), women who produced more stress hormones had more belly fat – the most dangerous kind – than women with lower hormone responsiveness. And not only were stress hormone levels directly correlated with waist circumference, but total and abdominal fat levels were also linked with prolonged raised blood pressure responses to stress.

Research has also shown that stress hormones make cells throughout your body less sensitive to insulin, leading to higher blood sugar levels. And another UCL study of 34 men who had suffered a heart attack or severe chest pain revealed that stress produced prolonged elevations in blood pressure and heart rate. Among the 14 men whose heart problem had been preceded by acute stress, anger or depression, stress also triggered the release of high levels of platelets, cells in the blood that are linked with clot formation. This may explain just how emotional stress can trigger heart attacks in vulnerable people.

In another study, people who scored highest on tests of anger and hostility had levels of c-Reactive Protein (CRP) – a marker of heart-threatening inflammation – two to three times higher than calmer study volunteers. The more negative their moods, the higher their CRP levels, and the greater their risk for future heart disease and stroke.

Can I undo it? Yes

You have to keep an open mind and do some work, though. Stress-reduction techniques have been proven to lower blood sugar, improve immunity, reduce depression, speed healing in people with psoriasis, ease chronic pain, lower blood sugar and possibly protect your heart, too. Plenty of research shows that people with heart disease linked to anxiety who lower their stress levels significantly cut their risk of a heart attack.

Plus benefits

More than you can count. A regained sense of joy and control is worth its weight in gold, and the physical health benefits will be substantial also.

Repair plan

● **Train yourself to stop getting stressed so easily** You've heard it often: stress isn't created by people or situations – it's entirely caused by how you react to them. You can let an obnoxious child or boss get to you or you can take a deep breath and decide not to let yourself react strongly or emotionally. So next time you feel a stressful situation emerging, work hard at managing it and staying cool. In time, you'll succeed.

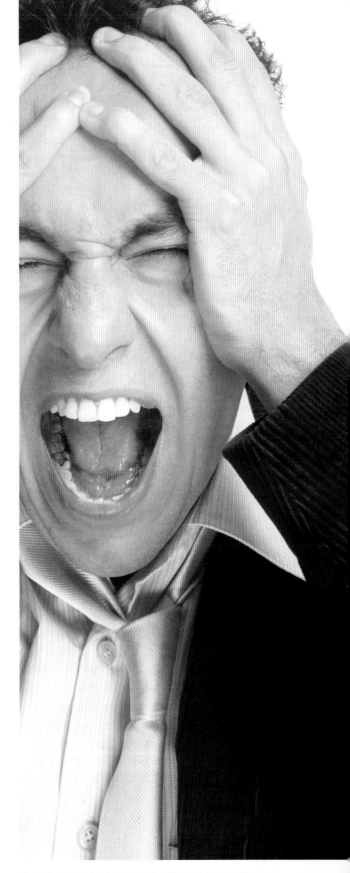

● **Learn a formal stress-relief process** Among the most proven techniques are yoga, meditation and deep breathing.

● **Try progressive relaxation** Close your eyes, breathe calmly and release tension in each part of your body, beginning with your feet and working up to your neck and head.

● **Learn to be optimistic** Whether you view the glass as half-full or half-empty makes a huge difference to your outlook on life, and perhaps to your health. Psychologists believe it's possible to learn to adopt a more optimistic outlook – simply by mimicking what optimists would say and do, even if you don't (yet) believe it.

● **If stress is taking a significant toll on your attitude and health, talk to a cognitive therapist** You'll learn how to see yourself and your thought process in a new, more objective light.

● **Eat healthily and exercise** A healthy lifestyle does wonders for your ability to manage stressful situations.

● **Enjoy a relaxing hobby** Knitting, building model aeroplanes, making pottery ... whatever you love and that you can immerse yourself in will calm you down.

● **Rediscover silliness** One of the secrets to achieving happiness is to acknowledge that in every grown man resides a young boy, and in every mature woman, a young girl. Our bodies may age, but our spirits needn't, and on some matters, shouldn't. So don't suppress your sense of fun and silliness. At any age, it's perfectly appropriate to laugh at comedians, have a pillow fight, make silly faces at each other and get a little saucy with your intimates. If you have lost your sense of humour, you need to do whatever it takes to bring it back, even if it's just renting silly films. Treat it as a doctor's prescription for your health. ▥

● FOR MORE ON A HEALTHY ATTITUDE, SEE PAGE 239.

I rarely get a full night's sleep

Damage done

Skimping on rest can have far-reaching effects on your health, whether you're an insomniac who cannot sleep or someone who gives in to the temptation to use sleep time to catch up on work or TV. Studies of both men and women have shown that people who get less than 6 hours of sleep a night have an elevated risk of diabetes.

But that's not all. If you wake up feeling as though you've barely slept – and if your bed partner has told you that you snore – you may have obstructive sleep apnoea, a breathing problem that raises your risk of high blood pressure, heart attack and stroke. And sleep apnoea is also linked with diabetes, according to a study at Angers University Hospital in France. Among nearly 700 men with suspected sleep apnoea, tests showed that half had signs of insulin resistance, a pre-diabetic condition. What's more, in men with confirmed apnoea, almost a third had actual diabetes, often previously undiagnosed, and the severity of the diabetes correlated with the severity of the sleep apnoea.

Of course, not getting enough rest can also fog your thinking skills, slow your reaction time – raising your chances of traffic accidents – and leave you vulnerable to anxiety and depression.

Can I undo it? Yes

Just a night or two of refreshing sleep can lift your mood and clear your thinking. Just a few good nights begins to reverse metabolic changes that raise your odds of diabetes. And fixing sleep apnoea can immediately lower your blood pressure.

Plus benefits

Sleep is like a universal healer. Getting enough will provide you with numerous benefits such as more energy, a better mood and clearer thinking. Sleep can even lower your risk of apnoea-related heart problems and diabetes.

Repair plan

● **Sip some herbal tea after dinner** Avoid caffeinated coffee and teas, which block the brain chemical that makes you feel drowsy and fall asleep.

● **Do something soothing before bed** Don't work, watch lively TV programmes or pay bills. Try a warm bath or a quiet hobby such as knitting, reading or listening to music.

● **Turn off the computer** Working on a computer seems to affect the body's sleep/wake cycle and biological rhythms, so stay away.

● **Change beds** Women who sleep with snorers are three times more likely to have insomnia than those sleeping with non-snorers (there are no studies on the effect of a snoring partner on men).

● **See your doctor if you snore** There may be a simple solution, or you could be referred for a sleep apnoea investigation.

● **Sort out common symptoms** See your GP if you have sinus trouble, indigestion, breathing problems or acid reflux, all of which can interfere with sleep.

● **Have a medicines review with your doctor** At least eight classes of drugs, including antidepressants and blood pressure drugs, could be responsible for keeping you awake at night. ■

● FOR MORE ON REMEDYING SLEEP TROUBLES, SEE PAGE 301.

I rarely exercise

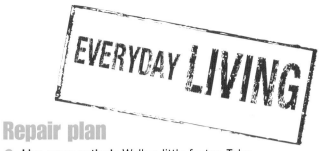
EVERYDAY LIVING

Damage done

Less muscle strength and density. Lowered metabolism. Weight gain. Balance problems. Higher blood pressure. Higher levels of 'bad' LDL cholesterol and lower levels of 'good' HDL cholesterol. More depression, stress and memory problems. And that's just the start of the damage caused by sedentary living.

All over the world, people are sitting more and moving less. A good name for it is 'sitting disease' – a sedentary lifestyle that diminishes muscle mass and ages your cardiovascular system while it weakens your immunity and leaves you vulnerable to stress, low moods and thinking problems associated with ageing. If you change just one damaging habit, it should be this one.

Can I undo it?
Yes, at any age

Studies of people in their 80s and 90s have found that adding walking and strength-training to their daily routines improves strength, balance, energy levels and more. And that's just the beginning. Just six months of exercise can improve memory and thinking, boost self-esteem, lessen depression, ease stress, increase immunity, improve your sex life, cool off chronic inflammation and strengthen your muscles so that you burn more calories.

Plus benefits

Moving more makes you less tired, less stressed and less apt to have bodily aches and pains. You can count on being in a better mood and having a trimmer, stronger, more energetic body. Of course, exercising results in better heart health but it also helps strengthen your immunity and sharpens your memory skills.

Repair plan

● **Live more actively** Walk a little faster. Take the stairs, not the lift. Park in the farthest spot from the supermarket. Stand while talking on the phone. Don't think that exercise can only be had during formal exercise sessions. Every moment of every day provides an opportunity to move in healthy, life-affirming ways. You'll find that high-energy living on its own can spark your energy and health.

● **Start slowly. Resolve to walk for 10 minutes a day** In a week or two, move up to 15 minutes if your feet, joints, legs and lungs are feeling good when you walk. Continue slowly increasing your time and distance until you're walking 30 to 60 minutes every day.

● **Add strength-training** It builds muscle, increases circulation and speeds up your metabolism.

● **Find a friend** Walking, swimming or exercising with a friend is more fun – and you're more likely to stick with it if you have an arrangement with someone.

● **Have 'active fun'** Join in the badminton game at picnics. Ask a friend to join you for a walk in a nearby park instead of going for a coffee. Take your grandchildren to the local pool instead of to the cinema. It bears repeating: formal work-outs are just one way of becoming active and stronger.

● **Wear comfortable clothes and supportive shoes** You don't need expensive athletic gear. Well-fitting walking shoes will protect your feet from injury, and trousers (or shorts) and a shirt that breathes will keep you cool while you're active. ■

● FOR MORE ON GETTING STARTED WITH EXERCISE, SEE PAGE 174.

I rarely go on holiday

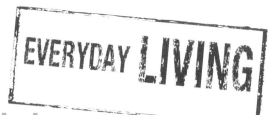
EVERYDAY LIVING

Damage done

Yes, damage can be measured, including a higher risk for heart disease.

When researchers from the State University of New York at Oswego surveyed 12,000 men aged 35 to 57, they found that those who didn't take at least one week-long holiday a year boosted their risk of dying from heart disease by 30 per cent during the course of the nine-year study.

Can I undo it? Yes

If you've been leading a high-stress lifestyle with few opportunities for relaxation, stay on top of your heart health.

How holidays help: any stress reduction, even for a few days, gives your heart and blood pressure a break. In one small New Zealand study, researchers found that holidaymakers slept about an hour longer than they did at home and got three times more deep, rejuvenating sleep afterwards than they got before their time off.

Even making relaxation a priority over the weekend can help. When Finnish researchers tracked the health habits of 800 women and men for 28 years, they found that those who didn't take a break from work-related stress over the weekend were three times more likely to have a fatal heart attack than those who got plenty of rest.

Plus benefits

This is your opportunity to spend time with and get reacquainted with your spouse, family and/or friends. Sharing good times with people you like helps you to feel less stressed. Get back in touch with the feeling of deep relaxation. In addition, you will enjoy better heart health overall.

Repair plan

● **Don't work this weekend** Skip home repairs, major lawn and garden work (unless it's a hobby you really love), and any other stressful obligations. Pretend you're on holiday. Eat a leisurely breakfast. Go for a walk. Visit a local attraction that you like. Take in a concert. Dine out with friends. Then, plan to do the same on one day of every weekend from now on.

● **Plan a real holiday** Half the battle of taking a holiday is committing to a time. So get out your calendar and pick a week (or more). Commit to it at work and among your family. Then get to the task of finding some great options, based on the budget you can afford. Merely looking for a perfect week-long sojourn can be relaxing and heart-healthy.

● **Make sure your next trip is relaxing** Even if you take holidays, you may be missing out on the health benefits if you try to do too much or agree to do activities that others like but that you simply don't enjoy. Put activities you like on the agenda, including time for relaxation beside the pool, lake or sea ... or get a massage, a spa treatment or take a long nature walk.

● **Move! See the sights on foot** Take advantage of outdoor attractions such as landscape gardens, nature trails, lakeside paths or a stretch of beautiful beach and take a long walk. Exercise releases feel-good endorphins: using your feet makes for happy holidays.

● **Consider rural over urban** City breaks are loud, exciting and exhausting. Holidays in the country are quiet, peaceful and recharging. For your health, the latter is what you need most. That doesn't mean choose a boring trip – just one that gets you away from the hustle and bustle you face at home. ■

● FOR MORE ON ACHIEVING BALANCE IN LIFE, SEE PAGE 238.

I work the night shift or have a changing shift pattern

Damage done

If you've ever spent a year or more on the night shift or on a changing shift pattern, you may be at higher risk of cancers of the breast and colon as well as cardiovascular disease, gastrointestinal problems and sleep disorders. Experts say that the night shift's health damage rivals the problems caused by smoking a pack of cigarettes a day.

The culprits? Stress and altered melatonin levels. Normally, melatonin levels reach their peak during sleep. But if you're exposed to light at night, levels decline sharply. The cancer connection: this sleep hormone also seems to inhibit the growth of tumours. At low levels, researchers suspect, it may not be able to do its job. Surprisingly, a changing shift pattern, or 'swing shift', may throw things off even more than a steady night job. In a study of 45 oil rig workers, researchers from Cardiff University in Wales found that those whose work schedules changed every few days had lower, more erratic melatonin levels and higher levels of heart-threatening fatty acids in their bloodstreams than men assigned to steady night work. 'Swing shift is a killer,' one researcher noted.

And then there are the unhealthy habits that are linked to night-shift work. Because few restaurants are open in the middle of the night, eating habits tend towards fast food and vending machines. And because of the night-time hours, late-night workers often skip on exercise.

Can I undo it? Yes

Altered melatonin levels seem to return to normal once night-time or shift work ends. But the added cancer risk may not go away. Be sure to report any symptoms to your GP promptly.

Plus benefits

Being diligent about getting your sleep and taking care of yourself will give you more energy and less chance of gaining weight while you're working nights. Talking to your GP about any health symptoms will catch problems early, when they're most treatable.

Repair plan

● **Establish a consistent sleep routine** Your body chemistry will adjust to some extent to your night-time work if you keep a regular schedule that includes plenty of rest. Go to bed at a consistent time and don't let errands and household chores interfere. You can do them when you wake up.

● **Bring your own healthy meals to work** Eating healthy foods has no shortage of benefits, and one of them includes better sleep. A diet of sugar, caffeine and fat – which is what you get from fast food and vending machines – not only hurts your health but also disrupts your natural energy/rest cycles.

● **Carry healthy drinks and lots of fruit or vegetable snacks** Having something healthy to crunch on or sip can help you to avoid two of the biggest dangers of shift work: drinking extra caffeine (as noted, it'll keep you awake when you finally have time to sleep) and smoking cigarettes.

● **Take an exercise break** Walk around the building, use the company gym if you have one or do sit-ups in the break room. You'll burn calories and feel more alert. ■

LIVING

3

Am I leading a healthy life?

Ready, set … slow!

Eat to feel good

Move to feel good

Live to feel good

Take charge of everyday health

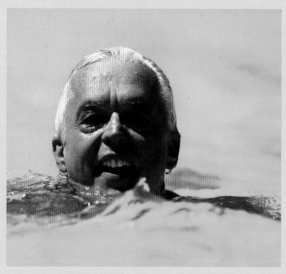

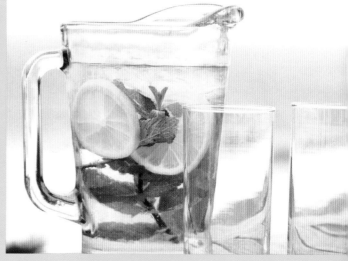

HEALTHY TODAY

The best way to ensure that you are healthy and energised in 20 years' time is to become healthy and energised right now. Here's how to feel great today, tomorrow and for the rest of your life

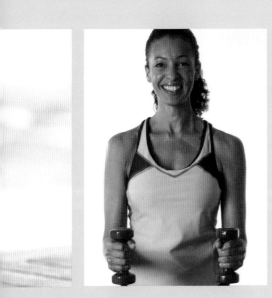
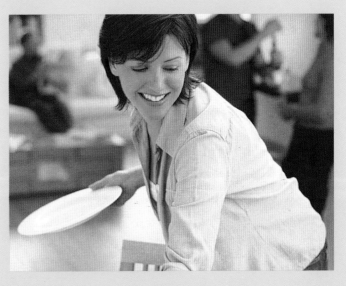

Did you floss your teeth yesterday?

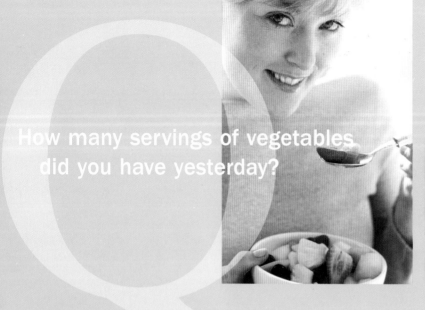

How many servings of vegetables did you have yesterday?

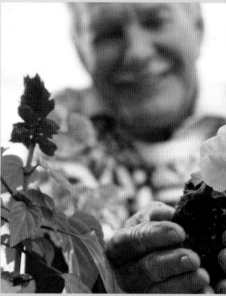

Have you had a cholesterol test?

Am I leading a
healthy life?

Y ou've just spent a lot of time exploring your past – the habits and lifestyle choices that have brought you to where you are today. Now it's time to talk about the present. What is your health like at this very moment? Are you fit, well-fed, in good spirits, energised?

Here are 35 questions that probe all aspects of your well-being. Give yourself at least 30 minutes to go through them. Some of the questions will ask you to get up and do something, so make sure you're dressed and prepared for activity, such as testing your balance and flexibility. Along the way, record your answers on the Score Sheet on page 105. The results are likely to speak for themselves.

But if you are the type of person who likes to keep a tally, the Score Key provides a points system that allows you to add up your marks and rank how well you are ageing.

Answer the questions honestly. No one is judging you, and you're the only one who will know the results. The purpose of this questionnaire is for you to identify the areas in which your health needs work, and to help you to understand whether you are treating yourself the way you richly deserve. ■

1 Pinch the skin of the back of your hand for 5 seconds, then release. How long does it take the skin to snap back into position?

   a My skin is tight enough that I can't really pinch it

   b Less than 2 seconds

   c 3–4 seconds

   d 5–6 seconds

2 Stand so you could grasp a chair back or worktop if you wobble. Fold your arms across your chest, shut your eyes and raise one leg, bending at the knee to as near a right-angle as you can manage. How long before you have to put your foot down?

   a 25 seconds or longer

   b 15–24 seconds

   c 5–14 seconds

   d Less than 14 seconds

3 Lean over as far as you can without bending your knees. How far can your fingertips reach?

   a To my toes or the floor

   b Within a few inches of my ankles

   c Not much past my knees

4 How much sleep did you average over the past five nights?

   a Less than 6 hours

   b 6–8 hours

   c More than 8 hours

5 Do you usually feel rested when you wake up in the morning?

   a Yes

   b No

6 How many servings of vegetables did you have yesterday?

   a One or two

   b Three or four

   c Five or more

7 When was the last time you had a pleasant conversation with a friend?

   a Today or yesterday

   b Three to seven days ago

   c More than seven days ago

8 How much of your free time yesterday did you spend in a chair or on a couch, watching television, using a computer, reading, talking or just passing the time?

   a Less than 4 hours

   b More than 4 hours

9 Over the past seven days, have you spent more than 4 hours outdoors?

a Yes

b No

10 The last time you were in a public building or shopping centre and had to go up or down one or two floors, did you take the stairs, escalator or lift?

a Stairs

b Escalator or lift

11 If you took a poll among your friends or co-workers, how would they rate your attitude of late?

a Happy, engaged, optimistic

b Stable, even-keeled, guarded

c Worried, frustrated, pessimistic

12 Did you floss your teeth yesterday?

a Yes

b No

13 The last time you flossed, did your gums bleed?

a Yes

b No

14 Think for a moment about the state of your overall health. How would you rate it?

a Great

b Fair

c Poor

15 Think about this past weekend. Were there things you wanted to do but couldn't or didn't because of physical or health-related limitations?

a Yes

b No

16 Think over the past week. Did you have any lapses in memory that you found annoying or troubling?

a Yes

b No

17 When you woke up this morning, were you in a good mood?

a Yes

b No

18 Over the past three days, did you engage in a hobby or activity that you really enjoy, such as cooking, hiking or attending a class?

a Yes

b No

19 Do you have a person you could talk to tonight about your personal problems, concerns or hopes?

a Yes

b No

20 Over the past week, how much exposure did you have to cigarette smoke, car exhaust fumes, fertilisers or insecticides?

a None that I can remember

b A few exposures

c Regular exposure

21 Have you had a cholesterol test?

a Yes, within the last two years

b Yes, more than two years ago

c No

22 Over the past seven days, how many times have you eaten fish/seafood?

a Three or more times

b Twice

c Once

d Not at all

23 Over the past three days, have you prayed, meditated or engaged in any form of deliberate relaxation?

a Yes

b No

24 As you are reading this question, do you have a cold, a headache or any other noticeable pain, symptom or health condition?

a Yes

b No

25 How many fizzy or other pre-sweetened drinks did you have yesterday?

a Three or more

b One or two

c None

26 Over the past two days, how long would you say you felt totally relaxed?

a Not at all

b Less than 30 minutes

c More than 30 minutes

27 Did you eat breakfast this morning?

a Yes, and it was very healthy

b Yes, but it wasn't that healthy

c No, skipped it

28 If a stranger did something very rude to you this morning, would you be angry and still talking about it tonight?

a Yes

b No

29 Sit in a strong, stable, armless chair. Hold the chair with each hand right next to your hips. Can you lift your body off the chair with just your arms?

a Yes

b No

30 As you read this, do you have a glass of water within arm's reach?

a Yes

b No

31 Since yesterday morning, how many servings of raw fruit have you eaten?

a None

b Two or three

c Four or more

32 Stand up and sit down rapidly, seven times. How difficult was that?

a I couldn't finish it

b It was challenging to my thighs and I'm breathing harder, but I did it

c Not very challenging at all

33 When was the last time you washed your hands?

a Within the past hour

b Within the past 3 hours

c It's been more than 3 hours

34 The last time you became really frustrated, what did you do?

a Ate some 'comfort food'

b Got angry, maybe even lashed out verbally at someone

c Did something healthy to relieve the frustration,
  such as walking or a relaxation exercise

35 Can you take your own pulse?

a Yes

b No

The answers

1 If you answered *a* or *b*, give yourself **1 point.** You are taking good care of your skin, and will continue to look young for your age.

2 If you answered *a*, give yourself **2 points.** Congratulations – you have the balance of a 25 year old. And if you're over 60, give yourself 1 point for a *b* (your balance is younger than you are). This is a good test of your balance, which is a key factor in preventing falls. If you have trouble with this exercise, turn to page 264 for advice on improving your balance.

3 If you answered *a*, give yourself **1 point.** But if the Internet had yet to be invented the last time you touched your toes, then you're facing some serious issues with flexibility. Flexibility is important if you want to remain physically active, which is critical to overall health. See page 191 for exercises designed to keep you flexible.

4 If you answered *b*, give yourself **2 points.** If you're having trouble falling asleep or staying asleep, turn to page 301 for tips on combating insomnia. And while answer c doesn't really signify a problem, some evidence suggests that people who sleep more than 8 hours don't fare as well as they age. Sleeping too much could also be a sign of depression.

5 If you answered *a*, give yourself **1 point.** Waking feeling rested is not only a sign that you had a good night's sleep but also an indicator of your overall health.

6 If you answered *c*, give yourself **3 points.** With the exception of exercise, perhaps nothing is as important to your overall health and well-being as your diet. If you think of vegetables as the garnish on your plate, then you need to pay particular attention to the chapter 'Eat to Feel Good', beginning on page 110. Vegetables are without question the most important food for you to eat for disease prevention.

7 If you answered *a*, give yourself **3 points.** As mentioned elsewhere, there is strong evidence to support the importance of social relationships for healthy ageing. It's vital to maintain the social connections you have and to continue to make new friends and join in social events. Numerous research studies show that shared activities, having someone to confide in and relationships that offer mutual support keep you healthy in mind, body and spirit. You'll find tips on building social networks throughout this book.

8 If you answered *a*, give yourself **2 points.** Sedentary living is a serious health problem, and its antidote, physical activity, is literally the backbone of healthy ageing. Without lots of movement, your muscles weaken and you put yourself at risk of frailty, not to mention a whole host of medical conditions including cardiovascular disease and Alzheimer's. Check out the chapter 'Move to feel good', beginning on page 174.

9 If you answered *a*, give yourself **2 points.** Being outdoors is a strong indicator of whether you have active hobbies such as sports, hiking or gardening. Not only is physical activity important but being able to enjoy the sheer pleasure of your body in movement and the joy of many productive and fun activities has been shown to keep you vital and young. It also keeps you socially connected and can recharge your spirit.

10 If you answered *a*, give yourself **1 point.** There's more to fitness than just formal exercise routines. Living life energetically, which in large part means keeping your body moving, ensures that you get the blood circulation and oxygen you need, as well as stretching your muscles in every corner of your being, including your mind.

11 If you answered *a*, give yourself **2 points.** A cautious approach to life isn't bad – in fact, being averse to risk can help you to live longer. But study after study shows that optimism and happiness are powerful healers and age-extenders. And life is so much more fulfilling for positive thinkers. An overly guarded, concerned or worried approach limits your opportunities for learning and personal growth. Plus, people who are happy are more fun to be around, and those who are optimistic just seem to find the good in life.

12 If you answered *a*, give yourself **2 points.** Taking care of your teeth means more than an attractive smile; it could make a difference to your cardiovascular health as well. Adults should floss their teeth daily. You can learn more about what good dental health is all about on page 273.

13 If you answered *b*, give yourself **1 point.** Healthy teeth and gums are the proverbial 'canary in the coal mine' when it comes to levels of inflammation in your body.

14 If you answered *a*, give yourself **4 points.** Numerous studies worldwide have shown that people who rate their health as only 'fair' or 'poor' have worse health outcomes, more disability and a higher mortality in the ensuing years – and this applies even after taking account of their actual starting level of health. In one Australian study of more than 12,000 women aged 70 to 75 at the start of the study, 52.3 per cent of those who rated their health as 'poor' died over the nine-year follow-up period, compared with only 11.5 per cent of those who said they were in 'good' health at the start.

15 If you answered *b*, give yourself **3 points.** Different people respond in different ways to various health problems in terms of the effect on their lifestyles. For example, as we age, nearly everyone develops some degree of arthritis, but only for some people does it significantly limit daily activities. The less you allow your health problems to get in the way of your life, the better you will age.

16 If you answered *b*, give yourself **2 points.** However, the mere fact that you had a lapse in memory tells you nothing about your brain's health or age. Memory problems are rarely a sign of ageing; more commonly, they are a sign of a hectic, stress-filled lifestyle. See page 340 for more on protecting your memory as you age.

17 If you answered *a*, give yourself **4 points.** The simplest definition of ageing well is waking up feeling refreshed and optimistic each day. For a long time, doctors who worked with older people struggled to understand why so many older adults reported being generally satisfied with their lives despite such obvious signs of poor quality of life, such as illness, disability or bereavement. Scientists now understand that the ability to make the best of our situation is one important component of successful ageing.

18 If you answered *a*, give yourself **2 points.** Even among centenarians, maintaining an active involvement in social, recreational or productive activities is an important predictor of decreased disability and of a lower risk of death.

19 If you answered *a*, give yourself **3 points.** As we've shown, older people who have at least one close relationship with someone in whom they can confide tend to have much better health and survival than those who are isolated.

20 If you answered *a*, give yourself **2 points.** Exposure to environmental toxins not only has potentially detrimental effects on our physical health but can also limit our enjoyment of life.

21 If you answered *a*, give yourself **2 points; if you answered *b*, give yourself 1 point.** You don't need to have in-depth medical knowledge, but it's important to understand how factors such as high cholesterol and high blood pressure affect your overall health. And knowing when to have certain issues (including suddenly losing weight, losing your balance or having unusual pain) medically evaluated can help you to stave off problems before they permanently affect your health.

22 If you answered *b*, give yourself **1 point; if you answered *a*, give yourself 1 point** (but only if you made sure the seafood was raised and harvested from healthy waters – sadly, it's a proven fact that fish from open seas contain high levels of toxins). Fish is an excellent source of anti-inflammatory omega-3 fatty acids, which studies find can help to maintain a healthy heart and keep your brain young. They can also help to reduce the inflammation that contributes to the aches and pains many of us experience with age.

23 If you answered *a*, give yourself **2 points.** Any form of calm contemplation, meditation or relaxation gives our minds a chance to wind down and our bodies the opportunity to combat the toxic effects of stress that so easily build up during daily living.

24 If you answered *b*, give yourself **1 point.** On average, most people spend most of their lives healthy. If you're having repeated headaches, chronic pain or more than one cold or other infectious illness a season, something is wrong. You need to reevaluate how you live your life, including taking a close look at your diet, exercise routine and stress management.

25 If you answered *c*, give yourself **2 points.** There is just nothing to be gained from drinking fizzy or other pre-sweetened drinks except weight. Stick to water, unsweetened iced tea (try green tea for a change) or the occasional glass of wine. If you do want to drink juices, dilute them with sparkling water.

26 If you answered *c*, give yourself **2 points.** The first person you need to take care of in your life is you, and that means finding time to relax, de-stress or, as some like to call it, chillax (short for 'chill and relax'). Doing so will stem the damaging effects of stress hormones, adding years of life to your heart, keeping your memory sharp and even reducing your risk of conditions such as insulin resistance and obesity.

27 If you answered *a*, give yourself **2 points.** You wouldn't drive a car with an empty petrol tank, would you? So why would you start your day on empty? If you don't get some glucose into your brain, and some fat and protein into your stomach, you're going to find yourself desperate for chocolate and crisps. And that's not good for anything – particularly your waistline. Many studies show huge health benefits from having a small, healthy breakfast each day.

28 If you answered *b*, give yourself **1 point.** Learning to let go of frustrating events, rather than ruminating on them, protects you against mental health conditions such as depression and anxiety, as well as the ageing effects of stress-related chemicals.

29 If you answered *a*, give yourself **1 point.** You have good arm strength and also good abdominal or 'core' strength, which is critical to reducing the risk of falls and back pain. Maintaining strength is crucial to remaining healthy and active in your future.

30 If you answered *a*, give yourself **1 point.** Staying hydrated becomes more difficult as you age because your thirst mechanism fades. And yet it also becomes more important for your overall health. If you always keep a bottle or glass of water nearby, you won't have to worry about it.

31 If you answered *c*, give yourself **2 points; if you answered *b*, give yourself 1 point.** Raw fruit provides valuable fibre and healthy glucose for cellular energy, not to mention disease-fighting antioxidants (even the best vitamins in the world can't compare). Consider fresh fruit a crucial part of a healthy, long-life diet.

32 If you answered *c*, give yourself **2 points.** You're managing to stay in shape quite nicely. This test challenges your aerobic fitness – that is, how well your heart and lungs can deliver oxygen quickly to your muscles. It also tests your thigh and abdominal muscles.

33 If you answered *a* or *b*, give yourself **1 point.** Frequently washing your hands with hot, soapy water is the best way to avoid becoming infected with cold, flu and other viruses or bacteria. Many people don't realise how often they touch their faces with their hands. And it's often your hands that pick up other people's germs from counters, doorknobs or other often-touched surfaces.

34 If you answered *c*, give yourself **2 points.** While you can't necessarily eliminate or even reduce stressful events in your life, you do have control over how you let them affect you. Finding healthy ways to cope (and no, that leftover chocolate cake doesn't count) will add years to your life.

35 If you answered *a*, give yourself **1 point.** An overlooked but important part of good health is constantly monitoring yourself. If you know how to take your pulse, it's indicative that you have invested a little time and thought into understanding your body's signals.

Am I leading a healthy life?

SCORE SHEET

Answer all 35 questions first, then score your results and tally up all the points you've earned in the 'Total points' box below. Check your score against the key on the left to see how you fare.

1		**19**	
2		**20**	
3		**21**	
4		**22**	
5		**23**	
6		**24**	
7		**25**	
8		**26**	
9		**27**	
10		**28**	
11		**29**	
12		**30**	
13		**31**	
14		**32**	
15		**33**	
16		**34**	
17		**35**	
18			

TOTAL POINTS:

The score key

55–65

Congratulations! You are doing most of the things you should to be healthy today – and many years from now. Be proud of yourself, but don't be complacent. With your healthy mindset, it should be easy to take on some more health-enhancing lifestyle choices that will make you even more likely to thrive for the rest of your life.

40–54

You're not doing badly in terms of your ageing potential, but there is definitely room for improvement. Look back at the questions and see if there are patterns to your answers. For example, did you do particularly poorly on the diet questions? Fitness questions? Attitude questions? Make a commitment to start there, then revisit this quiz in a few months.

Below 40

This quiz should be a wake-up call. It should have made clear, for example, that good health is not merely the absence of disease. It's time to ask yourself, 'What do I want the next 20, 30 or 40 years to look like?', then make the changes necessary to get there. If you keep going the way you're going, you'll face a host of age-related issues, ranging from frailty to memory loss to chronic health conditions, all of which will make your later years a burden, rather than a joy. ■

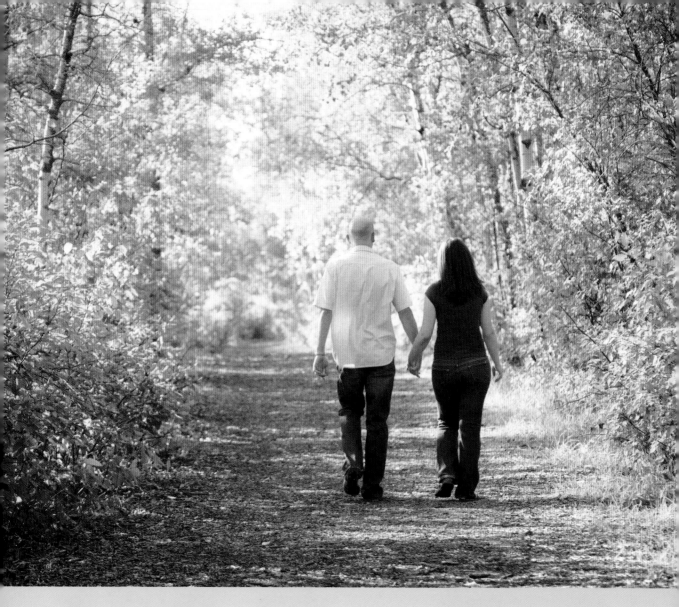

Ready, set ... slow!

So, how did you react to your healthy life
score? Maybe you feel there are so many things you have to fix
that you don't know where to begin. Or perhaps you're thinking: if those
are the changes I need to make to achieve long health, that's easy, so
let's get started.

Hopefully, you're ready to get started on a life of long health, but even if not, the message is the same: go slowly. Make one change at a time. Be patient and mindful of what your body's telling you.

The truth is that slow change can create a health revolution. When you make one change at a time in important areas affecting your health, you're setting yourself up for success. You won't feel overwhelmed. You'll have the time to fit a new habit into your life, no matter what else is going on. You'll see real benefits and build a foundation for making more changes successfully, too.

Starting with the next chapter and for much of the rest of the book, you'll discover the exciting, research-proven core concepts of a long and healthy life – that is, the ways to eat, move, de-stress and prevent disease that keep the world's longest-lived people vibrantly healthy for decades into old age. And the processes are broken down into lots of easy, small steps. Our hunch is that you'll want to try lots of them, and quickly.

Some experts would advocate that you overhaul your whole life with dozens of new rules to follow for what to eat, when and how to exercise and required relaxation techniques. And honestly, for a few people, it works.

But when US researchers at Baylor College of Medicine in Houston compared the success rates of people who took an all-or-nothing approach to health (they stopped smoking, cut back on sodium and started exercising, all at once) to that of people who adopted one healthy new habit at a time over an 18 month period, just 6 per cent of study volunteers in the all-or-nothing group could maintain all of their new habits. In the same study, the 'slow change' group had more success at exercising (they added far more steps to their days) and lowered their cholesterol levels more than the all-or-nothing group.

A prescription to move

The benefits of an active lifestyle are so great compared with other forms of health intervention that some GPs are actually prescribing exercise as an alternative to drugs. And a poll commissioned by Natural England showed that 94 per cent of people would welcome this if their GP thought that outdoor exercise would work instead of prescription drugs. So if you're having trouble getting started, ask your GP what kind of exercise would be best for you.

For most of us, starting small is smart, practical and most likely to help to ensure that you succeed. And, there's plenty of cutting-edge research on how our brains adapt to change that suggests it really does work best.

Experts who work with older people agree, too. It takes time for your body to adapt to a new level of activity, and you need to feel enthusiastic about the changes you make, not intimidated or discouraged. It's important not to rush at things so fast that exercise feels uncomfortable or painful – but even a few short, gentle exercises can build up to a habit that offers impressive health benefits. In one study at London's Royal Free Hospital, older people taking a 12 week exercise programme had a 30 per cent increase in muscle power – that's equivalent to regaining three decades of lost strength.

Small, it turns out, is big when it comes to changing your health habits.

THE POWER OF ONE SMALL CHANGE

Don't think little changes mean small health benefits. A little tweak – such as switching from white bread to whole-grain bread, ordering unsweetened iced tea instead of a fizzy drink or fitting 10 minutes of exercise into a busy day – can add up to big health bonuses. Consider:

- A brisk walk three times a week can reduce mild, moderate and even severe depression, researchers have found.
- If you watch TV for several hours a day, cutting out just an hour could reduce your risk of a serious pre-diabetic condition called metabolic syndrome by 19 per cent, according to one study.
- Switching to whole-grain bread, brown rice and whole-grain breakfast cereal could lower your risk of diabetes by up to 33 per cent, say German scientists.
- Drinking two glasses of skimmed milk a day could cut your risk of insulin resistance by 62 per cent and cut your risk of heart disease by 50 per cent, say British researchers who followed 2,375 men for 20 years as part of the United Kingdom's landmark Caerphilly Prospective Study.
- Losing just ½kg (1lb) lightens the load on your knees by 2kg (4lb) with every step – that translates to 2,200kg (4,800lb) less pressure every time you walk a mile.

Most experts agree that making small, slow changes is the best way to maintain new healthy-eating patterns. Aim for one change each week – but no more. Add an extra portion of vegetables and cut down on potatoes with dinner, have fruit instead of biscuits for a mid morning snack, cut back on sugar in your tea – it doesn't take long for the changes to add up. Within a few weeks your digestion will improve, and you may have more energy. And things you can't see will be improving, too – such as your immunity, blood fats and blood sugar.

And never believe it's too late to start. When researchers at the Medical University of South Carolina tracked health-negligent, middle-aged adults who began eating five or more fruits and vegetables every day, exercised for half an hour five days a week and didn't smoke, they reduced their risk of heart disease by 35 per cent. After four years, they even got their risk down to the same safe level as people who had always been active and eaten a healthy diet.

So where do you begin? Read the eating, exercise and everyday living chapters that follow and choose the changes that appeal to you most. Perhaps these are the things that sound fun or delicious or as if they'd feel really good. Maybe they're the smart ways finally to overcome a not-so-healthy habit that's been bothering you (perhaps fruity iced tea in place of gallons of sweet drinks, grilled fish rather than a cheeseburger, or a walk with your best friend instead of meeting for coffee and cake). Try one change in each important area … then commit to sticking with it for the next four weeks.

TRAIN YOUR BRAIN FOR HEALTH

Forming a new habit – one that you'll do automatically, as your 'default' setting – takes at least two weeks of faithful repetition. The reason: you're rewiring your brain. Researchers have discovered that giving up bad habits such as overeating, watching TV instead of exercising or anything else that may feel good but isn't great for your health works against the brain's pleasure systems. Your brain may actually go into withdrawal when you swap bad habits for good habits, because you're no longer supplying the activity or foods that send surges of the feel-good chemical dopamine washing through your brain cells.

Outsmart withdrawal by substituting another feel-good food or activity – the kind you'll find throughout the coming pages. Experts suspect that sticking with a new, healthier pleasure for long enough will teach your brain to release dopamine when you experience it – so that you actually look forward to that walk or slice of whole-wheat cinnamon toast in the morning.

It's not received wisdom, but change doesn't have to hurt to be good for you. That's especially true for exercise – 'no pain, no gain' is a myth. If it hurts, don't do it. Exercise that causes you pain will be very difficult to stick with. Instead, look for exercise options that make you feel energised, that match your body type and personality, your likes, dislikes and interests.

That's where mindfulness comes in. As you make changes, check in with yourself throughout the day. A change that's right for you will help you to feel energised yet relaxed. You may feel a little tired if you've just taken a walk or performed a few strength-training moves, but you shouldn't feel achy or exhausted. You may feel a little lighter in the tummy if you're eating more moderate portions, but you shouldn't feel starved. And if you're trying to add more relaxation, more hobbies and more socialising to your day, you should expect to feel excited and busy, but never overwhelmed.

Why? Change shouldn't become a source of stress. Research shows that when it does, stress hormones impel us to do whatever we've always done to calm down. That might mean eating a cake or smoking a cigarette, having a glass of wine or complaining. Stress, then, could interfere with your efforts to change.

Remember this point: if you start with changes that are easy to make, and stick with them for a few weeks, you'll find that the next wave of changes is even easier. And suddenly, you are well down the path towards the long health you desire. ■

4 traits of successfully healthy people

1 They're patient It takes at least two weeks – and probably more like four to eight weeks – to turn a new strategy into something that's second nature. You have to stick with it long enough to face all the challenges you meet regularly in your life and find a way to fit it in, no matter what. If you can do something for three weeks in a row, you've established a good habit. You'll know it's working because if for some reason you can't get your usual exercise, you'll miss it, or suddenly realise that you're not feeling so good because you haven't had your usual exercise 'dose'.

2 They take it seriously Buy the healthy foods you need. Set aside time for socialising. Schedule exercise. Don't leave change to chance. Make your new-found habits a regular part of your day, or log them in your diary and treat them as a commitment.

3 They get support Tell other people about your new routine and ask them to help – by reminding you, encouraging you or coming along with you. You can get even better motivation by joining or creating an exercise group or finding an exercise chum – someone with whom you can walk or work out, or just communicate by phone or via an online support group.

4 They know that small changes lead to big things Once you start making changes, you'll find that one move leads to another. When you start to see the benefits and feel the rewards, you'll be encouraged to carry on, and to make more changes to multiply the gains.

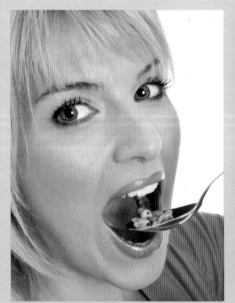
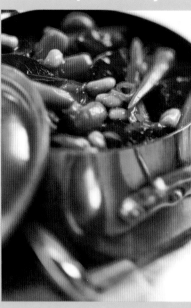
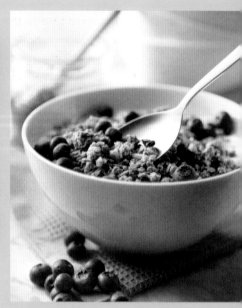

... more food but fewer calories

... food cupboard and fridge makeover

Eat to feel good

Imagine a place where joints ache less; minds and memories remain stronger; digestion problems are few; a good night's sleep is the norm; and energy levels stay youthful – even at the age of 90 and beyond.

Here, cancer is virtually unknown. People's arteries function as well at 85 as they did at 18 – and their odds of having a heart attack or stroke are the lowest in the world.

Places like this do exist today – on the sun-drenched Mediterranean island of Crete, in Okinawa, Japan, and even in the modern Seventh-Day Adventist households of America. What do these people have in common? Primarily, a healthy attitude and an even healthier diet. The foods people eat every day in these Shangri-las of longevity might amaze you. In the course of a single day in Okinawa, the average person eats nearly a dozen helpings of fruit and vegetables, seven servings of noodles, rice and grain, plus tofu, fish, seaweed and green tea. Dairy foods and red meat are rarely seen – or eaten. At night, friends knock back a glass or two of a fiery alcoholic drink made from hot peppers.

The menu is similar on Crete, where poultry and fish replace soya-based foods as the primary protein, and locals sip homemade red wines. The story is the same with Seventh-Day Adventists, except much of their protein comes from eggs and nuts. Many are vegetarians who also abstain from alcohol, tobacco and coffee.

Notably absent from their diet: salty, sweet, processed foods; buttery treats; juicy steaks; ever-flowing fizzy drinks; super-sized portions.

The payoffs for a life free of cheese-drenched chips, cakes and huge drinks? Healthy-eating Seventh-Day Adventists live up to 9.5 years longer than other Americans, say researchers who tracked the diets and health histories of over 34,000 members of this Christian denomination. Okinawans have the longest life expectancies in the world – the average man lives to be 77, the average woman to 85. And more people on Okinawa have celebrated their 100th birthdays than people from anywhere else – around three or four times as many, proportionately, as in the USA. On Crete, the healthiest eaters were 25 per cent less likely to die during a four-year study than their fellow countrymen who opted for more modern meals.

Even if your diet has been pretty unhealthy up to now, you can make up for it with relatively small changes. According to an eight-year study of over 26,000 Greek men and women, those who followed a traditional Mediterranean diet more closely – using olive oil, eating plenty of fruit and vegetables, more fish and less red meat, and drinking moderate amounts of alcohol – were less likely to develop cancer. The study, reported in the *British Journal of Cancer*, found that adopting just two aspects of the Mediterranean diet could cut the risk of cancer by 12 per cent. Using more olive oil alone reduced the risk by 9 per cent. It shows just how important diet is in cancer risk.

'We think diet plays an extremely important role in how long people in these parts of the world live and in how long they remain healthy, active, independent and happy,' says Bradley Willcox, MD, of the Pacific Health Research Institute in Honolulu and lead researcher of the Okinawa Longevity Study. 'A low-calorie, low-fat, plant-based diet is the key to maximising life expectancy and minimising the risk for all of the debilitating health problems that come with ageing.'

In fact, what you put on your plate and in your mouth counts even more than whether or not you were born with longevity genes. 'You could have Mercedes-Benz genes,' says Dr Willcox, 'but if you never change the oil, you are not going to last as long as a Ford Escort that you take good care of.'

The 7 choices of full-life eating

Here's the important point: you don't have to be born into one of these cultures to get their kitchen-table health benefits. Anyone, anywhere, can eat for health and long life. If you really wish, you can start from this moment forward, with your very next meal or snack. The benefits would be immediate. You'll feel more energetic, have better digestion and even sleep better in just two to four weeks. It's exciting how quickly you can feel the difference.

That's just the start of the benefits, too. You'll have fewer colds as your immune system improves. Your body will naturally get to its proper weight. And you'll take bold steps to prevent the diseases that plague our later years the most. Four of the ten leading causes of death – heart disease, cancer, stroke and diabetes – have a huge diet component to them. What we eat – and how we eat it – makes a big difference.

... you'd be surprised how much food many healthy people eat. Their secret: eating the right foods

The challenge is that if you ask 100 doctors the specifics of a healthy diet, you'll get 100 different answers. We're here to help. After taking a close look at the diets of the world's healthiest people, matching up those practices with the best scientific research, and then talking at length with many top experts on nutrition and health, what emerged were seven golden choices for eating for energy, disease prevention and long life. We call them choices rather than guidelines, laws or rules because we want *you* to be the one to decide that they are right for you. Only if you decide in your heart that they are worth doing will you take action.

Here they are in a nutshell; in the pages ahead, we'll be far more specific on how to make each choice super-easy to achieve.

Choice 1

Make more than half of your diet fruit and vegetables

Human beings evolved on a diet that was mainly composed of fruit, vegetables, fish and lean meats – and your body hasn't altered its nutritional expectations much over the past million years. That's how most people ate – until the advent of agriculture gave us a higher calorie intake from potatoes, cereals and beans. Then, a few decades ago, breakthroughs in convenience foods steered our diet towards processed 'food products' packaged in boxes, cans wrappers and freezer containers. It's no coincidence that these dietary changes have been paralleled by a massive rise in diseases linked to food, from heart disease to diabetes.

A mountain of research shows that making fruit and vegetables the centrepiece of meals and snacks – as they once were – is a powerful health-insurance policy. There are several reasons why, but one of the biggest is that plant matter is packed with compounds called phytochemicals that disarm free radicals. These are rogue oxygen molecules, created naturally in the body and also ingested with toxins and pollutants, that damage cells and raise the risk of cancer, heart disease and many other health problems.

One study at Sweden's Karolinska Institute involving almost 25,000 postmenopausal women followed for six years showed that those with a diet high in fruit and vegetables along with whole-grain foods, fish and beans and moderate amounts of alcohol reduced their heart attack risk by 57 per cent. Those who were also non-smokers, had a healthy waist/hip ratio and were physically active were a stunning 92 per cent less likely to have a heart attack than women who did not have all these 'low-risk' characteristics. Although only 5 per cent of the study group had the full combination of healthy dietary and lifestyle factors, the researchers concluded that most heart attacks in women 'may be preventable by consuming a healthy diet and moderate amounts of alcohol, being physically active, not smoking and maintaining a healthy weight.'

A more natural diet goes a long way towards protecting you from cancer as well. An extra helping or two of fresh produce at each meal could cut your odds of stomach cancer by 21 per cent, lung cancer by up to 32 per cent, ovarian cancer by as much as 40 per cent and prostate cancer by 35 per cent (even higher if you include lots of broccoli, cabbage and brussels sprouts – and we'll show you how to make them taste great). Researchers have shown that even a modest intake of fruit and vegetables protects against breast cancer – and the more you eat, the lower your risk. Those who consume six portions of vegetables a week (that's less than one a day) have a 21 per cent lower risk of breast cancer than those who eat only one. Six portions of fruit a week lowers the risk by 17 per cent compared with just one.

Choice 2

Eat more whole-grain foods

Dietary fibre – also called bulk or roughage – is simply the parts of plant foods that your body cannot absorb or digest. Whole-grain foods are filled with it. Eat more fibre, and you'll fill up faster, making weight control a breeze. Fibre also eases constipation and diarrhoea. In the long term, fibre can help to control cholesterol, balance your blood sugar and lower your risk of haemorrhoids, irritable bowel syndrome and diverticular disease (the development of small pouches in the colon).

But whole grains deliver so much more than just fibre. When you add whole-grain breads and pastas, brown rice and other grains to your diet, you're getting not only the chewy, high-fibre hulls (the bran) that cover the grain, but also the nutrition-packed germ and endosperm found in each grain. This grain package is a rich source of niacin, thiamin, riboflavin, magnesium, phosphorus, iron and zinc, as well as protein and a little bit of good fat. This extra nutrition may be one reason why people who eat whole grains have a reduced risk of diabetes and heart disease.

Choice 3

Eat more 'good' fats

Learn the phrase 'omega-3 fatty acids'. This is the one type of fat in our diet that is truly great for our health. Omega-3s are best obtained from oily fish, but are also found in green leafy vegetables, walnuts, pumpkin seeds and olive, linseed (flaxseed), rapeseed and hemp oils. They are the building blocks for hormone-like compounds that reduce chronic inflammation – a modern health problem fired up by too much belly fat, too little exercise and a diet full of the wrong types of fats. New studies show that your body also uses good fats to make inflammation-fighting chemicals called resolvins.

Yet most of us eat far too few omega-3s and far too many omega-6s – a fat found in high levels in corn, safflower, soya bean, sunflower and sesame oils. Omega-6 fats help the body to produce compounds that *increase* inflammation. In prehistoric times, people ate omega-3s and omega-6s in nearly equal proportions; today we consume as many as 30 times more omega-6s.

Yes, pork and beef fats taste wonderful. But for long life, the best fats come from plants and fish

Eating tasty foods such as salmon, peanut butter, walnuts and good-for-you oils can correct this balance. You'll slash your risk of heart attack and stroke, and possibly cut your odds for arthritis pain and depression, too.

Choice 4
Eat calcium-rich foods

Calcium's not just good for your skeleton. While 99 per cent of the calcium in your body is hard at work maintaining the strong, internal scaffolding that supports the bones and teeth, the remaining 1 per cent is a major player in keeping your cardiovascular system happy and your blood sugar control mechanisms healthy. A growing pile of research proves that calcium helps to lower blood pressure, keeps arteries flexible and assists your kidneys in flushing blood pressure-boosting sodium out of your body.

In tandem with other minerals such as magnesium and potassium, calcium can also lower your risk of insulin resistance – a potent risk factor for heart disease, diabetes and even some cancers – by up to 71 per cent. It may also guard against memory loss and cut colon cancer risk by 36 per cent.

Choice 5
Enjoy lean protein

Protein is your body's basic building material – used to make everything from muscles, bones and the tissues of internal organs to hormones, enzymes and even red blood cells. Putting lean protein on your plate delivers an immediate payoff: meats, low-fat cheeses, eggs and nuts linger longer in your stomach than bread, rice, fruit or veg, so you feel full for longer. Protein also slows the absorption of sugar

into your bloodstream, eliminating cravings that occur when sugar soars, then crashes after a carb-heavy meal.

Lean protein is also a rich source of the B vitamins that can help you to feel more energetic, since the Bs help to guide metabolic reactions throughout the body. You also get zinc, which builds strong immunity, and niacin, vital for clear thinking and efficient processing of blood sugar.

Protein's biggest bonus is preserving lean muscle mass. We all lose muscle mass at the rate of 3 to 5 per cent per decade starting in our mid 20s. By our 50s and 60s, we've lost plenty – and may be weaker, have poorer balance and a slower metabolism. Protein contains an amino acid called leucine that helps to preserve more muscle mass, studies show.

Choice 6
Eat fewer calories

Note that we didn't say 'eat less food'. Fruits, veggies and beans are filling and satisfying yet contain far fewer calories than fatty foods. That means you can usually eat them to your heart's content and still consume fewer calories.

But it's appropriate to face the hard question of whether you do eat too much food overall. Okinawans don't eat till their buttons burst. Instead, they practise a form of natural portion control called *hara hachi bu*, which literally means '80 per cent full'. In other words, they stop eating before they feel completely filled up.

'*Hara hachi bu* is sort of an insurance plan against feeling deprived or overeating,' says Dr Willcox. 'It takes about 20 minutes for the body to signal the brain that there's no need for more food. *Hara hachi bu* gives the brain a chance to catch up.' That restraint, plus a diet filled with low-calorie, high-satisfaction foods – and cooking techniques that use water (steaming and boiling) rather than frying or sautéing with oil – means that Okinawans eat about 1,800 calories a day, which is hundreds less than the typical Westerner consumes in a day.

Don't get us wrong – we don't advocate extreme calorie restriction. So far, no one's proven that drastically cutting calories extends human life (all those headline-grabbing studies only show it works in fruit flies and laboratory mice). And when people try it, super-low-calorie eating seems only to lead to irritability and potentially dangerous nutrient deficiencies.

But experts such as Dr Willcox believe that cutting back *a little*, without denying ourselves the nutrients we need and the eating pleasure we desire, is an important reason Okinawans and others live to a vibrant old age. Why? Fewer calories mean lower body weight and less of the dangerous abdominal fat that raises the risk of heart disease, stroke, diabetes, high blood pressure and some cancers – even Alzheimer's disease. Living at a healthy weight also puts less stress on the joints and may reduce the levels of cell-damaging free radicals in your body.

Choice 7
Enjoy eating

Sharing mealtimes with family or friends, and enjoying the smells and tastes of foods, all help to make life worth living. Meals among the world's healthiest people are long, happy occasions, not something to rush through or gobble while watching TV. In Greece, the nation's official dietary guidelines include advice to 'eat slowly, preferably at regular times of the day, and in a pleasant environment'.

Enjoying food is almost as important as the nutrients in the food itself. And meals need not be fancy to be cherished and savoured. It's

more an attitude of life-enhancing reverence and celebration. Small wonder that one way Greeks identify someone as a friend is by saying 'we have shared bread together'.

Beyond food

Then there's the reality of the modern diet: huge helpings of meat, mountains of grains stripped of key nutrients, and processed food filled with sweeteners, flavours, colours and preservatives. Not only does the modern diet give you lots of what you don't need, it also shortchanges you on what you *do* need.

Many of the classic signs of ageing – including fatigue, aches and pains, memory lapses, fuzzy thinking, balance problems and more – may be symptoms of unrecognised yet easily reversible nutritional shortfalls. A good diet can help older people to stay in good health, according to the British Nutrition Foundation. Yet national surveys consistently show that older people tend to have higher intakes of saturated fat, cereals and protein than is recommended, along with lower fibre, vitamin and mineral intake.

What do we mean by nutritional shortfalls? Well, take vitamin D: in your 70s, your skin synthesises 60 per cent *less* vitamin D than it did when you were a child. One recent British study of 7,437 people showed that 60 per cent of middle-aged adults have less than optimal levels of vitamin D – and the proportion rises to 90 per cent in winter and spring. The risk is higher the farther north you live and the fatter you are – obese people and those living in Scotland were twice as likely to have low vitamin D than others.

Lead researcher Dr Elia Hypponen comments, 'during the winter, no vitamin D is produced by the sun in the UK, so one has to rely on intake through dietary supplements and foods'. He recommends spending more time out of doors, eating oily fish and maintaining a healthy weight. It may also be sensible to take a supplement. 'Cod liver oil and many multivitamin products contain vitamin D, but the concentration in these is typically quite low,' he warns. Therefore, these alone may not be sufficient to allow you to maintain summer levels during the winter months. Single

antidepressants, cholesterol-lowering statin drugs, diabetes drugs, diuretics, pain relievers, laxatives and tranquillisers.

The combination of a less-than-healthy diet and nutrient-draining medications may help to explain why two landmark studies, the Framingham Heart Study and the Baltimore

... having a good diet can help older people to stay in good health

vitamin D supplements are available through the internet.

Again, healthy foods to the rescue, in the form of skimmed milk, fish and seafood and greens. But that multivitamin is also the perfect form of insurance.

Or take a look at the curious case of calcium. Many older people think that they don't need as much calcium. They assume it's important only early in life, during the bone-building years of childhood, teens and early 20s. But the fact is, women and men need even more calcium after the age of 50 than before because absorption drops with age. Studies show that nine out of ten older people don't get enough calcium from food, and plenty take no calcium supplements. But research confirms that inexpensive calcium pills can bridge the gap for women and may help men, though some experts warn that extra calcium from dairy products (but not non-dairy sources) could raise prostate cancer risk.

In addition, many prescription medicines and over-the-counter remedies can also create nutritional shortfalls by blocking absorption or speeding up the excretion of vitamins and minerals, or interfering with the action of vitamins in the body. In fact, drugs, like other chemicals and toxins, have sometimes been described as 'anti-nutrients'. Particular culprits are acid-suppressing drugs, antibiotics,

Longitudinal Study on Ageing, found that older people often face these health-threatening nutritional shortages as well.

- Thirty per cent of people aged 67 and older don't get sufficient folic acid, a vitamin that may play a role in heart health.
- Twenty per cent are low in B_6 – a vitamin that plays a role in sleep, appetite and mood.
- In addition, most older women and men may not get enough magnesium – important for healthy blood pressure – and zinc – significant in wound-healing, immunity and maintaining your sense of smell and taste.

For all these reasons, we are sure that certain supplements – a multivitamin, calcium, vitamin D and omega-3s – offer sufficient benefits to justify adding them to a daily routine. Studies show that they can fill real nutritional gaps.

We'll cover these three supplements in more detail later in this chapter. But let us reiterate our key point: for long life and ongoing health, it's mostly about food. Supplements may help to fill in gaps, but the best way to get the nutrition you need is from the foods you eat.

And so, go to page 120 for the first of the seven choices for full-life eating, along with hundreds of tips and tricks to make each an easy part of your daily meal routine. ■

5 foods
to protect your arteries

These amazing foods can: reduce your risk of atherosclerosis • whittle down your cholesterol • lower your blood pressure • cool inflammation • neutralise damaging free radicals • reduce your chances of developing metabolic syndrome by keeping your blood sugar lower and steadier • keep your heart pumping at a healthy beat.

1 **Roasted almonds – with the skins** One handful of almonds packs a whopping 9g of monounsaturated fat to help to slash bad cholesterol and boost good cholesterol. Simply choosing almonds instead of a cake or crisps for two snacks a day could cut 'bad' cholesterol by nearly 10 per cent. Natural vitamin E in the almond's 'meat' plus flavonoids in this nut's papery skin help to halt the development of artery-clogging plaque – be careful not to overdo it, though, or you'll pile on the calories.

2 **Tomatoes – fresh, sun-dried and in a sauce** Eating seven or more servings a week cut the risk of cardiovascular disease by 30 per cent in a study of more than 35,000 women. And according to a study from the University of Oulu in Finland, 30g of ketchup and 400ml of tomato juice a day cuts levels of 'bad' LDL cholesterol by 13 per cent after three weeks. How? It could be the antioxidant lycopene, or the tomato's stellar levels of vitamin C, potassium and fibre. Cooking tomatoes for 30 minutes or longer raises levels of available lycopene. And 15g of sun-dried tomatoes has more blood pressure-lowering potassium than a medium banana.

3 **Avocados** In a study by Mexico's Instituto Mexicano del Seguro Social, women and men who ate one avocado a day for a week had a reduction in total cholesterol of 17 per cent. Their levels of unhealthy LDL and triglycerides fell, and good HDL levels rose – thanks, perhaps, to the high levels of 'good' monounsaturated fat. The fruit is also full of cholesterol-cutting beta-sitosterol.

4 **Salmon** Among omega-3-rich fish, salmon is king: one serving contains about 1.8g of eicosapentaenoic acid (EPA) and docosahexaenoic acid (DHA), omega-3s that help to cut your risk of deadly out-of-rhythm heartbeats, reduce bad cholesterol, cool inflammation and discourage atherosclerosis and the formation of blood clots.

5 **Oatmeal** Betaglucan, the soluble fibre in oats, acts like a sponge, trapping cholesterol-rich bile acids in the intestines and eliminating them. The result is lower 'bad' LDL because there's less cholesterol to be absorbed into the bloodstream. A big bowl of oatmeal (what we usually eat as porridge) a day – about 225g – could cut cholesterol by an extra 2 to 3 per cent, suggests a study published in the *Journal of the American Medical Association.* ■

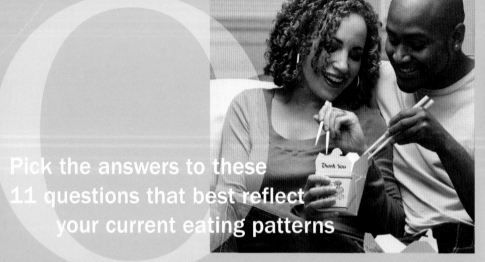
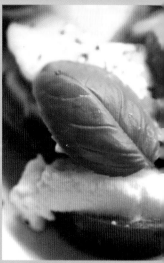

Is your diet making you old?

1 **My usual breakfast is:**

a Oatmeal or high-fibre cereal with semi-skimmed milk and some fruit.

b Sausage or bacon, an egg and a roll.

c A cup of coffee and maybe a slice of white toast.

2 **My favourite fruits:**

a Change with the seasons: I love berries, peaches, watermelon, apples, mangoes and more.

b Are the occasional apple, orange or banana.

c Are the cherries in chocolate-and-cherry ice cream.

3 **On a typical day, I eat this many vegetables:**

a Loads – a salad or soup with lunch, several helpings at dinner and even a helping as a snack.

b Two – a salad or side dish with dinner and maybe some lettuce or tomatoes at lunch.

c One – do chips count?

4 **Whole grains are a _____ part of meals in my house:**

a Big. We eat whole-grain bread and brown rice and have tried other grains, too.

b Small. I get brown bread sometimes or wheat crackers.

c Non-existent. I prefer the comforting, smooth texture of white bread, white rice and white noodles.

5 **My beverage of choice is:**

a Water.

b Coffee or hot tea.

c Fizzy drinks or squash.

6 **When I eat chicken, I:**

a Usually have it sliced (without skin) into vegetables, salads or other dishes.

b Have it grilled with the bone and skin.

c Have it battered and fried.

7 **My regimen for supplements is:**

a Consistent – I take a multivitamin every day, plus one or two other smart choices.

b Inconsistent – I've got lots of vitamins in my kitchen cabinet, and once in a while, I might even take one.

c Non-existent – vitamins are not a part of my life.

8 **When it comes to dairy foods, I:**

a Make sure I have several low-fat servings a day.

b Have an occasional pot of yoghurt, glass of milk or piece of cheese.

c Add milk to my coffee – that's about it.

9 **When I do my grocery shop, my trolley is mostly filled with:**

a Unprocessed foods, such as fruits, vegetables, eggs, orange juice and raw meat.

b A mix of fresh foods, packaged foods and frozen meals.

c Boxes, cans, jars and precooked meals.

10 **My typical dinner is:**

a Slow and social. I eat with my family or, when possible, with relatives or friends.

b Quiet. I often watch TV or read while dining.

c Expedient. I just grab whatever's at hand and don't make a formal sit-down meal of it.

11 **If I were hungry at 3pm, I would probably:**

a Have a piece of fruit or a handful of nuts.

b Tell myself that dinner is just a few hours away.

c Have a chocolate bar, biscuit, bag of crisps or scoop of ice cream.

Your score

If you circled mostly (a) answers: your meals – and your way of eating – are in line with the age-defying traditions of long-lived, healthy people in places such as Crete and Okinawa. You can take your nutrition-packed good habits to new heights by trying new fruits and vegetables, adding more types of whole grains to your cooking repertoire, snacking on good fat-rich nuts and savouring mealtimes even more.

If you circled mostly (b) answers: you're modestly healthy, but you're not doing much to prevent disease or add healthy years to your life. Your diet's too low in fruits, veg, whole grains and bone-building calcium. And it's also too high in sugars, refined carbs and artery-clogging fats. As a result, you may be feeling tired and moody, and have digestive problems. Choosing to eat well could help you to feel better in just a few short weeks – and lay the foundation for years of better health ahead.

If you circled mostly (c) answers: not only have you put yourself at greater risk of many serious diseases, but you are eating in a way that saps you of energy, reduces brainpower and makes you susceptible to colds, flu and other everyday challenges. The seven choices of full-life eating should become a top priority. Start by making small changes such as adding a multivitamin and calcium supplements to your daily routine, substituting fruit for sweets and starting meals with a salad. You'll soon discover that healthy eating is filling, flavourful and hugely pleasurable. And you'll feel better immediately. ■

CHOICE 1

Make more than half of your diet beans, fruits and vegetables

Want to slash your risk of everyday health problems such as migraine headaches, colds and flu and slow-healing wounds, as well as big medical problems including heart disease, cancer and dimming vision? Skip the pharmacy – and visit your local farmer's market instead.

'Eating lots of fruit, vegetables and legumes – foods high in antioxidants and other phytochemicals – is the cornerstone of the diets of healthy, long-lived populations around the world,' says Dr Willcox. 'It's one reason their rates for heart disease and many cancers are so low. When we compared the Okinawan diet to the typical Japanese diet, we found that Okinawans ate so much of these foods that they had three times the recommended levels of vitamin C, almost double the vitamin E, and their antioxidant intake was really high, too. So were calcium, magnesium and phosphorus – important for bone health and high blood pressure prevention. It's the power of good carbohydrates.'

A glass of red grape juice at breakfast, a big spinach-and-bean salad at lunch and a fruit salad after dinner provide immediate gratification, too. In one Australian study of 453 women and men aged 70 and older, those who ate the most healthy foods had the fewest signs of wrinkles. Treating yourself to the hundreds of disease-fighting compounds found only in plant foods boosts immunity, speeds wound-healing, and cuts your odds of everyday annoyances such as easy bruising, nosebleeds, yeast infections, haemorrhoids, gout and attacks of asthma caused by physical activity.

At work are thousands of beneficial compounds collectively known as phytochemicals. Among the best known are antioxidants, which protect cells from damage by free radicals (notice how often these rogue oxygen molecules are mentioned?). As we've discussed, free radicals damage cell membranes as well as the DNA that encodes the cell's operating instructions. Free radical damage has been linked to many major diseases. What neutralises them best? Antioxidants found in plant-based foods.

Other important phytochemicals include:
- Carotenoids that help cells to communicate better (possibly cutting cancer risk)
- Lutein, zeaxanthin and other compounds that act almost like sunglasses to protect your eyes from vision-robbing sun damage
- Flavonoids that can attack invading viruses and bacteria
- Building blocks for vitamin A that improve immunity by promoting the growth of the thymus gland, bolstering the functioning of white blood cells and keeping the delicate tissues inside your mouth and nose strong to deter disease-causing invaders better.

In a study of 30 volunteers at Ninewells Hospital and Medical School, Dundee, just one 100g serving of dark chocolate significantly inhibited platelet aggregation, a measure of blood-clotting potential – whereas white or milk chocolate had no effect.

So eating small amounts of dark chocolate is probably a heart-healthy habit – as long as you don't eat too much and avoid milk chocolate, which is high in fat with fewer of the beneficial nutrients of dark chocolate. Pair your chocolate with the right red wine (read on for our own full-life wine list) or a steaming cup of tea for even more phytochemical prowess.

TRUE SUPERFOODS

Low in calories, high in satisfaction and simply delicious (who can say no to a perfectly ripe peach in summer or a steaming bowl of bean soup on a snowy winter evening?), fruits, vegetables and legumes – beans, peas, soya beans, peanuts and lentils – deserve a starring role on your plate. Eat them to your heart's content, suggests Dr Willcox, one of the lead researchers for the Okinawa Longevity Study. 'I never limit [fresh] produce or legumes,' he says. 'When I'm hungry, I'll have some ripe pineapple or strawberries. I don't count my servings of legumes, either. They're higher in calories but so satisfying that you really can't overdo it, as long as you watch the added fat.'

This is a vital point, worth reiterating. As long as you don't use lots of oil or high-calorie add-ins, you can healthily eat as much fruit, vegetables and beans as you like. The exceptions are people who have diabetes or are prone to big blood sugar swings; then sweet fruit should be eaten in moderation.

Beans in particular are antioxidant superstars. When researchers analysed the antioxidant concentrations in more than 100 foods, small red beans came in first, followed by red kidney beans and pinto beans in second and third place, respectively. And as you'll discover later on, beans are packed with fibre and are a terrific source of protein. No single food can help you to fulfil the full-life eating guidelines as well as beans.

But let's not undersell vegetables. You can't go wrong if you shop in season. Just-ripe fruit and veg have the highest levels of vitamins and antioxidants; levels decline as fresh produce sits on the shelf. And don't assume that raw is better than cooked. Some phytochemicals are actually more available for absorption when veggies are processed, such as the prostate-protecting lycopene in tomato sauce and the carotenoids in lightly steamed spinach and carrots.

But you don't have to shy away from convenience products, either. Look for prepackaged, single-serving bags of baby carrots or raisins, precut melon chunks or fruit salads – and don't forget all the salad stuff easily selected from the deli counter. ■

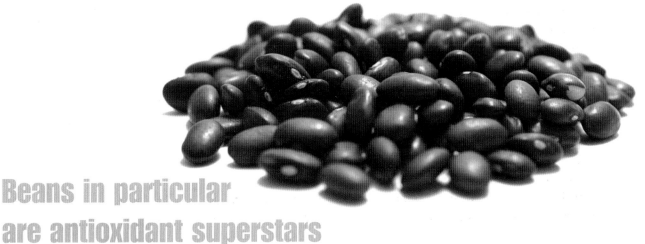

Beans in particular
are antioxidant superstars

smart ways TO EAT MORE Beans

FULL-LIFE EATING GOAL: at least five servings a week

Make beans your main ingredient on Tuesdays and Thursdays For those who don't eat beans that often, it's hard to think up many interesting meals in which beans are the star. But a glance at a bean cookbook will be a revelation. Beans are the successful centrepiece of many stews, soups, cassoulets, wholemeal salads and even sandwich spreads. Find a few recipes and give them a try.

Always have beans on hand Your cupboard should contain a large assortment of beans canned in water (no salt) and plenty more dried beans for overnight soaking and cooking. Both are healthy, but dried beans have more crunch and texture. We suggest using dried beans when you're cooking a bean dish from scratch (change the water before simmering to remove indigestible sugars that cause bloating and embarrassing personal gas!). Remember that kidney beans and soya beans must be boiled for some time to remove toxins – always follow the instructions on the packet. Canned beans are great for mixing into other types of dishes.

Add beans to everyday dishes Beans go well in rice dishes and even better in soups. They work fine in pasta sauces and add texture to roasts. Every time you cook a dish, ask yourself, 'Can I add some beans to this?'

Make dips and spreads No need to keep their original form. Blend with herbs, garlic, olive oil or other flavourings and use as dips for vegetables, spreads for sandwiches or hors d'oeuvres.

Mix plain canned beans with baked beans The tasty sauce in canned baked beans is full of sugar and calories. Keep the taste and lose some of the sugar by mixing in small red beans or kidney beans. Serve at lunch with a low-fat sandwich or whole-grain toast.

Make this marvellous lunch Just toss together black beans, baby spinach, mandarin orange sections and spicy vinaigrette. Add other high-antioxidant veggies left over from last night's dinner, such as steamed broccoli.

Use beans as a garnish Keep chickpeas in a sealed bowl in the refrigerator and put it on the table at every meal. Get in the habit of adding a few to your salads, vegetables or pasta. Or just nibble on them as you would if a bowl of olives or almonds were on the table. ■

Great combinations

Not sure which bean's best? Try these flavour suggestions.

Black beans: great with brown rice and in Mexican dishes.

Black-eyed peas: good in casseroles and curries or paired with ham and rice.

Chickpeas: toss into minestrone or mash with garlic and a touch of sesame seed paste (tahini) for a classic hummous dip.

Broad (fava) beans: add to stews or serve alone as a side dish.

Butter (lima) beans: good to mix with canned baked beans or add to salads.

Haricot beans: stir into soups.

Pinto beans: pair with rice.

Red beans and kidney beans: good in three-bean salads, chilli and other spicy dishes.

White beans (cannellini): delicious in chicken broth-based soups.

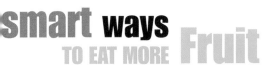

smart ways
TO EAT MORE Fruit

FULL-LIFE EATING GOAL: three to five servings a day

Have a piece of fruit with breakfast every day Toast and an apple. A roll and a banana. A bowl of cereal and berries. Yoghurt with cantaloupe melon. Fruit is the perfect breakfast food. Make it a mandatory part of your day's start.

Have citrus as your midmorning snack Most of us have a midmorning snack. Make your choice an orange. One serving a day of citrus cuts the risk of mouth cancer – the seventh most common cancer – by 67 per cent, according to an Italian analysis of 16 studies. Like variety? Try a different citrus fruit every week, from blood oranges to sweet-tart Mineolas, juicy clementines to luscious navel oranges, tart yellow to sweet red grapefruit.

Eat fruit for dessert six nights a week When scientists measure antioxidants in fruit, the winning choices read like the perfect shopping list. For example, research in Hong Kong published in the *British Journal of Nutrition* ranked the 'top ten' fruits by antioxidant potential as: strawberries, lemons, plums, oranges, kiwi fruit, grapefruit, persimmon, apples (especially green), mandarins and mangoes. And according to scientists at the Scottish Crop Research Institute, the humble British blackcurrant – often overlooked in such studies – contains higher levels of vitamins, minerals and antioxidants than 20 other fruits tested. Lead researcher Dr Derek Stewart explains that, generally, the darker the fruit the higher the antioxidant content. Having a brimming fruit salad after dinner most nights of the week equals at least two fruit servings and a huge

variety of good-for-you phytochemicals. Cut fruit will keep for six to nine days with minimal loss of vitamin C, carotenoids or other phytonutrients, say researchers. Just store it in a covered container.

Always keep frozen fruit on hand Visit a farmer's market or pick-your-own fruit farm, get a large quantity of your favourite berries or tree-grown fruit, take it home, clean it and pack it up for the freezer. Then you'll have year-round local produce, perfect for blender drinks, sauces, salads and dessert toppings. Don't want to do the work yourself? Most food shops sell frozen fruit.

Stock up on canned fruit, too It's nearly as nutritious as fresh, and you'll avoid 'overripe banana syndrome'. Canned foods can provide similar amounts of vitamins and minerals to fresh equivalents, and are often a good source of fibre, according to the British Nutrition Foundation. Most canned fruits are canned immediately or very soon after harvest, when nutrient concentrations and quality are at their highest – canned fruit may actually contain more vitamin C than fresh equivalents that have been on the shelf for a while. So canned fruit and vegetables count towards your recommended 'five a day' portions. But choose fruit canned in natural juices, not sugar-laden syrups.

Shop Continental-style That is, stop at a fruit market every few days, buy small amounts of what looks the very best, and eat it within a day or two. This is so much more pleasant than buying large bags of the same old stuff at the supermarket every two weeks. And even if the fruit costs more at the small market, you'll probably save money by eating everything you buy. Sadly, when you buy infrequently, you tend to throw out more than you realise due to spoilage.

Stock up on kitchen gadgets such as an apple slicer, a mango slicer and a sharp box grater With one push, an apple slicer divides your favourite Granny Smith or Golden Delicious into delectable slices and separates the core. It does double duty as a pear corer, too. Build on your repertoire with a mango slicer, to turn these fiddly fruits into sweet, ready-to-enjoy sections, and a sharp box grater for grating apples to mix with oatmeal.

Freeze bananas Frozen bananas are a delicious, sweet snack, better than an ice lolly. You don't need to peel them before freezing as long as they are slightly speckled/brown.

Savour a glass of real juice every day Many packaged fruit drinks are laden with sweeteners and flavoured artificially. But enjoying a glass of real orange juice (from a carton or from concentrate) or pure red grape juice every day is a healthy pleasure with a big payoff, experts say. One study found that people who enjoyed three glasses of fruit (or vegetable) juice a week had a 76 per cent lower risk of Alzheimer's disease than those who had less than one glass a week. And researchers at Glasgow University say that grape, grapefruit, cloudy apple and cranberry juices contain the highest amounts of the beneficial chemicals thought to underlie this protection against Alzheimer's and other chronic diseases. Indeed, red grape juice contains as many polyphenolic antioxidants as red Beaujolais wine. ■

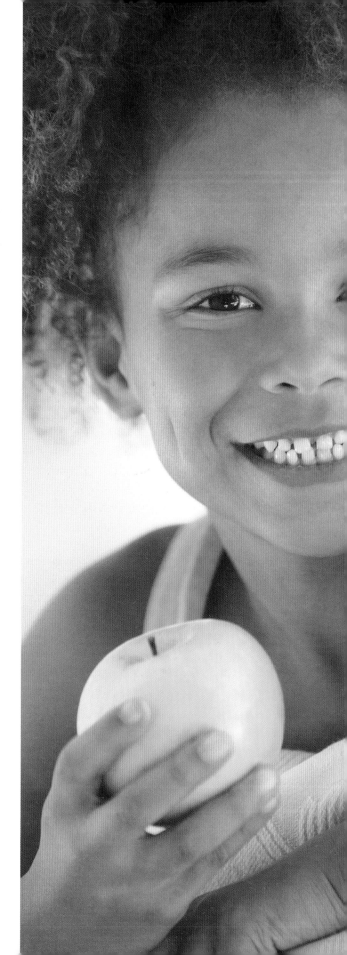

smart ways
TO EAT MORE Vegetables

FULL-LIFE EATING GOAL: four to seven servings a day

Serve yourself a double portion – every time It's the simplest way to get more vegetables into your diet – and if you're trying to lose weight, doubling the greens and losing the potatoes will help. At first, it'll seem odd to have your plate so full of green, but in time it will be a welcome habit. Make sure you haven't 'de-healthed' your vegetables with excess butter, oil or fat or your calorie count will surge. Also, don't double up on high-starch vegetables such as sweetcorn, peas or beans since they're higher in calories – have one portion and one of green, leafy veg instead.

Flavour your vegetables the tasty, healthy way Don't smother your steamed or raw vegetables in butter or sauté them with bacon to give them more flavour. There are many ways to make vegetables delicious without pushing up the calorie count.

- Drizzle with a little honey.
- Grate on a light sprinkling of cheese.
- Toss with olive oil, lemon, salt and pepper.
- Mix with a small amount of soy sauce and sesame oil.
- Sprinkle with a vegetable-friendly herb such as coriander, rosemary or basil.
- Grill with just a light coating of olive oil, salt and pepper.
- Add a few drops of a favourite hot sauce.
- Stir-fry with a little oil and curry powder.

Add microwaved baby carrots and frozen peas or chopped green beans every time you heat up soup Microwaving carrots allows you to add them to soup fully cooked; otherwise, they need simmering time to soften. And you get more vitamin A from cooked carrots, too. Frozen vegetables only need to be heated through, so you can add them directly to the simmering soup. In a few minutes, you'll have a hearty lunch or light supper.

Use veg in place of pasta Most sauces that work well on pasta work well on vegetables, too. Serve spaghetti sauce over steamed green beans, for example. Make lasagne with strips of aubergine or use courgette in place of noodles. Make 'cauliflower and cheese' in place of 'macaroni and cheese'.

Get into a raw-vegetable habit Tomatoes, cucumbers, carrots, celery, radishes, broccoli and peppers are just a few examples of vegetables that are outstanding to eat raw. Try to get in the habit of a daily raw-vegetable snack – if you eat them unadorned, you can eat as many as you wish. Also, put out a plate of raw vegetables at every dinner. You and your loved ones will naturally nibble them throughout the meal.

Start every dinner with a salad That's at least one serving – and if you fill your bowl with your favourite salad veg, you'll start the meal with a smile. Be choosy. If you dislike iceberg lettuce, try a beautiful green salad mix or baby spinach. Add juicy fresh produce such as tomatoes, sliced red peppers or even strawberries or raspberries. For more flavour, sprinkle chopped fresh herbs such as basil and coriander on top. Drizzle with a teaspoon each of olive oil and lemon juice.

Sip vegetable juice with your afternoon snack A glass of low-sodium, low-sugar vegetable juice counts as a full serving of ▶

making greens sweet

It's the strangest conundrum in the garden patch: many of the healthiest vegetables taste unappetisingly bitter because of natural chemicals that give them their healing oomph.

Human tastebuds are wired to detect minute amounts of bitterness in food. Thanks to a genetic quirk (and up to a sixfold higher concentration of tastebuds), one in four adults is a 'super-taster' – particularly sensitive to bitter chemicals, even if they're good for you. As a result, they frequently skip proven heart-protecting, cancer-defying foods such as beetroot, broccoli, brussels sprouts, cabbage, aubergine, kale and spinach – all of which earn high marks on official lists of high-antioxidant vegetables.

BEETROOT Mix grated raw beetroot with lemon juice, golden raisins and celery. Or roast with balsamic vinegar. In animal studies, the pigment responsible for the beetroot's purplish-red hue, called betacyanin, disarmed cancer-triggering toxins. The earthy taste of beetroot comes from geosmin, a chemical that also has cancer-fighting powers.

BROCCOLI Mash steamed florets with potatoes or shred peeled broccoli stems and sauté with garlic and a dash of olive oil. One antioxidant that makes broccoli bitter, called sulphoraphane, whisks cancer-promoting substances out of the body. Another, dubbed indole-3-carbinol by scientists, discouraged tumour growth in laboratory studies and reversed suspicious precancerous changes inside cervical cells in women.

BRUSSELS SPROUTS Roast them with onion chunks, then toss with rice vinegar. These cousins of broccoli have plenty of bitter sulphoraphane as well as compounds called isothiocyanates, which detoxify cancer-causing substances in the body. In one Dutch study, men who ate brussels sprouts daily for three weeks had 28 per cent less genetic damage (gene damage is a root cause of cancer) than those who didn't eat sprouts.

CABBAGE Cook red cabbage, chopped apples (leave the skin on for more antioxidant power) and raisins in apple juice; season with ground cloves. Eating cabbage a few times a week can cut your risk of cancer of the breast, prostate, lungs and colon. In one study of 300 Chinese women, those with the highest blood levels of cancer-fighting isothiocyanates (found in cabbage) had a 45 per cent lower risk of breast cancer than those with the lowest levels.

AUBERGINE Brush with olive oil, sprinkle with oregano and grill. All types of aubergine are rich in bitter chlorogenic acid, which protects against the build-up of heart-threatening plaque in artery walls (and fights cancer, too), say scientists. In studies, aubergine lowered cholesterol and helped artery walls to relax, which can cut the risk of high blood pressure.

KALE Braise in apple juice or cider to offset bitterness. Kale has compounds called glucosinolates, which seem to fight cancer by activating liver enzymes that help to disarm carcinogens.

SPINACH Eat it fresh and raw. Create a salad dressed with puréed raspberries, raspberry or balsamic vinegar and a dash of olive oil. Possibly the healthiest veg in the world – thanks to high levels of vitamins A, B_6, C and K, and riboflavin, plus manganese, folate, magnesium, iron and calcium – spinach also contains the antioxidant lutein, which protects your eyes from damage or vision loss.

vegetables. Tomato-based juices are high in the antioxidant lycopene.

Ask for a plain vegetable in place of potatoes or noodles when you eat in a restaurant Choose one that's not fried or served in a creamy or oil-based sauce, and ask for your veg with no butter, otherwise many restaurants add it automatically. If nothing fits the bill, request a green salad instead.

Instead of cheese, add a thick layer of vegetables to your sandwich Give dark green lettuce, fresh herbs, sliced tomatoes and onion a go. But leftover vegetables from last night's dinner can be delicious, too: how about a chicken sandwich with grilled courgette?

Turn cold cooked vegetables into a side salad Don't let leftover green beans, peas, carrots, beetroot, asparagus, corn or other vegetables go to waste. Simply serve with lunch as a cold salad, topped with a splash of lemon juice and a dash of coarsely ground black pepper.

Use shredded vegetables in cooking Finely shredded carrots, cabbage, lettuce, squash and other vegetables add wonderful texture to many dishes that might not otherwise include such healthy ingredients. Add to soups, pasta sauces and even rice dishes. Or use the vegetables as a bed for your chicken or fish. Smart habit: keep a tightly sealed container of shredded vegetables in your refrigerator with the goal of using it up over the next three to four days. If you have a lot left after a few days, just sauté it with a bit of olive oil, lemon juice and herbs for a terrific side dish. ■

The two-colour rule

It is simple always have fruit and veg of at least two different colours on your plate. This holds for breakfast, lunch and dinner. Start breakfast with a berry/citrus salad or have red and black berries with yoghurt. Have red and orange peppers in your lunchtime salad. Heap your plate with purple-skinned aubergine and tomatoes at dinner.

Why is this sensible? First, you'll automatically have two servings of fresh food. Second, they'll flood your body with a wider variety of beneficial antioxidants and other phytochemicals. Third, brightly coloured fruits and vegetables are often more nutritious than subtler-coloured versions. Two examples: red-leaf lettuce has three times more antioxidants than green-leaf lettuce, and yellow and orange peppers have more than red or green peppers, experts report.

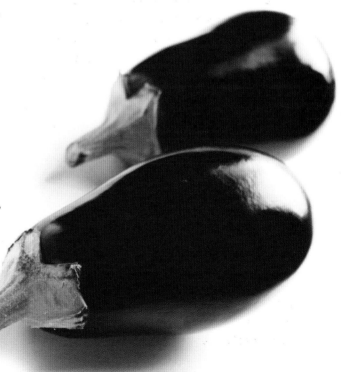

smart ways
TO EAT MORE Antioxidant superfoods

FULL-LIFE EATING GOAL: up to 30g of quality dark chocolate a day; one alcoholic drink a day for women, two for men; four cups of green or white tea a day

Pair chocolate with citrus Ascorbic acid in oranges, lemons, tangerines and other citrus fruits may release more of the healthy antioxidants locked in cocoa, research suggests. Try making a chocolate dip using a block of dark chocolate melted slowly in a metal bowl suspended over a pan half-filled with hot water. Use as a dip for peeled, segmented clementines, tangerines or sweet-tart Mineola oranges.

Blend equal parts of nuts, dried fruit and mini chocolate chips for a delicious, high-antioxidant snack mix Use dark chocolate, of course – it packs more antioxidants than milk chocolate. Include dates, raisins and prunes, the dried fruits with the highest antioxidant levels, as well as pecans, walnuts, hazelnuts, pistachios or almonds – all high-antioxidant nuts. Parcel out 2 tablespoon portions into tiny sealable bags and drop one in your bag or briefcase for a delicious snack when you're out and about.

End the day with a cup of cocoa When Dutch researchers studied the diets and health of 470 older men for 15 years, they found that higher cocoa intake was associated with lower blood pressure and a whopping 50 per cent drop in risk of dying from heart disease.

Have a cup of green, black, white or jasmine tea at midmorning and midafternoon 'Older, healthy people in Okinawa drank plenty of jasmine tea, which is rich in antioxidant catechins,' Dr Willcox notes. But skip the milk. A British study found that in your teacup, milk proteins bind to some beneficial compounds and could prevent absorption. A Swedish study of 61,000 women found that a cup of black tea a day lowered ovarian cancer risk by 24 per cent.

Toast your health with red wine Take advantage of high concentrations of artery-scouring compounds found in these red varieties: Zinfandel, Syrah (Shiraz), Pinot Noir, Merlot and Cabernet Sauvignon. (Tannat, a red wine variety big in southwestern France and Uruguay, is also super-high in tannins.) Or ask your wine seller for a wine that has been given extended contact with tannin-rich skins, seeds and stems. Australian research shows that for both younger people (aged 18 to 30) and older people (aged over 50), drinking 400ml red wine each day for two weeks significantly increases blood antioxidant status. And in a study in France involving 34,000 men aged between 40 and 60 at the start, the chance of death from heart and vascular disease 10 to 15 years later was reduced by 35 per cent among those who drank two to three glasses of wine daily, and by 30 per cent for those who drank three to five glasses. The risk remained lowered for men drinking up to seven glasses of wine a day, but increased above that.

Of course, the most important thing to know about sipping wine for its health benefits is when to stop. In the UK, government advice is that women can drink up to two to three units of alcohol a day and men up to three to four units a day without significant risk to health. ■

Toast your health with red wine

20 top antioxidants

Mother Nature tucked a medicine chest full of **disease-fighting antioxidants** into fruits, vegetables, grains and even spices. These beneficial compounds fight damage to cells from rogue molecules called free radicals – and can help to reduce your risk of heart disease, cancer and dozens of age-related health problems.

Until recently, experts didn't know which foods had the highest levels. According to Hong Kong scientists who tested the antioxidant power of equivalent portions of 34 fruits and vegetables, these are among the ones that pack the most antioxidant power:

1 Strawberry
2 Lemon
3 Plum
4 Orange
5 Kiwi fruit
6 Grapefruit
7 Persimmon
8 Apple (green)
9 Pak choi
10 Spring onion
11 Mandarin
12 Mangetout
13 Onion
14 Apple (red)
15 Turnip (green)
16 Cabbage (long)
17 Broccoli
18 Cauliflower
19 Garlic
20 Tomato

Once, high-fibre eating was perfectly natural because we ate mostly unprocessed foods. Then the rise of the processed food industry stripped our diet of fibre. What happened next was even worse. Once the need for fibre was recognised, manufacturers introduced a new crop of high-fibre health foods that made for less-than-pleasant eating – 'bran' cereals that made you feel as if you were chewing on pebbles, gritty wholewheat pasta and health bars with the texture of sawdust. The alternative wasn't very appealing either: mixing gluey fibre supplements with water, to be downed as quickly as possible.

No wonder the concept of 'high-fibre' foods scares people. But fear not. Shop shelves are crammed with high-fibre cereals and wholewheat breads that taste good and have a great texture. Delicious whole-grain pastas, brown rice and more exotic grains are commonplace. Despite this bounty, though, the average British adult manages to get just 12g of fibre a day – far short of the average 25g experts recommend.

Fibre becomes more important with each passing birthday, simply because with age, food moves more slowly through the digestive system. Partly, it's a natural slowdown, but often, getting less physical activity and drinking less fluid play a role, too. Fibre helps by making your stools bulkier, which stimulates your digestive tract to keep things moving.

Supplements work, but nothing beats the fibre in real food. You can get all the fibre you need from fruit, vegetables and whole grains. Although fibre supplements will help with constipation, they don't include all the other wonderful nutrients you get from natural foods – the vitamin E, good fats, protein and antioxidants that help to protect against heart disease and diabetes and even cancer.

HOW MUCH IS ENOUGH?

If you're trying to ensure that past dietary lapses don't catch up with you, perhaps take even more fibre than the recommended intake. To reduce your risk of the disorders above, plus high blood pressure and intestinal disorders, your goal should be 30–40g of fibre a day.

According to the UK Women's Cohort Study, involving 35,792 women aged 35 to 69 years, a fibre-rich diet – over 30g a day – halved the risk of a premenopausal woman developing breast cancer over the seven year follow-up. And in a large study of the eating habits of more than half a million people in ten European countries, those in the top 20 per cent for fibre intake – consuming an average of 35g of fibre daily – had their risk of bowel cancer slashed by 40 per cent, compared with those eating only 15g fibre daily (still more than the UK average intake). To get 30–35g fibre daily you need seven portions of fruit and vegetables a day – similar to the amounts eaten by Mediterranean populations, who have a lower overall cancer risk – plus the equivalent of five slices of wholemeal bread.

Getting fibre from a wide variety of sources yields the most health benefits, say French researchers who analysed the diets and health of 6,000 people. They found that whole grains worked best for weight control, lowering blood pressure and reducing levels of heart-threatening homocysteine in the bloodstream; fruits controlled tummy fat and cut blood pressure (thanks in part to all the fibre in the tiny seeds packed into berries); vegetables lowered blood pressure and homocysteine; and fibre in nuts had the strongest effects on weight control, tummy fat and controlling blood sugar.

fibre. And all that fibre, plus the protein, means beans are low on the glycaemic index, a measure of food's impact on blood sugar.

Beans aren't the type of food you eat several times a day, though. More likely, you'll turn to breads, cereals and pasta for much of your fibre intake. According to a survey by the Medical

Fibre becomes more important with each passing birthday

Switching to whole grains is one of the easiest eating upgrades you can make. You probably already eat bread, rice and pasta, so there's no need to add or subtract anything from your diet. Just reach for a different type.

But if you increase your fibre intake too quickly, you are likely to get intestinal gas, bloating and even cramping pains. Take things slowly – and keep up your fluid intake to soak up the extra fibre, or you may get constipated. So in week one, switch to wholewheat bread and aim for four daily servings of vegetables and fruit. The second week, have six portions of fruit and veg daily and add brown rice. The third week, go to nine servings of fruit and vegetables and give whole-grain pasta a try. Eat more beans, too. They're a great source of fibre.

HIGH-FIBRE SUPERFOODS

We have already extolled the virtues of beans as antioxidant powerhouses, but their fibre content is among the best of any food. Beans have both kinds of fibre: insoluble, which helps your gastrointestinal system to eliminate waste products more quickly, and soluble, which forms a gel in your intestines that helps to lower levels of 'bad' LDL cholesterol by whisking it out of your body. Research shows that 175g of beans a day can lower cholesterol by up to 10 per cent in just six weeks. No natural food has more

Research Council, wholemeal bread and breakfast cereals account for more than three-quarters of all servings of whole-grain foods. But most people don't eat nearly enough – in fact, one in three British adults eats no whole-grain foods at all on a daily basis, and less than 5 per cent eat three or more servings a day.

And although brown and wholemeal breads are growing in popularity, traditional 'sliced white' is still Britain's favourite, accounting for 71 per cent of all the bread we eat. Yet British consumers have a stunning choice of breads – over 200 varieties are on offer.

So how do you make the switch to healthier bread? Check the fibre content on the label – don't go on the amount per portion or slice, as this is often misleading; look for the amount of fibre, in grams, per 100g of bread. On average, white bread has 1.9g, brown 3.5g and whole-grain 5g – nearly three times as much as white.

Not a bread eater? Then how about whole-grain cereal or oatmeal? Both are health superfoods. Betaglucan, the soluble fibre found in oats, acts like a sponge, trapping cholesterol-rich bile acids in the intestines and eliminating them. The result is lower LDL cholesterol because there's less cholesterol to be absorbed into the bloodstream. Having a big bowl of porridge a day (about 225g) could cut cholesterol by an extra 2 to 3 per cent.

Healthy, filling and ready to eat, whole-grain cereal is a perfect convenience health food. One study found that participants who ate whole-grain cereal every day were 17 per cent less likely to die over the next several years from any cause and 20 per cent less likely to die from cardiovascular disease than those who rarely or never ate whole-grain cereal.

Want whole grains for other parts of the day? Add brown rice and other fibre-rich grains such as barley or bulgur wheat to your plate. So, what's wrong with white rice? Milling and polishing rip off more than the chewy coating on rice; they also steal fibre and nutrients that make brown rice a delicious, satisfying, disease-battling superfood. Compared to white, brown rice packs four times more insoluble fibre as well as good amounts of niacin, vitamin B_6, magnesium, manganese, phosphorus, selenium and vitamin E. Best of all, it's easy to find in supermarkets these days – even in quicker-cooking forms for nights when you just don't have 45 minutes to wait for dinner to cook. ■

Toast your health – with water

Sparkling or still, bottled or straight from the tap, good, old-fashioned water could cut your risk of a deadly heart attack by as much as 54 per cent – and at the same time ease constipation, boost flagging energy and perhaps even lower your risk of cancers of the breast, prostate and large intestine, research suggests.

In a study of 20,000 women and men, researchers found that those who downed at least five glasses of water every day had a significantly lower risk of heart attacks than those who whet their whistles with coffee, orange juice and other beverages. Why? Water is absorbed readily into the bloodstream, keeping blood diluted and less likely to form heart-threatening clots. Other liquids, the researchers say, require digestion, a process that draws fluid out of the bloodstream, thickening the blood and increasing clot risk.

Are you getting enough water? After the age of 60, don't rely on feelings of thirst to tell you the answer. That's because sensations of thirst decline as we get older – unfortunately, just at the time when many people drink less water to avoid dealing with urination problems such as stress incontinence in women or prostate problems in men.

The best way to know if you're fully hydrated? Examine your urine – if it's pale and has only a faint odour, you're probably drinking enough. If it's dark, scanty or has a strong odour, you probably need to drink more water and other fluids.

What you need: about six glasses a day

The standard advice to have eight glasses a day is now considered by many experts to be overstated. And tea counts, too – indeed, a recent study showed that drinking tea is just as hydrating as water. So have tea, coffee and juice, but try to include plain water as well. If you're eating a lot of juicy fruits and vegetables, you'll get fluid from them, too.

smart ways
TO EAT MORE Whole-grain bread

FULL-LIFE EATING GOAL: two to four servings a day

Say a permanent goodbye to white bread
Steer clear of giving yourself or your loved ones a choice. When your current bag of white bread is finished, don't buy another one. Use wholewheat bread in all the same ways you'd use white. For French toast, with eggs, for a sandwich and with dinner, wholewheat bread can replace all the white bread you've used in the past. It's that simple. Even if you love crusty French loaves or baguettes, there are whole-grain alternatives that have a lovely texture and mix well with Mediterranean foods.

Create a bakery habit You and your family deserve individually made, freshly baked bread. So why settle for a loaf made on an assembly line at a bread factory? Make it a habit to stop at a good-quality bakery, say hello to the proprietor and pick up healthy, whole-grain bread. Eat it over the next two days, then head back for a new loaf. Make it a never-ending cycle.

If you buy packaged bread, study the label
Look for wholewheat flour as the first ingredient, then check the nutritional facts label for the fibre content. Your goal: buy a loaf with at least 3g of fibre a slice.

Another clue is to look for products that display this health claim: 'People with healthy hearts tend to eat more whole-grain foods as part of a low-fat diet and healthy lifestyle.' Any product displaying this claim must contain at least 51 per cent whole grains by weight.

What if the fibre's high, but the bread's not made from whole grain? Put it back and keep looking. Some breads made mainly from white flour have added fibre, which can help with digestion (and prevent constipation), but the loaf won't have the phytochemicals and nutrients of real whole-grain versions.

Crunch it Look for whole-grain crackers that supply at least 3g of fibre a serving. Choose a lower-fat, low-sodium variety, such as Scandinavian-style crispbreads that taste great with hummous or peanut butter or as a bread substitute for open sandwiches. Five or six crackers count as one grain serving.

Make your own Replace the white flour in bread, muffin and quick-bread recipes with wholemeal flour. Start with half wholemeal and half white. If you totally replace white with wholemeal, for every 125g of plain flour use 115g wholemeal, since wholemeal flour has a heavier texture. In bread recipes, use a tablespoon to transfer the wholemeal flour to the scales instead of scooping or pouring; this introduces extra air into the flour, which makes the loaf lighter. You can also replace some of the liquid in baked goods recipes with orange juice to temper the sharper, tannic-acid taste of wholemeal flour. ■

Say a permanent goodbye to white bread

smart ways TO EAT MORE Whole-grain cereal

FULL-LIFE EATING GOAL: have for breakfast at least three times a week

Make cereal your breakfast default That means starting most of your mornings with a bowl of whole-grain cereal, milk and fruit. You can't get much healthier than that. But don't assume that all cereals are automatically healthy. A recent survey by consumer watchdog *Which?* analysed the content of 275 different types of processed cereals and reported that more than 75 per cent were high in sugar. The two worst offenders had a staggering 55g of sugar per 100g, and some even contained as much sugar as a chocolate bar.

What's more, nearly a fifth of all cereals tested had high levels of salt – sometimes more per portion than a packet of ready-salted crisps – and 7 per cent contained high levels of saturated fat, in the most extreme case, at 20.3g per 100g, as much fat as sausages.

And to satisfy British tastes, some global manufacturers add more salt and sugar to the UK versions of their cereals – even to supposedly healthy high-fibre products – than they do to the American versions!

So don't imagine that you're automatically improving your diet simply by swapping a greasy breakfast fry-up for a bowl of bran flakes – check the labels on your cereal packets before you buy. Look for less than 5g sugars, 0.5g salt and 1.5g saturated fat per 100g (not per portion).

Use cereal as a topping Keep a small box of high-fibre cereal in the cupboard to use as a crunchy topping on yoghurt, oatmeal, fruit salads and green salads. It almost acts as a fibre supplement.

Be sure to finish the milk The B vitamins added to cereals leach into milk quickly. Be sure to spoon up the milk at the bottom of the bowl to get the cereal's complete nutritional offerings.

New to higher-fibre cereal? Mix it half and half with an old favourite You'll get loads more fibre than before, yet at the same time ease the transition to a new breakfast habit. The next week, fill your bowl with two-thirds higher-fibre brand and one-third old favourite. The week after, try sprinkling a little of your old standby over your new favourite cereal as a topping.

Put oatmeal on your breakfast table at least twice a week – more often in chilly weather To eat more, start with old-fashioned porridge and add a little brown sugar or maple syrup, dried or fresh fruit, chopped nuts and skimmed milk. You'll get about 4g of fibre in 40g of raw oats.

Try this quick cooking method for old-fashioned oats Bring a saucepan of water to a rolling boil, add the oats and bring the water back to a boil. Turn off the heat, cover the pan and take a shower. In 10 minutes, the oats will be ready to eat. Or use your microwave to make super-quick porridge.

Or try long-cooking Irish oatmeal This delicious, stick-to-your-ribs porridge takes 45 minutes to cook, unless you know this chef's secret: the night before, bring the oats and water to a boil, cover and turn off the heat. In the morning, simply simmer for 5–10 minutes, until the oats are as tender as you like. ■

smart ways
TO EAT MORE Whole-grain dinner dishes

FULL-LIFE EATING GOAL: two to four servings a day

Serve no-worry brown rice in place of potatoes tonight Yes, classic brown rice does require 45 minutes of cooking time, so you have to plan ahead a little. Make the cooking process easier by investing in a rice cooker (toss in rice and water and turn it on – no need to worry about a burned pot) or cook a big batch of brown rice at the weekend and freeze meal-sized portions in sealable freezer bags. Reheat in the microwave on weeknights.

Stock instant, boil-in-the-bag or quick-cooking parboiled brown rice, too These grains are cooked, then dried. They do lose some texture along the way, but they retain most or even all of brown rice's fibre and nutrients. Their star quality: they cook in 5–20 minutes, making this convenience food great as a once-in-a-while fallback. You can also cook up quick brown rice to use in place of the ubiquitous tub of white that comes with a Chinese takeaway.

Replace white rice in recipes with brown It works as well – or better – in chicken-and-rice dishes, stuffed cabbage, soups and casseroles. You'll love pudding made with brown rice, too, for its nutty flavour and chunky yet tender texture.

Shop for another great grain this week Other whole grains you may find in your local grocery shop or healthfood shop include amaranth, barley, couscous, millet, quinoa and wild rice. Each has a unique flavour and texture. Try a new one each week. Give it the sniff test before purchasing to be sure the oils in the germ don't have a stale, rancid odour. Refrigerate or freeze grains to retain freshness.

Keep a supply of fast-cooking favourites on hand Pearl barley is great for its creamy texture, its 6g of fibre per 200g – including cholesterol-lowering soluble fibre – and its fast cooking time: just 30 minutes. It's a delicious side dish replacement for rice and gives soups and stews a soft, thick texture. Bulgur is just wholewheat that's been steamed, dried and cracked. Think of it as a whole-grain convenience food; it cooks in 20 minutes. Traditionally used for Middle Eastern tabbouleh (a salad with bulgur, tomatoes, cucumber and parsley), it also makes a delicious side dish. Couscous is really a tiny-grained pasta made from wheat flour. The catch: some is refined, some is whole wheat. Your assignment: look for wholewheat couscous in the supermarket or healthfood shop. It's the fastest-cooking whole-grain product of them all: just add boiling water and cover, and in 5 minutes it's ready to serve. Switching to wholewheat couscous means getting 7g of fibre a serving, compared with just 2g in ordinary couscous.

Stir it in Add 60g of cooked bulgur wheat, brown or wild rice or barley (not pearl) to stuffings, soups, stews, salads or casseroles. Add a cooked whole grain or whole-grain breadcrumbs to minced meat or poultry for extra body. Make risottos, pilaus and other rice-type dishes using grains such as barley, brown basmati rice, bulgur, millet, quinoa or sorghum.

Popcorn counts! Use a popcorn maker for a high-fibre, low-fat snack. Each 8g of air-popped popcorn has 1.2g of fibre (and just 31 calories). ■

CHOICE 3 Eat more 'good' fats

Food is not the only cause of chronic inflammation in your body, and it isn't the only cure, but it certainly plays an important role. Research shows that even a standard-sized fast-food breakfast quickly floods the bloodstream with inflammatory compounds and keeps levels high for the next 3 hours. If you have a fast-food meal for lunch as well, you start the cycle all over again.

Equally dangerous is the fact that most modern adults no longer eat a healthy combination of two important fats – omega-3 and omega-6 fatty acids. We need both for healthy brain function. But while two important omega-3s (eicosa-pentaenoic acid – EPA – and docosahexaenoic acid – DHA) reduce inflammation and prevent chronic health problems such as heart disease and arthritis, omega-6s tend to *increase* inflammation. Yet while early people ate these two fats in more or less balanced proportions – a ratio of 1:1 or 2:1 omega-6 to omega-3 – today we eat 15 to 30 times more omega-6s.

Why? In part because we eat lots of processed foods, often dripping with corn, sunflower and soya bean oil, all top sources of omega-6s. We eat grain-fed beef and poultry instead of free-range meats (grass-fed animals have more omega-3s in their fat stores). Just as dangerous is skimping on good fats – the omega-3 fatty acids found in cold-water fish such as salmon and also in nuts, leafy green vegetables and olive oil – as omega-3 deficiency can also promote inflammation.

The solution? Rebalance your fats by eating more fish, more nuts and more good-for-you oils. This could help to ease arthritis pain, relieve asthma, lessen symptoms of eczema and psoriasis and even cut your risk of depression.

In the long term, good fats may cut your risk of dangerous heart arrhythmias (out-of-sync heartbeats that can lead to a heart attack), high blood pressure, stroke, cancer, diabetes and even Alzheimer's disease.

ANTI-INFLAMMATORY SUPERFOODS: FISH, NUTS AND SEEDS, AND OILS

Fats equal bad. Carbohydrates equal good. Not too many years ago, those were the basic rules of healthy eating. How simplistic they were! In the previous section, we showed that the story isn't nearly that simple for carbs. Now it's whole grains equal good, refined grains equal bad.

Our understanding of fats has changed similarly. In the past 20 years, we have learned that certain fats are indeed among the most unhealthy foods you can eat, but other fats are among the most healthy. Don't worry, though – it's still pretty easy to separate the good fats from the bad. Here's the basic breakdown.

How good are good fats? Well, good enough that you should go out of your way to have plenty in your daily diet. We've already had one big reason: healthy fats reduce inflammation in your body, greatly reducing your risk of many major diseases. Another reason is that they help to shore up levels of 'good' HDL cholesterol, which may become more important than keeping 'bad' LDL low after about age 60.

Get started today by putting good-fat superfoods on your plate. And don't forget

BAD FATS: fats from pork, beef and other land animals and 'trans fats' artificially created in factories.

GOOD FATS: fats from plants, such as those in nuts, olives and beans, and fats from most fish.

fruit and veg. They contain a natural form of salicylic acid, the same inflammation-cooling compound found in aspirin.

Here are the good-fat superfoods.

● No other food comes close to delivering the high-quality, high-concentration omega-3s you'll find in **salmon, sardines, herring, mackerel and other oily, cold-water fish.** They're the richest sources of the two most powerful omega-3s, EPA and DHA. Fish is so powerful that even just three servings a month could cut your risk of stroke by 40 per cent; two meals a week could slash your heart attack odds by 59 per cent. Yet most of us manage just 115g of fish a month.

Often, we are scared away by reports of environmental toxins like methylmercury, PCBs (polychlorinated biphenyls) and DDT (dichlorodiphenyl-trichloroethane) lurking in fish. In 2002 researchers reported results of a study part-funded by the British Heart Foundation of more than 1,400 men from eight European countries, which found that men who had been hit by a heart attack had mercury levels 15 per cent higher than those who hadn't. As fish consumption is believed to be the principal source of mercury exposure in adults, this suggested the toxin could counteract the heart benefits of fish.

However, scientists think that any risk applies only to larger, predatory fish that accumulate especially high mercury levels – such as shark, swordfish and marlin and, to a lesser extent, tuna. Because of potential risks to the developing nervous system, the UK Food Standards Agency advises that pregnant

women, women intending to become pregnant and children under 16 should avoid shark, marlin and swordfish, and adults should eat no more than one portion of any of these fish once a week. Pregnant women should also limit the amount of tuna they eat to two fresh tuna steaks or four medium-sized cans a week. In addition, because toxins are especially concentrated in fatty tissue, it's not a good idea to overdose on oily fish. Generally, men, boys and women past child-bearing age can eat up to four portions of oily fish a week, but girls and younger women are advised to limit consumption to two portions weekly.

Other than these precautions, most people can eat most types of fish quite safely and the benefits generally far outweigh the dangers. The best plan is to eat a wide variety of fish so you're not exposed to one potential source of toxins over and over again.

● Crunchy, tasty **nuts and seeds** are rich sources of heart-healthy monounsaturated and polyunsaturated fats and even, in a few cases, of plant-based omega-3s that may play a special role in preventing cancer and heart disease. With nuts, a little is good, but more isn't better. All that fat makes them high in calories. For a 100 calorie snack, all you need are 8 walnut halves, 16 to 20 almonds, 10 to 12 cashews, 10 pecans, 7 or 8 macadamia nuts, 15 hazelnuts or 1 tablespoon of peanut butter.

● Move over sunflower, soya bean and corn oil. The good fats found in **olive, grapeseed, walnut and pumpkin oil** have proven health benefits and can help you to establish a healthier, more natural balance between omega-6 and omega-3 fatty acids. ■

smart ways
TO EAT MORE Fish

FULL-LIFE EATING GOAL: at least two servings a week

Have no-mess baked fish for dinner on Friday – and then have a double-good-fat fish sandwich for lunch on Wednesday
Just place a fish fillet on a large sheet of foil and top with your choice of flavoursome additions (how about sun-dried tomatoes and chopped garlic with salmon, or slices of fresh lemon over flounder?) plus a splash of water, wine or fruit juice. Bake at 180°C until cooked through, usually about 20 minutes.

On Wednesdays, mix canned salmon with a bit of low-fat mayonnaise and grated carrots and apples. Enjoy on high-fibre bread with a leafy green side salad.

Stocking up? Look beyond the fish counter
It's a misconception that frozen and canned fish isn't as healthy as fresh, wild fish. In fact, because it's frozen soon after being caught, frozen fish is often 'fresher' than fresh, which may have spent several days in transit and sitting in the shop. Just let the fillets thaw in the fridge during the day, then grill with lemon or poach lightly.

And don't overlook canned fish. Oily fish are very suitable for canning and retain much of their nutrients – just avoid fish canned in brine (because of the high salt content) and make sure that fish in oil is drained well before serving. There's even affordable wild salmon hiding in the canned foods aisle. Canned red or pink salmon is usually wild, not farmed – full of omega-3s and low in contaminants.

Love prawns? Don't wait for company
Prawn cocktail and peel-and-eat prawns are fun and easy ways to work more low-fat protein into your week. And don't be swayed by the high-cholesterol prawn scare. Prawns quirky cholesterol count – about 200mg in 12 large ones, about the same as in one large egg – could make you pass up this low-calorie delicacy. But for most of us, prawns should get the green light. In fact, the 'bad' cholesterol in your blood mostly comes not from cholesterol in foods but from saturated fat – and prawns have exceedingly low levels of this. What's more, research shows that although prawns raise 'bad' LDL cholesterol by 7 per cent, they also boost 'good' HDL cholesterol even higher and decrease heart-threatening blood fats called triglycerides by 13 per cent. The bottom line is that they are a heart-friendly food. ■

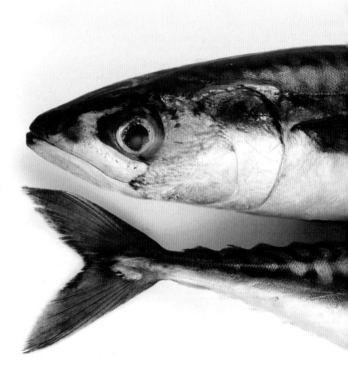

smart ways
TO EAT MORE Nuts and seeds

FULL-LIFE EATING GOAL: at least three snack-sized servings a week

Sprinkle chopped peanuts on your brown rice tonight Or spread a tablespoon of peanut butter on a slice of wholewheat toast for breakfast (top with banana slices for natural sweetness). In five big population studies, nut consumption cut heart risk by up to 35 per cent. Peanuts pack an extra nutritional bonus that may explain why: they've got beta-sitosterol, which blocks cholesterol absorption and, in scientific studies, discouraged growth of tumours of the breast, colon and prostate. Peanuts can also help you to feel full and satisfied for longer. Studies show that although they are high in fat and energy-dense, they actually boost energy utilisation so that peanut eaters weighed less than peanut avoiders.

Scatter sunflower seeds on top of muffins or hot cereal; add to a green salad Sunflower seeds also provide linoleic acid, an essential fatty acid your body cannot produce and must obtain from food. In studies, women who got the most had a 23 per cent lower risk of heart disease. As the seeds' fats turn rancid fast, store in the fridge, for up to three months, or in the freezer for up to a year.

Munch 22 almonds tonight 'Bad' LDL levels dropped 6 per cent and 'good' HDL levels rose 6 per cent in a University of California study of people who ate almonds and used almond oil in place of half the regular fats in their diets.

Instead of a chocolate bar for a snack, carry nuts in a breath-mint box You need to wash it out first, but one of those little boxes is the perfect size to hold about 20 almonds – the perfect snack size – and it really couldn't be more portable.

Add a dusting of ground walnuts or flaxseed to your cereal, veg or salad every day Both contain impressive amounts of another beneficial omega-3 oil called alpha-linolenic acid. Getting some into your diet is a good idea, nutritionists say; plenty of studies show that eating walnuts or flaxseed can help to cut heart disease risk.

Coat fish with sesame seeds before baking A portion of 35g packs 144mg of phytosterols – super-healthy chemicals that help to block cholesterol absorption. ■

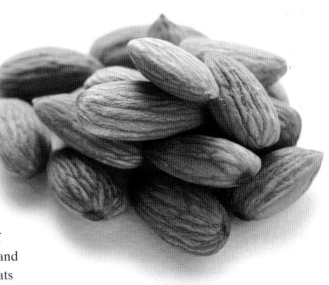

Munch 22 almonds tonight

smart ways
TO EAT MORE Healthy oils

FULL-LIFE EATING GOAL: 1 to 2 tablespoons a day

Flavour with olive oil One of the richest sources of monounsaturated fats, olive oil seems to cool the inflammation that leads to heart disease, diabetes, cancer and worsening arthritis. In one Spanish study of 755 Canary Islands women, those who had 9g a day were the least likely to get breast cancer.

Watch the calories, though. A tablespoon of olive oil – or virtually any oil – packs around 100 kilocalories, so use a light hand. Drizzle 1 to 2 teaspoons on veg such as squash, asparagus and green beans instead of butter. Buy an oil mister to use on your pans rather than an oil spray, which is heavier on the oil. Get only what you'll use in the next two months and store it in a cool, dark spot. Old olive oil goes rancid and tastes like soggy cardboard.

Splurge on extra-virgin This is the fruity, full-bodied good stuff to use in situations where taste is important, such as in salad dressings; it also has the most antioxidants. In a Spanish study comparing the effects of extra-virgin olive oil with olive oil that had all of its antioxidant phenols filtered out, the arteries of people who had the extra-virgin oil expanded and contracted easily in response to changes in blood flow – a trait that cuts heart attack risk.

Make the most of speciality oils There are plenty of other oils that can boost your health and spice up your recipes, and an increasing selection is available in supermarkets as well as from healthfood shops. Try pumpkin seed oil, high in omega-3s and vitamin E and delicious drizzled on salads and cooked vegetables, or shaken with balsamic vinegar for a different salad dressing. Walnut oil is low in saturates, high in monounsaturates and contains a healthy balance of omega-3 and omega-6. It has a strong nutty flavour, so use sparingly in salad dressings and when baking, or lightly brush it onto chicken or fish. Rapeseed oil is low in saturates, high in omega-3s and vitamin E, and has a high smoke point so can be used for frying. So can groundnut oil (also called peanut or arachis oil), which is high in healthy monounsaturates. Sesame oil, which is rich in omega-3s and monounsaturates, also contains powerful antioxidants called lignans, and cholesterol-busting phytosterols. It's especially good for oriental recipes and can be used in salads, cooking and sauces, and for low-temperature sauté recipes, but avoid high-temperature frying.

Try grapeseed and linseed oil Grapeseed oil, also rich in healthy fats, is perfect for high-temperature cooking. Linseed oil, which breaks down in high heat, is best used at room temperature as a salad dressing. Dress leafy greens by shaking up a smart vinaigrette with linseed oil, balsamic vinegar and your favourite herbs and spices. Then store the extra in the fridge: heat destroys the essential fatty acids in this fragile, light-tasting oil. Think oil's too much of a luxury on your salad? It's time to rethink fat-free dressing. New research shows that none of the cancer-fighting alpha or beta-carotene antioxidants found in salad greens are absorbed unless oils are present. (You could add nuts or avocado instead.) ■

Olive oil is one of nature's greatest gifts: its extraordinary flavour is matched only by its healthiness

Eat calcium-rich foods

Once, the equation for avoiding brittle bones was simple: get more calcium. After all, your bones do need it – and when your body doesn't have enough for other functions, it draws more from your skeleton. Lack of calcium contributes to osteoporosis, the brittle bone condition that underlies fractures sustained at some point in their lives by one in two women and one in five men over the age of 50. There are more than 200,000 osteoporotic fractures each year in the UK, and the consequences can be disastrous: half of all those who fracture a hip are never again able to live independently, and around a third die within a year.

Getting more calcium is important to help to prevent osteoporosis – but calcium is only part of the story. The best bone-protecting equation begins with adequate calcium but doesn't stop there. You also need vitamin D, magnesium and potassium to help your body to absorb and use calcium, and you need regular bone-protecting resistance moves to build or maintain bone density.

According to the Food Standards Agency, an adult needs 700mg calcium a day. And calcium is important not just for your bones. There's plenty of evidence that getting enough can also help to control your blood pressure, lower your odds of developing a pre-diabetic condition called insulin resistance and even help to prevent memory loss and colon cancer. So try to get two to three servings of low-fat dairy foods a day as part of your diet. Combine that with the smaller amounts of calcium in other foods you eat, and you should be getting enough. If you don't eat dairy, add a calcium supplement daily or increase your intake of other calcium-containing foods, such as green leafy vegetables, soya beans, nuts, bread (fortified with calcium) and fish such as canned salmon, sardines and pilchards eaten with the bones.

CALCIUM SUPERFOODS: MILK AND BEYOND

Skimmed milk, low-fat cheese and fat-free yoghurt are among the richest sources of calcium on the shelf at your local supermarket. Each serving of one of these provides about 350mg of calcium along with the minerals and vitamins you need to absorb and use it. If you love milk, that's great news. It's just another reason to pour some over your morning cereal, end the day with a steaming mug of cocoa or enjoy cheese and whole-grain crackers for a midafternoon snack.

What if you don't like milk, though, or simply can't drink it? Some people feel bloated and uncomfortable after eating dairy foods, because their bodies are missing the enzyme needed to digest the milk sugar lactose. If you're lactose intolerant or just prefer not to consume much dairy, we've got lots of calcium-rich alternatives, from leafy green salads to nuts to fortified soya milk and orange juice and even yoghurt.

It's true – many people whose systems are intolerant of milk can have yoghurt without any problem. Why? Enzymes in yoghurt convert milk sugars into a digestible form. So if milk makes you uncomfortable, yoghurt may be a good alternative.

As a food, yoghurt is a multi-tasking marvel: it works as a breakfast food, a frozen dessert or a dip; you can also use it as a base for smoothie drinks and salad dressings and as a sauce for chicken or seafood. It's packed with calcium and protein as well as magnesium, riboflavin and vitamins B_6 and B_{12} – plus beneficial bacteria that improve digestion and boost immunity.

Be sure to read about calcium supplements later in this chapter. Nutrition experts agree that they're one of the smartest supplements women – and possibly men – can take.

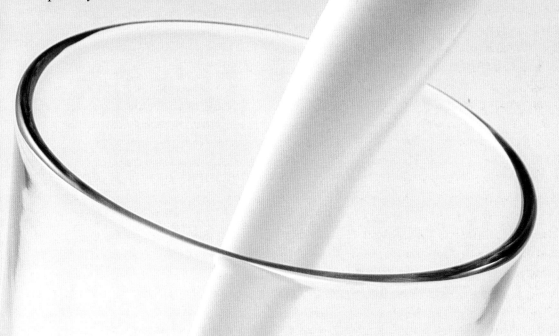

If you love milk, that's great news. It's just another reason to pour some over your morning cereal and end the day with a steaming mug of cocoa

smart ways
TO EAT MORE Milk and cheese

FULL-LIFE EATING GOAL: one to two servings a day

Close your eyes and switch to skimmed
If you're drinking whole-fat milk, switch to semi-skimmed. If you're already on semi-skimmed, make the move to skimmed. Here's an easy way to make the switch: buy a small container of the next level down, shut your eyes and sip. Creative researchers say that when thousands of consumers put on sunglasses so they couldn't tell what kind of milk they were drinking, nine out of ten said that they liked the taste of either semi-skimmed or skimmed milk better than that of higher-fat milks. Why it's worth it: each glass of skimmed milk you drink instead of whole milk saves you 5g of saturated fat, a quarter of your recommended daily maximum.

Sip delicious 'hot vanilla' or hot chocolate on a cold morning Mix 250ml of skimmed or semi-skimmed milk, two packets of sugar substitute (or 2 teaspoons of sugar or honey if you prefer) and your choice of ¼ teaspoon real vanilla extract or 2 teaspoons unsweetened cocoa in a small saucepan or microwaveable container. Heat for about a minute.

Cook with milk instead of water Instant hot cereals and low-sodium instant or canned soups mix easily with milk, which lends extra body and flavour to these quick comfort foods.

Make milk your fast-food drink Most fast-food restaurants sell the skimmed variety in cartons or single-serving bottles.

Order a skimmed-milk cappuccino Skip high-calorie coffee drinks at your favourite coffee shop. Skimmed milk makes cappuccino extra-foamy and fun to sip. Sprinkle with your choice of cocoa powder, cinnamon or nutmeg.

Make a healthy dairy pasta topping Purée fat-free or low-fat cottage cheese and fat-free evaporated milk with lemon juice and rosemary for a light pasta sauce.

Chose guilt-free cheese ... When the full-fat cheese in your refrigerator is all gone, resolve never to buy it again – and check the dairy cabinet for low-fat, cottage and cream cheeses. (They're worth a second look. As with whole-grain pasta, current supermarket offerings are miles better in terms of taste and texture than the first-generation low-fat cheeses on the market 15 years ago.) Full-fat cheese is one of the top three sources of artery-clogging saturated fat in our diets. Choose lower fat, and you can keep the flavour *and* spare your heart.

... Then savour it in small doses Grate a little over chilli or spaghetti or some veg. Have one slice on your sandwich. Have an individually wrapped piece of low-fat cheese with wholewheat crackers as a snack. As long as you're not worried about your weight or your cholesterol level, a little cheese is very pleasurable and can make all kinds of foods taste even better. But if you are overweight or have high cholesterol, think twice. Cheese is high in saturated fat, and its richness makes it easy to overeat. Each 30g of full-fat cheese has 4 to 6g of saturated fat. How much cheese is that? Something like the amount you'd find melted on a slice of a medium pizza. Going low-fat (or fat-free) and reducing your portions could save you a significant 5g of heart-threatening saturated fat a day.

Choose pizza and other cheesy dishes with less cheese and more sauce and vegetables UK cheese consumption is on the increase, mainly as a result of the cheese used in ready-meals and takeaways. We eat around 10kg of cheese per person a year in Britain. That's low compared with, say, the French, but most of that 10kg is hard or semi-hard cheeses, laden with fat. Along with an increase in cream consumption, this means that many of us are losing the benefits of switching from full-fat milk and butter to healthier options. So go for less cheese and healthier low-fat options on your pizza.

Lighten up your Italian cooking Choose light mozzarella instead of standard for half the fat, and reduce the amount of Parmesan you sprinkle on top of dishes. ∎

Use milk or yoghurt as a secret ingredient in soups, desserts and sauces

smart ways TO EAT MORE Yoghurt

FULL-LIFE EATING GOAL: five servings a week

Buy one large container of plain yoghurt at a time rather than lots of pre-flavoured small versions If only shop-bought strawberry yoghurt were just yoghurt with slices of fresh strawberry. Instead, it's yoghurt with sweetener, more sweetener and a little bit of fruit. All those refined sweeteners double the calories of the yoghurt without any extra nutrition. Instead, buy plain yoghurt and use it creatively in your cooking. If you want to flavour some with fruit for breakfast, add a teaspoon of your favourite jam and some slices of real fruit, then mix it together. It will be equally delicious but far less calorie-heavy than the shop-bought version.

Make a breakfast smoothie a few times a week It's easy! Blend 225g plain, low-fat, or fat-free yoghurt with a banana, a handful of fresh or frozen berries, a splash of orange juice and a few ice cubes until smooth. An amazing breakfast in a glass. Once you master this basic approach, you can start experimenting with other fruit juices and fresh fruits.

Serve raw fruits and vegetables with a yoghurt-based dip Mix curry seasoning and honey into plain low-fat yoghurt for a sweet and spicy dip for carrots. Or add chopped fresh basil and lemon to yoghurt for a Mediterranean flavour that's great with sliced cucumber and courgette.

Have a yoghurt parfait at snack time or for dessert Layer low-fat or fat-free yoghurt, berries, mandarin oranges and granola or chopped almonds in a pretty wine glass or dessert bowl. It makes a treat worthy of royalty.

Buy frozen yoghurt ice lollies Buy the brand with the least sugar and saturated fat and keep them in the freezer. Or take a carton of frozen yoghurt, then whirl in the food processor with frozen or fresh fruit for a delicious dessert.

Skip yoghurts with built-in toppings Chocolate chips, crunchy biscuit, granola – many yoghurts come with their own fancy mix-ins in a special compartment. Skip these; they only add extra fat and sugar, raising the calorie count of that little tub of yoghurt to way over 200.

Check the calcium count on cultured soya yoghurts Dairy-free soya yoghurts have only the tiniest amount of saturated fat. If you're trying to avoid milk products or just want to get more soya into your diet, consider these products only after you check the calcium content. Many are lower than their made-from-milk cousins. Many are also lower in magnesium, protein and B vitamins.

Make your own cheese It's easier than you think, and you get a low-calorie, cheese-like spread that can be sweetened with honey or spiced up with pressed garlic and herbs as a sandwich spread. Simply line a strainer with paper towels, dump in plain yoghurt and set over a bowl or pot. Cover and refrigerate overnight. In the morning, you'll have a whey-like liquid in the bowl and thick yoghurt cheese in the strainer, ready for you to give it your own culinary twist.

Use yoghurt as a topping For example, spoon a dollop onto thick black bean or split pea soup, then sprinkle with black pepper or herbs. You'll never know it's not soured cream. ■

FULL-LIFE EATING GOAL: three to five servings a week

Check out fortified orange juice and soya milk Some contain as much calcium as a glass of skimmed milk, but be sure to read the label so you know how much you're getting. Don't shortchange yourself by thinking your juice or milk has more calcium than it really does. Shake soya milk well before pouring; the calcium added to it can settle to the bottom.

Go for 'green calcium' Yes, there is calcium in some vegetables. The levels aren't quite as high as in dairy foods, though. You'd have to eat 200g of cooked kale, 400g of cooked broccoli or 1.44kg of cooked spinach to equal the calcium in a glass of skimmed milk. Think of calcium-rich veggies as a nice add-on that can help you to reach your calcium goal and provides a range of minerals and vitamins. The best vegetable sources of calcium include kale, broccoli, spinach, pak choi and almonds.

Eat more rhubarb It takes a creative cook to figure out how to get more rhubarb into your diet, but it's worth it. Use 240g of cooked rhubarb and you get 348mg of calcium, making it one of nature's top sources of the mineral. Only the stalks of a rhubarb plant are edible, and they are quite tart. That's why rhubarb is primarily paired with sweet fruits in breads, cakes, crumbles, pies and ice cream.

Nibble on dried figs A serving of ten dried figs provides 269mg of calcium, a wonderfully large amount.

Some tofu counts, too Tofu made with calcium sulphate (check for it on the ingredients label) supplies a respectable 204mg of calcium in a 125g serving.

Eat more beans As we've said, beans are an anti-ageing superfood, and here's one more reason: they're good sources of calcium.

And have nuts and seeds, too Calcium can be found in healthy amounts in Brazil nuts, hazelnuts, chestnuts, sesame seeds, tahini (sesame seed paste), sunflower seeds and pumpkin seeds. A good idea: keep a canister of your favourite seeds on your kitchen table and add a teaspoon as a topping to cereals, vegetables, salads and soups. ■

Cooked rhubarb is one of nature's top sources of calcium

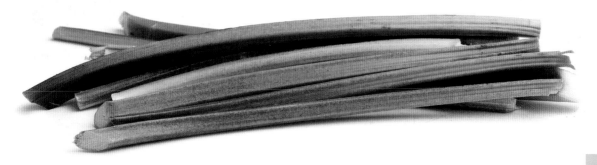

Enjoy lean protein

A juicy baked chicken breast. Beef stew studded with chunks of rich, lean meat. Turkey steak with a pile of steaming vegetables. These protein-packed dishes aren't just mouthwatering; they can help you to maintain strong muscles and strong immunity, keep you feeling full for longer after you eat and deliver key vitamins and minerals that become even more important for good health as the years pass.

You don't need more protein as you get older – but you do need to maintain your intake, and many older people don't, with the result that many are not getting as much protein and other nutrients as they need. Why? Food may seem less appetising if taste and smell sensations are blunted, dental problems may make chewing more difficult and the bother of cooking may seem simply too much. Your challenge: eating *enough* without getting too much heart-threatening saturated fat.

The solution to this protein puzzle is a delicious new eating strategy – similar to the way healthy older people in Okinawa and Crete eat: put more protein such as poultry or lean beef on the table, add fish and mix in plenty of other healthy foods that fill in protein gaps, such as dairy products, nuts, beans and even some vegetables. Our modern twist? Use healthy convenience foods such as skinless, boneless chicken breasts and make easy substitutions such as choosing skinless minced turkey instead of minced beef.

At the beginning of this chapter, we mentioned the key reasons why protein is so important to your diet. It provides essential body-building materials that are used to create muscle cells, bone cells, blood cells and more. And no matter what your age, your body is still generating new cells all the time. Protein also slows absorption of blood sugar, helping to keep hunger and food cravings at bay.

Plus, lean protein is a rich source of the B vitamins that can help you to feel more energetic. Why? The Bs help to guide metabolic reactions throughout the body. And they can help to protect against heart disease by controlling levels of a compound in the bloodstream called homocysteine.

With lean protein, you also get healthy doses of multi-talented zinc, a mineral important for maintaining strong immunity – it plays a role in the production of infection-fighting white blood cells. In one study of women and men over the age of 70, those who ate the most protein had significantly stronger bones over four years than those who ate the least. Another bonus: brain-protecting niacin. When researchers checked 3,718 people aged 65 and older, then tested their cognitive skills for six years, they found that those who got the most niacin from food were 70 per cent less likely to develop Alzheimer's. Vitamin B_6 and niacin can also help your body to process blood sugar more efficiently.

THE PROBLEM WITH MEAT

So why does meat get such a bad health press? Two reasons. First, protein and fat are closely bound together in most cuts of meat, and animal fat is among the most troublesome parts of your diet. That's why we keep using the word 'lean' in front of protein; it's important to choose meats that are as low as possible in visible fat. Second, we tend to eat big helpings of meat. Restaurants often taunt diners with the size of their burgers or steaks or racks of ribs. This can mean as much as eight times more than a healthy serving.

So how much protein do you need? Experts suggest 4.5g for every 10lb of body weight. Translation: if you weigh 68kg (10 stone 10lb), you need 67g daily. That's what you'd get if your day's menu looked like this:

- Cereal with 250ml skimmed milk for breakfast
- A tuna sandwich on wholemeal bread for lunch
- A medium-sized skinless chicken breast for dinner
- A cup of hot cocoa made with skimmed milk before bed

As you can see, that's not a whole lot of meat. Yet as women age, they tend to eat less and less protein. Roughly 10 to 20 per cent of women aged over 55 get less than 30g of protein a day – even if they're eating plenty of food.

PROTEIN SUPERFOODS: CHICKEN, TURKEY AND LEAN BEEF

What's not to love about chicken? A roast, skinless breast has just 120 to 140 calories, and it's packed with all the protein satisfaction you could ask for with less than half the fat of a trimmed T-bone steak. It's versatile – starring in everything from chicken soup at lunch to a plump, roast bird for Sunday dinner. In a hurry? You can find it ready to eat virtually everywhere – in sandwiches and pasta salads (minus the mayonnaise) from takeaway shops and even ready-roasted from supermarkets.

Meat meets greens

Here are two intriguing reasons why you should always eat green vegetables with meat.

1 A mysterious component of beef – known to scientists simply as **'the meat factor'** – helps your body to absorb more of the iron in vegetables.

2 **Cruciferous vegetables** such as broccoli or brussels sprouts help your body to disarm unhealthy carcinogenic compounds called heterocyclic amines that are produced when meat is grilled or chargrilled.

And turkey? This grand bird is not just for special occasions. A 115g serving of turkey breast provides 60 per cent of the protein you need each day without the fat you'd get in many cuts of pork or beef. And you don't have to buy a large bird to enjoy a delicious turkey dinner. Most supermarkets offer small cuts of boneless turkey.

As for red meats, there are more healthy choices than you might realise. Lean beef cuts such as sirloin and tenderloin are surprisingly low in fat – and their fat isn't all the artery-clogging kind. Half the fatty acids in a serving of lean beef are monounsaturated fatty acids, the same heart-healthy type found in olive oil that research shows may lower cholesterol.

What's more, a third of the saturated fat in beef is a unique fatty acid called stearic acid, which has been found to have a neutral or cholesterol-lowering effect. A serving of beef is an excellent source of five essential nutrients: protein, zinc, vitamin B_{12}, selenium and phosphorus, and a good source of four more: niacin, vitamin B_6, iron and riboflavin.

The story is similar with pork: the tenderloin is super-lean, luscious and perfectly healthy in moderate portions. ■

smart ways
TO EAT MORE Chicken and turkey

FULL-LIFE EATING GOAL: one serving a day

Grab fast, low-fat chicken Grocery shops typically stock skinless, boneless breasts; thighs; and fast-cooking breast fillets. Don't let price stop you from stocking up on them. These healthier, quicker-to-prepare alternatives to whole birds ensure that 100 per cent of what you buy ends up in your meal, as opposed to the waste inevitable with a whole chicken.

Buy a roast chicken Many food shops today offer roast chickens for sale. Go ahead and buy one! When you get home, strip off the skin, remove the meat from the bones and drain off any sauce or juice. That way, you get rid of the fat and the excessively high sodium levels of any shop-applied marinade. What's left is deliciously healthy, lean chicken meat, ready for instant eating. Serve it up on its own, shred it into soup or onto salad or add to vegetables.

Make a 10 minute chicken-and-veg meal Grab a pack of boneless, skinless chicken breast fillets and some precut vegetables, such as squash, broccoli, green and red peppers and onions. Dump them all in a pan with a splash of olive oil and some low-sodium stock, bring to a boil, then reduce to a simmer. Season with garlic, ginger, basil, tarragon or just a sprinkle of salt and pepper. Cook until the chicken's done and the vegetables are as crunchy – or soft – as you like. Voilà! Dinner's ready.

Create a marinade habit Marinades make your poultry amazingly tender, moist and flavoursome. The day before you intend to cook, place the raw chicken in a sealable container, pour on a marinade, cover and refrigerate until cooking time the next evening. Almost any liquid can be the base: orange juice, a vinaigrette, even yoghurt. Add your favourite herbs and spices for flavour. If you want even greater convenience, use a shop-bought low-fat marinade. Then cook your favourite way. One important rule: discard marinades once you've removed the chicken, or use to make a cooked sauce.

Leftovers? You've got lunch! Leftover cooked chicken will keep for three days in the fridge. Put some in a wholewheat tortilla; sprinkle with chopped tomatoes, diced avocado, onions and grated low-fat cheese; and grill for a healthy Mexican-style treat. Or combine chopped chicken with a dollop of low-fat mayonnaise, tarragon and grapes for an elegant chicken salad.

Make chicken chilli Add chunks of cooked chicken to a bean chilli to bump up the protein content.

Buy skinless minced turkey breast instead of minced beef Use it as you would minced beef in chilli, lasagne and other pasta recipes.

Grill or bake a turkey breast instead of a whole chicken Slice, then refrigerate or freeze leftovers for use later in turkey sandwiches or turkey salad (toss diced turkey with low-fat mayonnaise, chopped apples, walnuts, celery and grapes).

Make an autumn turkey salad Place cubed turkey, sliced cooked sweet potato, cranberries and walnuts on a bed of spinach and drizzle with your favourite olive-oil dressing.

Keep turkey in the freezer for quick meals Put skinless, boneless turkey cutlets in sealable bags and freeze. Thaw in the microwave, then sauté in a frying pan with a dash of olive oil. ■

smart ways
TO EAT MORE Lean beef and other meats

FULL-LIFE EATING GOAL: three servings a week

Look for 'lean' or 'extra-lean' on the label
These cuts will have 4.5g or less of saturated fat and 5–10g of total fat per serving. Or ask your butcher to provide you with lean cuts, such as sirloin or tenderloin.

Use lean meat as an *ingredient*, not a main course This may be the best trick of all when it comes to getting meat portions correct. Rather than thinking of meat as something to be served by itself, make it part of other dishes. Here are several smart ways.

- Add thinly sliced beef to your sautéed vegetables or wok stir-fries.
- Top a crunchy, robust salad with beef slices.
- Make kebabs with lean meat cubes and vegetables.
- Add small chunks of cooked pork and sautéed vegetables to cooked brown rice for a one-dish meal.
- Add lean minced beef to spaghetti sauce.
- Make bean, vegetable and meat combinations, such as chilli or cassoulet. Just be sure to add the meat to the beans after it's been cooked and drained; otherwise, the beans will absorb the fat.

Serve your beef sliced Typically, steaks and pork chops are served whole, and that makes for a giant portion, far beyond the healthy amount. The solution: slice the steak in the kitchen and fan out the slices on the dinner plates. This looks great and really reduces the portion sizes.

Garnish your steak Even better, sauté thinly sliced onions, peppers, tomatoes and garlic cloves and spoon a healthy portion over the steak slices. This will make the meat portion seem even larger and more inviting – without extra meat.

Cook roasts separately from vegetables Roasting makes fat melt away from meat. That's good. If potatoes, carrots, turnips or other vegetables are in the pan, they'll absorb the fat you're trying to avoid. That's bad. A better approach: cook the meat, decant the fat, *then* cook the vegetables in the remaining broth.

Use the 'see it, lose it' rule If you see fat on your food, remove it. For example:

- If there's fat on the meat, trim it off.
- If there's skin on the chicken, remove it.
- If there's liquefied fat on top of the stew or soup, skim it off.
- If there's a pool of grease underneath your meat, soak it up with a paper napkin.

Put meat-based soups or stews in the refrigerator overnight In the morning, it'll be super-easy to remove the hardened fat on top.

Use bacon as a flavouring, not a serving One piece of crumbled bacon goes a long way towards adding that wonderful smoky flavour to healthier dishes. ■

CHOICE 6 Eat fewer calories

When your meals are mostly vegetables and fruits, along with moderate portions of beans, whole grains, lean protein and good fats, you're harnessing an important longevity secret: more food but fewer calories.

The key is choosing the right foods in the right portions. You don't have to be stingy with the amount you eat or ever feel deprived or count a single calorie if you make the first five choices of full-life eating – namely, by feasting on fruit and veg and enjoying moderate amounts of other healthy foods such as yoghurt, salmon, olive oil, low-fat cheese and dark chocolate. On Okinawa, this strategy (minus the chocolate) allows people to eat *more* food by weight than people in other parts of Japan yet consume several hundred fewer calories a day because their choices are naturally lean.

This is an important point: you can eat heaped platefuls of veg and fruit for fewer calories than are in a small bag of crisps. And the vegetables and fruit pack several huge health bonuses. First is what they contain that packaged snacks don't: oodles of antioxidants, vitamins and fibre. Second is what they *don't* contain that packaged foods do: fat, refined carbohydrates and artificial additives that play a role in mem-ory loss, fatigue and so many killer diseases.

We've made these points before, in the chapter *Seven Keys to Ageing Well*. There we told you of two exciting keys to longevity: not obsessing about the bathroom scales and choosing foods that you can eat to your heart's content without overdoing the calories. In this section, we'll show you how to achieve these goals – and enjoy every luscious bite of this natural, never-say-diet approach to achieving a healthy weight. The bonus? Eating this way brings extra pleasure to your table because you never have to worry about eating the wrong things or 'cheating' on the latest weight-loss scheme.

SAY GOODBYE TO DIETS

Best of all, it's a great, natural, feel-good way to step off the crazy, unhealthy weight-loss roller coaster. Too many weight-loss gimmicks and gurus want you to believe that temporary deprivation and restriction are the keys to slimming down. They've demonised some foods as the cause of the world's obesity epidemic and often market highly processed alternatives (such as food-replacement milkshakes, bars and frozen meals) as the alternative. The truth is, when you rebalance your plate and choose from a wide variety of healthy foods (and treat yourself to the ones you love most), you've found a way to eat that helps your body to settle at its natural, healthy weight; give you the energy you need to be more active; and promote life-long health.

Should you worry about your weight at all? It depends. If excess weight is hurting your health, energy or mobility, then discuss weight loss with your family doctor (and if your doctor agrees that weight loss is a good idea, plan to lose pounds slowly). But if you're just hoping to fit into a smaller bathing suit next summer, reconsider. For many people, 'vanity' weight loss provides limited health benefits, and a growing stack of research suggests that after the age of 55 or 60, vanity weight loss is *detrimental* to your health. In one 12 year study of 1,801 people aged over 71, women who lost weight increased their risk of dying by 38 per cent, and men increased their odds by 76 per cent. (Of course, your best option if you'd still like to be trimmer and more fit is exercise.)

Whether or not weight loss is your goal, you can't go wrong with our approach to healthy eating. It's as simple as choosing a big fruit salad over a slice of chocolate cheesecake. Having a large piece of skinless chicken instead of a small cheeseburger. Or choosing a double portion of grilled veg instead of a handful of chips. It's delicious and satisfying – and it means never going hungry.

We've already extolled the nutritional wonders of healthy foods, from sweet cherries to hot red peppers, wholewheat bread to succulent lean beef. Now we can reveal their added full-life health bonus: each time you choose one of these natural wonders instead of a more processed food, you save a significant number of calories while you flood your body with important vitamins, minerals, antioxidants, fibre, anti-inflammatory compounds and satisfying components such as proteins and fats.

Some examples: a hot-fudge sundae with two scoops of ice cream plus fudge sauce, whipped cream, a cherry and nuts could contain 700 calories – or more. A generous bowl of fresh raspberries, strawberries and chunks of ripe mango and pineapple might have 150 calories.

A cheeseburger on a bun made from refined flour might have 600 calories. But a grilled skinless chicken breast and a wholewheat roll has just 300 calories. And if you add a side plate of green beans and a lettuce and tomato salad with olive oil vinaigrette, you've got a whole meal for less than the calories in a single cheeseburger. ■

smart ways TO EAT More food but fewer calories

FULL-LIFE EATING GOAL: make fruit or vegetables at least half of what you eat

Have unsweetened cereal for breakfast
You can enjoy a bigger serving of healthy whole grains for fewer calories. The reason: sugar is very high in calories yet has virtually no bulk. Add chopped fruit for flavour and sweetness.
Start every lunch with salad A big, fresh salad brimming with veg or fruit fills you up, fits in several vegetable servings and tastes great. Start with a generous bed of lettuce and top with chopped tomatoes, grated or sliced carrots, cucumber rounds, sliced green or red pepper and any of these: shredded courgette, sliced raw mushrooms, onions, fresh herbs (basil is heavenly), celery, fennel or shredded cabbage. Top with fat-free dressing, a dash of low-fat mayonnaise or a tablespoon of olive oil-based vinaigrette.
Add a first course of vegetable soup to dinner every night Research suggests that your body's satisfaction sensors are activated when a food is bulked up with water. Think of a bowl of low-fat, low-sodium chicken broth brimming with carrots, tomatoes, onions and green beans. For the quickest soup, heat a can of low-sodium vegetable soup, then add your favourite frozen veg and spices.
Dish up your food before serving Put food onto the plates in the kitchen rather than putting serving bowls of food on the table. The only serving bowl you should allow on the dining room table is the one holding the vegetables. That way, there's no temptation to take another piece of meat or an extra helping of noodles.

Keep chopped fruit at the front of the eye-level shelf in your refrigerator Studies show that cut fruit retains important nutrients for nearly a week. And it's easy and delicious to open the refrigerator door and indulge in chunks of watermelon, wedges of melon, pineapple slices, grapes and strawberries.
Eat a bulky, high-fibre food when you're hungry Would you rather have 19 tiny peanuts or a whole juicy apple adorned with a teaspoon of peanut butter? Both snacks are healthy, and each has about 110 calories. But the apple's size makes it much more satisfying and appealing.
Don't underestimate the power of bulk It's been suggested that 'portion distortion' plays a role in increasing obesity: we're getting fatter because portion sizes are getting bigger. In one study, students at a party ate 56 per cent more snack foods (an average of 142 more calories each) when snacks were served in large bowls rather than smaller ones. Make use of the knowledge by using tiny bowls for high-energy foods, such as peanuts, and large ones for servings of healthy, low-calorie, high-fibre foods, such as cherry tomatoes, salad greens (with a dash of dressing) and other high-fibre foods.
Designate healthy, low-calorie 'free foods' Sometimes we all just want to snack – and snack and snack some more. Keep some low-calorie, nutritious foods that you enjoy on hand, such as apples, frozen berries, carrots and sliced red peppers. Allow yourself to eat as much as you want.

Switch to zero-calorie beverages Water, still and sparkling, with a dash of lemon juice, iced tea and hot tea are all great choices. Getting away from sweetened drinks can save you hundreds of empty calories every day.

Make fruit your usual dessert To make it special, spend some time in the fresh produce section of your food shop. Look beyond your usual choices for something new or indulgent. If you usually skip berries, pomegranates or figs because of the price, for instance, consider buying them. If you usually buy just one type of fruit, buy two or three and plan to make a pretty fruit salad. After all, you're not spending money on biscuits and cakes. (And check out the choices in the canned-fruit and frozen-food aisles. Often, the best-quality berries are frozen. Just thaw gently in the microwave.)

Reverse dessert priorities Usually, people adorn calorie-dense, nutrition-light desserts such as cakes with a few berries. Next time you plan a nice dessert, do the opposite: make the bulk of your dessert berries or fruit sorbet and adorn it with a small biscuit or cake or a square of high-quality dark chocolate.

Create a pile Restaurants sometimes present appetisers and main courses in a neat pile, rather than spread around the plate. It looks dramatic, and makes it less obvious how much of each dish you're getting. So try this at home. The next time you serve up, say, steak, mashed potatoes and sautéed spinach, create a pile from the three. Make your bottom layer a large serving of vegetables (in this case, spinach spread into a circle in the middle of the plate). Put a modest-sized disc of mashed potatoes on the spinach. On top, put four slices of the beef. Then add sauce, herbs or other final touches and serve for a tasty, well-proportioned dinner.

Have salad for a snack Many people snack not out of hunger, but to satisfy a desire for flavour or texture. That's why so many snack foods are salty and crunchy. You can satisfy that desire for texture just as easily, and far more healthfully, with a salad. Use lettuce, carrots, cabbage, celery and peppers to give your mouth the robust texture it desires. If you use a light dressing, you can eat a whole bowl of salad before you get to the calorie count of a handful of crisps. ■

Make fruit your usual dessert

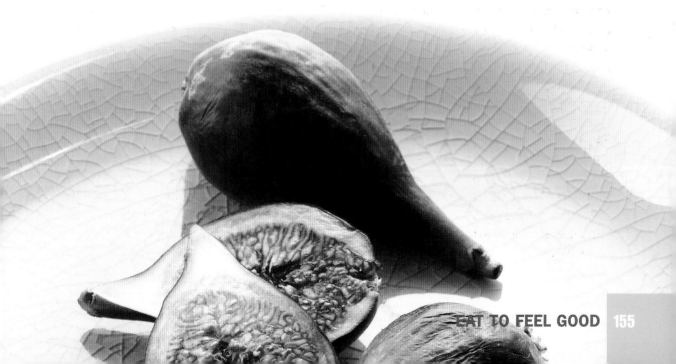

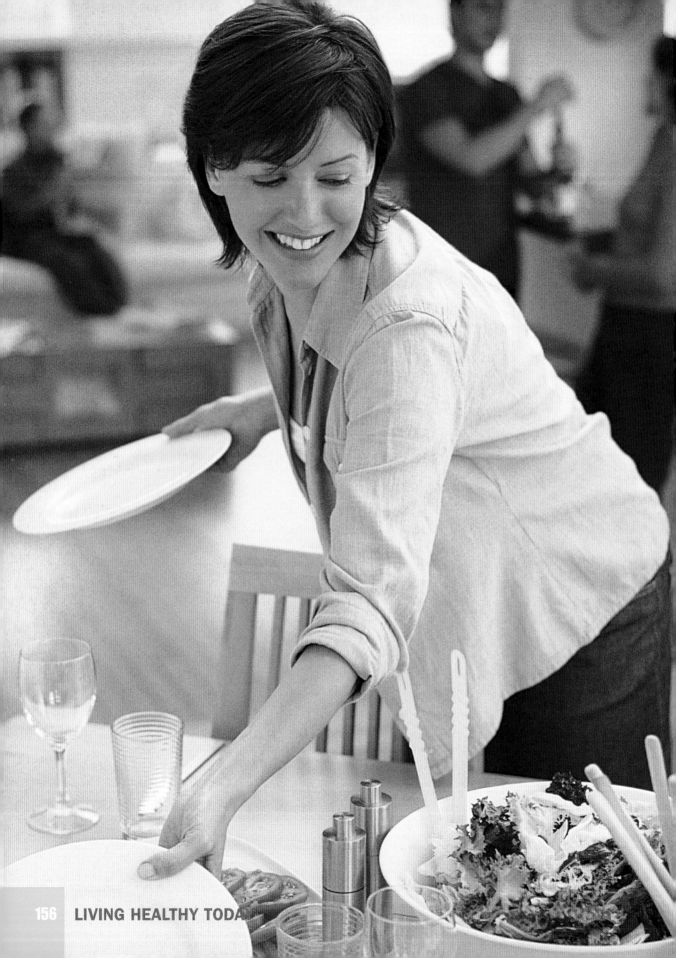

LIVING HEALTHY TODAY

smart ways TO IMPROVE Your eating patterns

FULL-LIFE EATING GOAL: eat small amounts of food six times a day, every day

Practise *hara hachi bu* This Okinawan eating practice translates as '80 per cent' and means that traditional Okinawans stop eating when they're 80 per cent full. This is a great way to avoid overeating because it gives your brain time to notice what's in your tummy and send an 'I'm full' signal. Instead of reaching for seconds, put your fork down and clear the table as soon as you feel the first slight twinges of fullness. (Return to the table for more conversation or take cups of tea into the living room with your dining companions to extend the pleasure of your meal.) 'When you start to feel full, your stomach really has become full,' Dr Willcox says, 'but physiologically, there's about a 20 minute delay before the stomach tells the brain.'

Downsize your dinnerware In recent years, many tableware manufacturers have increased the size of the plates and bowls they sell to keep pace with the larger portions to which we've grown accustomed. If you tend to overeat, serve meals on salad plates instead of dinner plates.

Never skip breakfast The first meal of the day revs up your metabolism and fills your belly with the fuel you need for energy. A good breakfast prevents excessive eating later in the day. If you're not a natural breakfast lover, wait till an hour after you wake up before eating. Or try an unconventional meal, such as a sandwich or bowl of soup.

Practise the 3 hour rule Don't let more than 3 hours pass between your meals and snacks. Eating regularly keeps you from becoming ravenous or experiencing the effects of low blood sugar: feeling lightheaded and low on energy. Moderate-sized meals and snacks can also help you to avoid overeating because it's comforting to know that there's another chance to eat coming soon.

Make lunch the big meal of the day In traditional European societies, the midday meal is the star. Not only do people take time to linger together over the food, but they also eat more of it than they do at dinner – giving their bodies more time for digestion and more fuel for the rest of the day. Eating a bigger lunch can also help you to avoid the late-afternoon slump that can lead to overeating and to poor food choices such as sweets and snack foods.

Set a new second-helpings rule Allow yourself second helpings only of fruit and vegetables, not of grains, fats or meats.

Eat 90 per cent of your meals at home You're more likely to eat high-fat, high-calorie, highly processed foods away from home than in your own kitchen or dining room. And you'll avoid the temptation of large restaurant portions, too.

Eat slowly and calmly Set aside at least half an hour to eat each meal of the day. Make the food last for that whole length of time by eating slowly and stopping frequently to enjoy the conversation of your companions, the view out of the window or the music on the radio. This slow-eating strategy gives your brain the opportunity to notice how much you've already eaten and send a signal that you're done.

Practise the grounded-fork rule To help to slow your eating, force yourself to put down your fork after every bite and do not pick it up until you've swallowed what you've just put in your mouth. ■

CHOICE 7 Enjoy eating

Welcome to the last choice of full-life eating: enjoyment. Seems a little redundant, doesn't it? We've mentioned taste and flavour countless times throughout this chapter, and we've repeatedly made the point that healthy eating is a celebration, full of pleasure and ritual. So why this particular topic again?

Simple. Many people don't eat for enjoyment or nourishment. They eat because they're nervous or bored or frustrated or because at 3.30pm, it's just second nature to take a break and have a chocolate bar. Or they eat because they feel they have to – Mum would be insulted, after all, if you didn't have seconds.

Other reasons why we eat are more positive, even if misguided. We show affection with food ('I love you so much, here are *two* boxes of chocolate!'). We celebrate with food. We assuage our guilt with food ('I'm really sorry. I brought you a cake as a peace offering.') We reveal our heritage and tradition with food. In this modern world, eating is habit, ritual, therapy and relaxation. All this is well intentioned, but at what cost to our health?

Sometimes the problem is merely hectic living. Do you eat so fast you can't remember what you've just consumed, mindlessly nibble while watching TV or find yourself gobbling fast-food meals in the car while you drive? While all of us eat on the run occasionally, if you make a habit of eating quickly and without pleasure, you will miss out on the profound life and health-enhancing joys of the table.

In cultures where people live long, healthy lives, meals are events. In Japan, for example, 'Okinawans look for meaning in food and in meals,' notes Dr Willcox. Instead of opening a packet of biscuits when guests arrive, Okinawans respectfully serve tea. Gathering around the table is a social time as much as a time for food. There's more conversation, more time between bites of rice or fish or vegetables. When this type of meal is over, you leave the table with a full belly and a full heart.

Eating slowly – and savouring the colours, textures, temperatures and flavours of foods – enhances digestion, discourages overeating and promotes relaxation. Sharing a meal or snack with friends is a stress-reducing opportunity to reconnect. Now take the pleasure a step or two further. Shop unhurriedly for fresh ingredients and enjoy the sensual experience of washing, chopping and cooking them to create a wonderful meal for yourself and others.

Each of us has deeply embedded habits and prejudices regarding food. Our message: reconsider the role of food in your daily life. Are you eating merely out of habit? Is food providing solace for insecurities or frustrations? How many times a day do you gobble down food mindlessly, without the flavour even registering?

Be a mindful eater. Don't focus just on the right foods but also on the right *reasons* to eat – for nourishment, health, social ritual and, of course, enjoyment. A bag of crisps may sound like the right medicine for a tough day, but we suggest hugs or a walk instead – followed by a healthy sit-down meal with someone you love. ∎

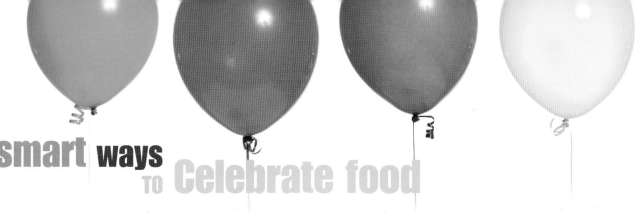

smart ways TO Celebrate food

FULL-LIFE EATING GOAL: enjoy laughter, conversation and relaxation at as many meals as possible

Give thanks Privately or as a group, give thanks for the fact that you're here and able to enjoy the company and the food. It need not be a prayer if you're uncomfortable with that. Come up with your own ritual. It could be a toast, everyone saying hello or a quick moment of silence, or even holding or shaking hands. Whatever you're comfortable with is the best choice of all.

Really taste the food and enjoy the moment Put your utensils down between bites. Use the time to chew and swallow. Note the flavours, colours and textures of the meal as well as the look of the table and the ambience around it. Look out of the window and enjoy the view. Think about ways the food fits into the scenery: are you having porridge because it's a cold, snowy day, just as you did as a child? Are you having a light, no-cook supper that features juicy fruits on a sweltering summer evening, just as you did on a tropical holiday a few years ago?

Make conversation Take turns sharing a positive or funny experience you had during the day, then discuss a challenge you faced and overcame – or are still confronting. Talk about the food and about enjoyable subjects from local or world news. Save complaints and controversies for another time. The table should be a happy place.

Turn off the TV and put away mobile phones, pagers and laptops Make mealtime inviolable. Friends and colleagues can reach you later.

Invite a friend or meet somewhere for a meal Make a meal even more social by sharing it with someone who's not in your household. Don't feel like cooking? Meet at a café or local cafeteria or bring packed lunches to a table at a park. The important part is being together.

Savour every nuance of your meal Think of a traditional Japanese tea ceremony, in which every sense has a role to play: you listen and observe as the tea is poured, feel the hot cup in your hand, smell and taste the tea. To focus your mind and slow things further, bring a meal to the table course by course and leave time between courses for relaxation and conversation.

Eat seasonally Enjoying local seasonal produce can make a meal more meaningful by linking your plate to the place where you live. Visit a farmer's market for seasonal vegetables or meats. As you prepare and eat them, think about how they grew in the same sun and rain you've experienced over the past few months.

Treat family like company Fresh flowers, a nice table setting, garnishes on the plates – you and your family deserve such niceties every day. Resolve never to eat at a messy table. ■

smart ways to Break bad food habits

FULL-LIFE EATING GOAL: never use food to cope with life's challenges

Figure out your stress-eating triggers
Experts estimate that 75 per cent of overeating is due to emotions. Do you eat when you're angry? Bored? Lonely? At a party when you're feeling nervous? Pay attention to the situations that prompt you to reach for extra helpings or snacks. Identifying your overeating triggers is the first step in fixing emotional eating problems.

Fix emotional eating Once you've discovered which emotions are behind your bad eating habits, you can fix the situation. If you're feeling angry, try putting on some music and dancing. Worried? Turn off the news and read a funny book or turn on a comedy programme. Sad? Read something inspirational, meditate or pray or call a friend. Lonely? Call or write to a friend or take a walk to a place where there are people, such as the library. Just be mindful that food can't soothe or solve your troubles; at best, it will mask them for a short time. That's not a benefit at all.

Chat more, eat less Never stand by the crisps and mindlessly eat while you talk with other guests at a party. Instead of letting conversation lead you into mindless eating, let socialising be the centrepiece of your experience by staying far from the buffet. When you arrive at a picnic or barbecue, grab a low-calorie drink and find a great seat at a table filled with friends, family or friendly strangers. Then approach the buffet table or grill with a purpose: grab a plate, add carefully chosen foods and carry it back to your spot at the centre of the real fun.

Write in your diary Paying attention to your feelings by writing them down is a powerful way to make yourself feel valued – and feel better – without resorting to soured cream and onion crisps. Keep a feelings diary and pay attention to situations that lead to overeating. That way, you'll learn how to spot dangerous situations sooner and take preventive steps.

Have more fun When life is busy and your to-do list long, it's easy to turn to food as quick entertainment and solace. In fact, you may be missing out on other healthy pleasures that would be more satisfying. When was the last time you enjoyed your favourite activities, such as going to concerts or dog shows, gardening or museum hopping, roller-skating or visiting antiques shops? Make time for fun, and you may find you don't need those biscuits after all.

Tune in to your true hunger level Before you take a bite, stop and rate your hunger on a scale of one to ten – with one meaning famished and ten being totally stuffed, the way you'd feel after a big Christmas dinner. The time to eat is when you're at about three. The time to stop eating? When you're at five to seven – feeling comfortably satisfied but not overly full. If you're reaching for food when you're not at three, pull back and remind yourself that it will be snack time, or mealtime, soon.

Get moving! Physical activity cuts stress and pumps feel-good endorphins throughout your body while burning calories. Make a new commitment to getting half an hour of activity most days of the week. Great options include walking, exercising to aerobics videos and DVDs, signing up for a class or doing strength training at a gym, or simply choosing active fun such as hiking, bowling, swimming or skating.

smart ways TO EAT Healthier snacks

FULL-LIFE EATING GOAL: replace junk food in your diet with healthy alternatives

Eat between meals Yes, you read that correctly. We believe you should eat every 3 hours or so to avoid severe hunger that leads to low blood sugar and overeating.

Snack on fibre-rich produce plus protein When snack time does come round, treat yourself right with a satisfying mini-feast of fruit or veg plus protein. Have a handful of cherry tomatoes plus a piece of low-fat cheese in the morning instead of a muffin. Try apple slices with peanut butter or a few slices of chicken or turkey on a slice of wholewheat bread in the afternoon. Target your morning snack to be about 80 calories and your afternoon snack to be about 150 calories. You can also have a serving of whole grains, such as a slice of wholewheat bread, instead of the protein or in place of fruit for an afternoon snack.

Good protein choices include one hard-boiled egg, 1 tablespoon peanut butter, 14g nuts (such as 12 almonds, eight cashews, eight pecan halves, 26 shelled pistachios or six walnut halves), two slices of roast chicken (about a quarter of a breast) and 125g yoghurt.

Easy vegetable choices include cherry tomatoes, baby carrots, sliced peppers, cucumbers and chopped broccoli. Fruit choices include a piece of any whole fresh fruit or 125g chopped or sliced fruit.

Plan for a treat Strive for balance on a big day out, such as at an amusement park or fair. You don't want to drive home regretting what you ate, but you also don't want to spend your special outing feeling deprived while everyone else slurps their lemonade and tosses back handfuls of chips. Your smart strategy: in advance, decide on one moderate-calorie treat a day.

Take your own snacks Head off a moment of hungry weakness by packing ready-to-eat veg, fruit (in a protective plastic container), a sealable bag containing nuts or a handful of whole-grain crackers and low-fat cheese, or half of a peanut butter sandwich on wholewheat.

Invest in a water-bottle carrier These carriers allow you to carry a bottle of water easily. Having water with you at all times will help you to resist fizzy and other sweetened drinks and keep you hydrated. Often, when we think we're hungry between meals, we're actually thirsty.

Keep an emergency snack in your bag or car A healthy cereal bar – look for one with less than 200 calories and at least 3g of fibre – could help you to avoid overeating or choosing high-calorie snacks if you find yourself away from home for longer than you expected.

Use snacks to fill nutritional gaps If you notice after lunch that you haven't eaten much fruit, for example, or haven't had any dairy products, plan your next snack strategically to fill the gap.

Sit down when you snack Put your snack on a plate or in a bowl and sit at the table to eat it. Have a glass of water or a cup of tea at the same time. This will make the 'mini-meal' last longer and feel more substantial.

Say no to vending machines For the rest of your life. Convince yourself that bags of salty, greasy snacks and bars of sugary processed sweets have no place in your life. After a month or two of successful avoidance, you'll forget that stuff ever appealed to you. ■

Foods that harm

When you eat for long life and lasting health, there's no room in your diet for these three health-robbing, age-accelerating food additives: sodium, sugar and bad fats. Packed into processed foods, fast food and manufactured treats, they seem to have an addictive power over us – and long-term health consequences such as high blood pressure, high blood sugar and a higher risk of heart disease and stroke.

Small wonder that top nutrition experts call them everything from 'the biggest food-processing disasters in history' to 'Frankenfoods' (referring, of course, to Dr Frankenstein's manufactured monster). Between 65 and 85 per cent of the total salt we consume every day

fresh, whole foods more and that you feel better. Moving away from processed foods full of these additives requires patience and perseverance, but it's worth while. The other key: eating outside the box – or wrapper. Opting for unprocessed foods, in their natural state (think fresh fruit, veg, whole grains and freshly brewed tea) automatically means you'll get less of the bad stuff. Here's what you should know.

SODIUM

Too much sodium raises your odds of developing high blood pressure – a condition that affects one in every three men and women in England. Most of them don't even know they have it – there are usually no symptoms. But it's often

... there's no room in your diet for these three health-robbing, age-accelerating food additives: sodium, sugar and bad fats

comes not from salt we add during cooking or at the table, but from salt already present in the foods we eat. No wonder either then that the Food Standards Agency has urged food manufacturers and retailers to reduce salt levels in a wide range of pre-prepared and processed foods, including bread, cakes, biscuits, pastries, breakfast cereals, ready-meals, bacon and cheese.

Breaking free of these health robbers can be a real effort. Sodium and sugar heighten the flavour of foods – especially low-flavour or tasteless processed foods. And saturated fats and trans fats lend a pleasing crunch to crackers and keep baked goods moist and tender. But it can be done. When people follow a low-sodium diet for 12 weeks, they start to rate lower-salt foods as just as appealing as ordinary foods.

It can take a while to retrain your tastebuds. But you'll notice that you enjoy the flavours of

dubbed the 'silent killer', because if you have high blood pressure you are three times more likely to develop heart disease or to have a stroke, and twice as likely to die from these conditions. Too much sodium prompts your body to hold on to more fluid (to 'dilute' the extra saltiness); this increases blood volume, forcing your heart to pump harder with every beat and putting extra stress on blood-vessel walls. Numerous studies have shown that reducing the amount of salt you eat can lower blood pressure and so reduce the risk of heart disease and stroke. What's more, a high-salt diet can thin your bones, boost your risk of gastric cancer and worsen lung function in people with exercise-induced asthma – a condition that plagues nine out of ten people with asthma, studies show.

The worst high-salt foods: condiments, smoked fish and meats, sausages, ham and bacon, cheese, pickles and olives. And the top sources of 'hidden' salt in processed foods: baked beans, breakfast cereals, bread products such as crumpets and bagels, pre-mixed sauces and stock cubes, crisps, pizza and other ready meals, prepared soups and sandwiches.

Automatically throw away 'flavour sachets' and 'spice mixes' that come with cook-at-home dishes They're mostly salt. Instead, invest in several sodium-free spice blends or make your own. Three we love: ground black pepper mixed with a dash of sodium-free dried lemon peel; oregano, ground cumin and a shake of red pepper flakes; and basil, marjoram and thyme. You can save about 500mg of sodium a serving.

Always buy natural – or better still, reduced-sodium – cheese A slice of pasteurised, processed Swiss cheese packs 435mg of sodium; a slice of real Swiss cheese contains 54mg; and a low-sodium slice has just 4mg. Same goes for grated Parmesan: a tablespoon of pre-grated Parmesan has 76mg, while the low-sodium version has 3mg. Choosing low-sodium cheese is a great strategy because it's so flavourful you won't miss the salt at all.

Never buy canned fish, beans or vegetables in salted water or brine If you have any in the cupboard, rinse them twice before using. Salt-added canned veg and beans may contain a fifth of your daily sodium allowance, up to 500mg per half cup. Drain off the liquid, dump the beans or veg into a colander or strainer and rinse, then rinse again. A good 'shower' can remove nearly half the sodium. A 3 minute rinse cuts the sodium in canned tuna by 80 per cent.

Make your own salad dressing Bottled salad dressings can contain up to 620mg of sodium in a single 2 tablespoon serving – and reduced-fat dressings often have more salt to offset the loss of flavour. Make your own dressing with

Learn to love labels

Let's be honest: you can't completely remove salt, sugar and 'bad' fats from your diet. But you can try to get them down to acceptable levels. We each eat, on average, 9g of salt a day – at least two and a half times as much as we need – and the government is urging people to reduce this to less than 6g daily. At the start of the 18th century we ate about 4lb of refined sugar annually; today on average we each consume nearly our own bodyweight in sugar every year. And Britons eat on average over 90g of fat a day, around 36g of it saturated. Nearly 14 per cent of our total energy intake comes from harmful fats, whereas a healthy level is more like the 6 per cent seen in countries such as Japan.

As many of these harmful ingredients are hidden in pre-prepared foods, it can be difficult to spot them. Sugar can pop up in the unlikeliest of places – ready meals and savoury snacks, for instance: the contents list may describe it using names such as glucose, sucrose, dextrose or fructose, but they're all sugar. Hydrogenated vegetable fat must be listed, but the really bad trans fats don't need to be labelled separately under European law, even though they're present in harmful quantities in many biscuits and cakes, fast foods and some margarines. The safest bet is to steer clear of anything that says 'hydrogenated'.

	LOW (per 100g)	MEDIUM (per 100g)	HIGH (per 100g)
Fat	0–3g	Between 3g and 20g	20g+
Saturated fat	0–1.5g	Between 1.5g and 5g	5g+
Total sugars	0–5g	Between 5g and 15g	15g+
Salt	0–0.3g	Between 0.3g and 1.5g	1.5g+

Source: Food Standards Agency

8 tablespoons olive oil, 4 tablespoons balsamic or cider vinegar or lemon juice, and your choice of herbs and spices (try crushed garlic, black pepper and oregano), then refrigerate. A 2 tablespoon serving packs less than 3mg of sodium.

Eat real meat instead of sliced meats, bacon and sausage A single slice of pre-packed ham contains 350mg of sodium; one slice of bacon, 192mg. Pretty much any meat product that's processed in a factory or cured or smoked for flavour is off the scale when it comes to sodium. Make sandwiches instead with unsalted turkey breast or lean beef.

Toss away the blood pressure time-bomb condiments Garlic and onion salts pack 1,480mg of sodium per teaspoon; soy sauce, 500 to 2,000mg per tablespoon; and stock cubes, 1,200mg per tiny cube. Throw them out – now. Safe alternatives include onion flakes, garlic powder and low-sodium soup stock. Don't bother with reduced or low-sodium soy sauce, as it still packs 300 to 830mg per tablespoon.

Shake less sodium in the kitchen – and at the table Use sea salt in recipes – it's coarser, so it doesn't pack as tightly in a measuring spoon. And it retains important minerals and trace elements that are often lost in the processing of ordinary table salt.

THE 'BAD' FATS

The damage caused by trans fats has been one of the biggest food scares of recent years. Trans fats are by-products of a chemical process called hydrogenation, developed to raise the melting point of oils to make them more stable. For nearly a century, the process has been used to make food oils from vegetable oils that otherwise go rancid too quickly to be useful, and to make these oils stay solid at room temperature – so they can be substituted for butter and lard in cooking. The theory was that hydrogenated vegetable oils would be a healthy (and cheap) alternative to artery-clogging saturated fats. But in a classic case of consumer science gone awry, trans fats are now estimated to cause 50,000 deaths a year by promoting heart disease and cancer as well as dementia and diabetes.

A recent review published in the *British Medical Journal* concluded that trans fats have 'no nutritional value' and have harmful effects even at low intakes of only 3 per cent of total daily energy intake (a mere 20 to 60 calories' worth). What's more, each 2 per cent rise in energy intake from trans-fatty acids is associated with a 23 per cent increase in heart disease.

Unfortunately, it took a long time before scientists discovered the damage that trans fats cause. Meanwhile, food manufacturers had already made them key ingredients. Today, they're in at least 42,000 food products. But a growing stack of research confirms that trans fats are health robbers – and in response, more and more trans fat-free processed foods are becoming available. As the dangers of trans fats have become apparent, many supermarkets and food manufacturers have reduced the amounts present in their products – and even if they're not labelled as such, there's a clue in the word 'hydrogenated'. (Keep reading labels, though. Some manufacturers have reverted to using saturated-fat rich palm oil or coconut oil. Those aren't healthy alternatives, experts warn.)

Here's how to steer clear of bad fats – and fill your fat quota with the good stuff every day.

Permanently ban factory-made biscuits, cakes and other baked goods from your diet Instead, snack on individually wrapped dark chocolates, crunchy nuts or raisins. Some experts estimate that up to 95 per cent of prepared biscuits and 100 per cent of crackers may contain trans fats. More trans fat-free options appear every day, though these snack foods provide tons of age-accelerating saturated fat, sweeteners, refined carbohydrates and

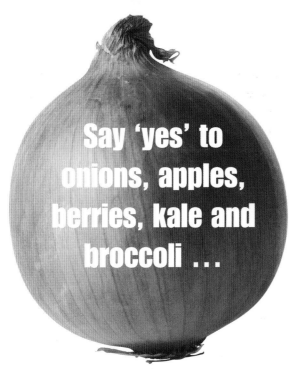

Say 'yes' to onions, apples, berries, kale and broccoli …

calories. But don't give up treats. A 30g serving of dark chocolate provides heart-healthy antioxidants. A small handful of nuts (20 or so, about the amount that would fit into a box of mints) or a small box of raisins provides lots of flavour and chewing satisfaction as well as a wealth of fibre and antioxidants, and, from the nuts, you get good fats that protect arteries.

Say 'no thanks' to commercially fried foods

Get a grilled chicken sandwich instead of the crispy fried version, and have a salad in place of chips. The fast-food industry has been slower than retailers and producers to adapt to the dangers of trans fats and, of course, you can't readily tell what your food has been fried in. One major chain uses EU-subsidised rapeseed oil that contains 16 per cent trans fats. And because hydrogenated oils stay stable for a long time, they can be reused again and again – some chip shops reportedly reuse the same oil for up to three months. And even restaurants that claim their foods are trans fat-free probably aren't using good fats – the fryers are usually filled with blends containing high amounts of omega-6 fatty acids, a type of fat we already consume way too much of.

The anti-cancer diet

Here are some of the ways to cut your cancer risk, based on recent studies.

Say 'yes' to onions, apples, berries, kale and broccoli Eating lots of antioxidants called flavonols – found in these foods – cut pancreatic cancer risk by 23 per cent. Among smokers, a flavonol-rich diet lowered the risk by 59 per cent, report researchers from the Cancer Research Center of Hawaii who studied 183,518 women and men.

Go to the limit with fruits and veg Study participants who got 12 servings a day lowered the risk of various cancers by 29 per cent compared with those who ate just three daily servings, a recent study of 500,000 people aged 50 and over found.

Choose the red wine Red-wine drinkers may reduce their risk of lung cancer by around 13 per cent for each daily glass, according to a study of 132 male lung cancer patients compared with 187 minor surgery patients at a hospital in Spain. Rosé, beer and spirits had no impact – and white wine seemed to have the opposite effect, though the number of white wine drinkers studied was too small to draw any conclusions. Researchers suggest that an antioxidant in red wine called resveratrol, together with the tannin, which is also antioxidant, may be able to stifle tumour development and growth.

Have fish more often Eating plenty of omega-3-rich oily fish such as salmon, herring and mackerel could reduce the risk of developing prostate cancer, according to a 30 year study of moe than 6,000 men at Sweden's Karolinska Institute in Stockholm. Men who ate no fish had a two to three-fold higher risk of prostate cancer than those who ate moderate or high amounts.

Bake – and spread – good fats If you've been eating margarine or spreads made with hydrogenated vegetable oil, the news about trans fats may find you rethinking your preferred spread. Don't throw in the towel and return to butter. Instead opt for products made with olive oil. These have heart-healthy monounsaturated fats and may come with added omega-3s.

Check your favourites online Many food chains – from fast-food places to coffee shops – list the trans fat content of their menu items on their websites. If you've got a favourite, check it out.

Drink coffee, not fat Love special coffee drinks? Order a latte or cappuccino with skimmed milk, then sprinkle cinnamon, cocoa powder and vanilla over the foam. You'll get a serving of bone-building, calcium-rich milk and avoid saturated fat: a mocha drink, for example, can pack nearly 500 calories and 16g of fat, much of it saturated.

Replace butter in recipes and sautéing with good-for-you oils Use olive oil for baking – a good rule of thumb is ¾ tablespoon of oil for every 1 tablespoon of butter called for. Keep an oil mister loaded with olive oil near the hob and spray pans before cooking – you'll get flavour but keep the calories down.

Have a fancy fruit salad deluxe instead of premium ice cream Fancy ice creams can contain as much fat as a fast-food double cheeseburger. Switching to an all-fruit sorbet is a better choice but will still flood your body with loads of extra sugar in most cases. The best choice: indulge in an over-the-top fruit salad. Layer frozen raspberries, sliced mango, super-sweet fresh pineapple (buy it precut in the fresh produce department), mandarin oranges packed in juice and whatever else you love. It's colourful, sweet and fun to eat – and gives you a bonus of age-defying antioxidants and fibre.

SUGARS

We all know that eating too much sugar can pile on the pounds (especially because many sweet foods are also high in fat), but did you know it

Processed-food manufacturers – not Mother Nature – encourage us to crave sweetness can also raise your blood sugar, increasing your risk of diabetes, heart disease and stroke? According to a review in the *British Medical Journal*, 'sugar is as dangerous as tobacco' – and far more important in terms of world health because the burden is life-long, whereas tobacco-related diseases tend to strike in middle age or later. 'Sugar should be classified as a hard drug, for it is addictive and harmful.'

How can we be addicted to sugar? The more we eat, the more we want. Why? A big shot of refined sugar makes blood sugar skyrocket, then plummet as the hormone insulin ushers the sugar into cells throughout the body. Sometimes it can fall to a lower level than before you drank that giant cola or ate those 35 jelly babies. As a result, you feel tired, hungry and cranky – and crave more sugar. But these tips can help you to break the sugar habit and get off the roller coaster.

Replace soft drinks with healthier sips As we've discussed, one of the best things you can do for your health is to replace fizzy drinks, sweetened teas, fruit drinks and other sweetened beverages gradually with water, unsweetened tea or diluted fruit juice. To start, try pouring some grape or orange juice into carbonated water for a low-sugar spritzer. Or add a squeeze of lemon or lime juice to filtered water. Visit the herbal tea section of your supermarket and bring home new flavours to drink hot or cold. Treat yourself to one glass of real fruit juice – without added sugar or sweeteners – each day, and venture beyond just orange. Yes, real juice has calories (between 100 and 140 per 0.2l glass), but it counts towards your daily fruit servings, and the full-bodied flavour and natural sweetness is intensely pleasurable.

Buy 100 per cent fruit juice Many ordinary fruit drinks are heavily laden with sugar – some fruit squashes are basically sugar water with a bit of added fruit concentrate. So don't assume the juice you buy is all juice. Read the label; if the ingredients include sugar, put it back and look for one that's 100 per cent pure fruit juice.

Look at other labels as well It's worth checking almost all packaged food you buy, be it biscuits, salad dressing or pasta sauce. If sugar is listed among the first five ingredients, it's probably sweeter than you need.

Have fruit for dessert six days a week, then indulge on the seventh Sometimes the best way to give something up is to have a little once in a while. You might not fall off the wagon when you pass the bakery on Wednesday if you know you can have two homemade chocolate biscuits on Saturday night.

Rediscover the tang of plain yoghurt Mixed with fresh fruit and topped with a dusting of nuts, plain yoghurt has half the sugar of sweetened vanilla yoghurt and 60 fewer calories.

Sensible supplements

You've got car insurance, home insurance, life insurance and perhaps even pet insurance. Isn't it time for affordable, proven and sensible *nutrition* insurance?

Maybe you think you don't need it. Or you're already taking a load of pricy, super-duper, top-end supplements. Or you have a single dusty bottle of something hidden somewhere in the medicine cabinet. In all these cases, it's time for a sensible new approach. Experts say that after the age of 50, your best 'nutrition insurance' is taking an inexpensive multivitamin plus a calcium and vitamin D supplement every day, with a few fish-oil capsules thrown in if you don't eat fish at least twice a week. These are all most people will ever need to cover any shortfalls. And you don't need high doses, fancy supplements or overpriced pills. Just the basics.

And it's worth saying it again: you don't need high-dose supplements for everyday good health (unless your doctor has a good reason to prescribe one). In recent years, study after study has shown that big doses of vitamins such as A, E and even C don't provide any health advantages – and could be dangerous. In the largest-ever analysis of antioxidants – a look at 68 studies involving 232,606 people conducted by researchers at Copenhagen University Hospital in Denmark – people who regularly took beta-carotene, vitamin A and vitamin E supplements had a 4 to 16 per cent *increased* risk of death. Some experts have criticised the study's design, but everyone agrees that getting disease-fighting antioxidants from fruit, veg and whole grains is a smarter move.

Even if you're among the 2 per cent of us who never, ever indulges in fast food or junk-food, your diet may no longer completely cover all the special vitamin and mineral needs that crop up in your 50s, 60s and beyond.

Convinced? Here's how to buy – and use – your new 'nutrition insurance' policy.

MULTIVITAMIN MAGIC

Our definition of supplement magic? Not crazy, pie-in-the-sky claims or extra ingredients – such as added minerals, herbs or antioxidant extracts. These sound promising but research shows that they probably don't deliver any discernible health benefits. To us, multivitamin magic means finding the right multivitamin at the right price – and not letting the vast array of nutritional supplements crammed on pharmacy shelves confuse you or tempt you to spend extra money for stuff you simply don't need.

Here's how to find, store and take the perfect multivitamin.

Spend like a cheapskate A multivitamin that provides sufficient levels of important vitamins and minerals doesn't need to be expensive. You don't need fancy brand names, tablets that can only be obtained from specialist suppliers or exotic extra ingredients. A moderately priced named brand or shop's own make is usually fine.

Trouble swallowing? Ask your pharmacist about alternatives Chewable multivitamins or children's liquid supplements may do the job just as well, though you may need to adjust the dose accordingly.

Look for 100 per cent of the Recommended Daily Intake (RDI) for the 'big nine' nutrients Look for 100 per cent of the Recommended Daily Amount (RDA – the amount a typical, healthy person needs in a day) for thiamin (B_1); riboflavin (B_2); niacin (B_3); vitamins B_6, B_{12}, C, D and E; and folic acid. You don't need megadoses – the goal is to get what you'd normally get from food, not to flood your body with extras that will usually just be excreted in your urine (for water-soluble vitamins) or stored in fat tissue (for fat-soluble vitamins). And there is some evidence of harmful effects from taking too many multivitamins, so stick to the recommended dose, usually one tablet daily.

Limit intake of retinol-based vitamin A More than 5,000 IU a day of vitamin A from retinol may increase the osteoporosis risk. Look for supplements containing no more than 2,500 IU of retinol-based vitamin A (it may be listed on the label or in the ingredients as vitamin A acetate or palmitate). Less risky: vitamin A that comes from beta-carotene, which your body converts to A as needed. A big caution: if you smoke, keep levels even of supplemental beta-carotene low since studies suggest high levels may raise lung cancer risk.

Go easy on iron You probably don't need any more than you're getting from a normal diet, and some studies have suggested that high iron intakes may be linked with an increased risk of heart disease. In the UK all flour and many breakfast cereals are already fortified with iron. The total recommended intake of iron from all sources is 8.7mg a day for men and postmenopausal women, and 14.8mg a day for women who are still menstruating. You should not take more than 17mg daily from supplements. Excess iron can cause constipation and, with exceptionally high doses, abdominal pain, nausea, vomiting and diarrhoea. Too much iron can also exacerbate or unmask a genetic disorder called haemochromatosis, which affects 1 in 250 people, for whom iron overload is potentially fatal.

Don't exceed 100 per cent of other minerals You just don't need more than the RDA for chromium, copper, iodine, manganese, molybdenum and zinc. And most of us take in sufficient quantities of chloride, magnesium, phosphorus and potassium from a healthy diet. Don't worry about sci-fi-sounding trace elements such as boron, nickel, silicon, tin and vanadium. Experts aren't sure we need them at all.

Consider getting more vitamin D from a separate supplement Many studies suggest that not getting enough vitamin D – from food, supplements or sunlight – could raise the risk of osteoporosis and broken bones, multiple sclerosis and a wide variety of cancers, including breast, ovarian, colon and prostate. More recently, an intriguing study suggested that getting more vitamin D could cut your risk. After following 1,179 healthy postmenopausal women for five years, researchers found those who got 1,400 to 1,500mg of calcium plus 1,100 IU of vitamin D from supplements every day had a 60 to 77 per cent lower risk of cancer than those who didn't get those amounts. The connection? Studies suggest that vitamin D helps to stop cancer from proliferating, promotes the death of tumour cells, and helps to stop tumours from developing blood vessels that allow them to grow larger.

Food sources alone can't raise the amount of vitamin D in your bloodstream to protective levels. A 100g serving of salmon, a top source, packs just 360 IU; a glass of fat-free milk, 98 IU; and fortified breakfast cereal has about 40 IU per serving. And while ultraviolet B (UVB) light in sunshine synthesises vitamin D in your body, rays are too weak from November to May in northerly climes – and not everyone can or should sunbathe in shorts or a bathing suit for 15 to 30 minutes a day anyway. (Plus, after the age of 50, your body simply makes less vitamin D.)

Your best bet? Look for D supplements. The safe upper limit for adults is 1,000 IU a day, experts say.

Read the label before buying a formula for older people – or any formula designed specifically for women, men or a particular ethnic group Judge these trendy 'customised vitamins' against our standards. Some may offer slightly more or less of certain nutrients, but in most cases, experts say, a low-cost multivitamin is just as good.

Don't be swayed by marketing ploys Your body doesn't care if the vitamin C comes from rose hips or was produced in a big vat somewhere. And unless you've got an allergy or sensitivity to ingredients such as wheat, lactose or rice, you shouldn't pay extra for allergen-free types.

CALCIUM SUPPLEMENTS

No multivitamin could possibly contain a day's worth of calcium, simply because this bone-building mineral is made of big molecules that couldn't be packed into a single pill small enough for a human being to swallow. Unless you faithfully get three to four servings of dairy products every day, plan to keep a calcium supplement on your shelf – and to take it. Research proves that it can cut your risk of developing brittle bones and of the debilitating fractures that change the lives of millions of people each year. Here's how to buy and take this important supplement.

Test it yourself Wondering about your pill's absorbability? Place one in a small glass of warm water for half an hour and stir occasionally. If it hasn't dissolved in 30 minutes, it probably won't break down in your stomach either.

Carbonate or citrate? It depends on your personality and schedule Both types potentially work equally well. Calcium citrate is more expensive, but is better absorbed and can be taken once daily on an empty stomach. You need more calcium carbonate to get the same effect, and there's a limit to how much can be absorbed in one go, so you need to take it twice a day, and it should be taken with food. Calcium carbonate tablets are generally bigger, which can be difficult for some people to take, and this form is less effective if you have the reduced stomach acid that's common in older people.

So choose citrate if you can afford it and need the convenience, especially if you're busy, forgetful, away from home a lot or have low stomach acid. But if you're happy with taking tablets more than once a day and remembering to take them with meals, cheaper calcium carbonate is fine.

What about other types of calcium? Supplements are available as calcium gluconate, lactate or phosphate, but they're not as effective. Avoid brands made with bonemeal, dolomite or oyster shells, because they may contain lead or other toxic heavy metals.

New to calcium supplements? Start with a comfortable 500mg a day Take this amount for one week and see how you feel. Some types may cause gas and constipation. If this happens, switch to a different type.

Never take more than 500mg at a time Your body can't absorb more than that. If you take a second calcium supplement on the same day, space them at least 3 hours apart for maximum absorbability.

Balance pills and food If you have a glass of milk and a slice of cheese with lunch, you've just got at least 500mg of high-quality calcium and don't need a supplement right now. If you have just a little calcium at dinnertime (say, a serving of broccoli sprinkled with almond slivers), and you haven't had much other calcium during the day, adding a supplement could bring you up to your daily goal of 700mg. Don't forget – calcium-fortified foods count, too.

Love cereal and milk in the morning? Do some maths before adding a breakfast calcium supplement Around 250ml of skimmed milk plus a bowl of fortified breakfast cereal could provide nearly a day's worth of calcium. If your morning calcium quota's being met in your bowl, don't bother adding a supplement—save it for lunch, dinner or snacks so you'll get the most benefit.

Take it in the daytime Plan to get most of your calcium in before dinner. That way, you'll have time to catch up in the evening if you've missed a supplement or somehow had a day without many high-calcium foods.

Create a lifelong calcium habit Calcium protects bone only when you take it faithfully—several times a day, every single day of every single month of every single year. When researchers followed women and men in their late 60s and early 70s for three years, those who took calcium increased bone-mineral density and slashed their fracture risk. But all those bone-guarding benefits disappeared when the volunteers stopped taking their supplements for the subsequent two years.

Don't mix calcium with medicines that must be taken on an empty stomach It can interfere with the absorption of antibiotics such as tetracycline, thyroid hormones, corticosteroids and even iron supplements.

FISH OIL

Fish-oil capsules are among the best ways of getting the benefits of omega-3 fatty acids quickly and easily. And as we've said, those benefits are substantial. Omega-3 fatty acids can cut heart attack risk by a whopping 73 per cent when consumed daily as part of a healthy diet. Omega-3s can also cut triglyceride levels by up to 40 per cent. There's some evidence as well that omega-3s from fish can reduce the stiffness and joint pain of rheumatoid arthritis and may also cut stroke risk.

Additional benefits found in some studies include a lowered risk of asthma, macular degeneration (a potentially blinding eye disorder), depression and memory problems, and possibly a protective effect against breast, colon and prostate cancers. Go for a supplement that provides at least 1,000mg of the two most powerful omega-3s – eicosapentaenoic acid (EPA) and docosahexaenoic acid (DHA). Higher levels may work better for cutting triglycerides and easing rheumatoid arthritis symptoms, but keep your intake below 3,000mg a day unless you discuss it with your doctor, since more could cause bleeding. Fish oil's anti-clotting powers could be dangerous for people with bleeding disorders and those taking anticoagulant medications such as warfarin. Here's how to buy and take these golden orbs of good fats.

Don't worry about pharmaceutical-grade capsules It's reassuring to know that two major tests of fish-oil supplements found no significant amounts of mercury in top-selling brands. That means you don't have to pay extra for pharmaceutical-grade fish oil: the stuff from the chemist shop is fine. The one good reason to pay for pricier pharmaceutical capsules is that you can get all you need from fewer capsules (they're more concentrated).

Decide on your dose, then find it on the label Most of us could use 500 to 1,000mg of supplemental EPA and DHA a day, though some experts say a great way to up your omega-3 intake every day is to go for 2,000 to 3,000mg. (Check with your doctor first if you take an anticoagulant.) A single 1,000mg capsule contains roughly the amount of these two fats found in a 115g serving of salmon. Since capsules vary in strength, read the label to figure out how many you'll need to reach your desired dose.

Don't confuse fish oil with cod-liver oil Fish oil is actually made from the bodies of fish, unlike cod-liver oil, which is made exclusively from – you guessed it – fish livers. The danger: cod-liver oil contains high concentrations of vitamin A; taking it in the same quantities recommended for fish oil could harm your kidneys. ◼

Fish-oil capsules are among the best ways of getting the benefits of omega-3

full-life
HEALTH PROJECT storecupboard and fridge makeover

When your cupboards and fridge are packed with delicious, convenient, healthy foods, eating the full-life way is easy. To get there, do this larder makeover project. Here's how to get started.

Supplies to have on hand: A sturdy step so you can access high cupboards and hard-to-reach spots at the backs of shelves safely. Rubbish bags. Sealable bags to contain messy items you're keeping – or throwing out. Cleaning supplies for cupboard and fridge shelves. A pencil and notepad to make notes about things you need to buy.

Best time for a larder makeover: The day before the bins are emptied, so discarded food won't sit around to attract pests or go bad.

How much time to set aside: Two to ten hours, depending on kitchen size. You can break the job into small, manageable chunks if it seems too big to tackle all at once. Do one or two shelves a day, for example. Or tackle the fridge today and save the freezer for next week. If you'd rather do all the cupboards or fridge in one day, start with the highest shelves and work down to the lowest.

What to do just before you begin: Clear your kitchen table and worktops so you have room to work. Designate one area for foods you'll keep and one for items you'll discard. If you can't bear to throw out food that's still edible, take it to a social event or donate to a local charity. Or designate a shelf for items you'll use up and not buy again.

Step 1 CLEAR OUT YOUR CUPBOARDS

As you remove foods from your shelves, put the following in the discard pile:

Out-of-date foods, as well as anything that's dried out, spoiled or rancid. Exposure to oxygen can make cooking oils and whole-grain products go bad even before the expiry date; give yours the sniff test and throw away any that smell stale or bad

Processed foods containing trans fats and/or saturated fats. Get rid of biscuits, crackers, baking mixes and shop-bought cakes and other processed foods that list hydrogenated or partially hydrogenated oils or saturated fats as one of the top four ingredients

High-sugar and/or refined-grain cereals, breads, baked goods and pastas. You'll replace these with whole-grain, low-sugar versions

Empty-calorie snack foods. Throw away. When you snack for long life, you'll be eating crunchy, juicy fruits, veg, nuts and whole-grain crackers instead of high-sodium, high-fat, low-fibre crisps and crackers

High-sodium condiments and processed foods. Throw out or give away any items that contain more than 20 per cent of the Recommended Daily Amount of sodium per serving (roughly 300mg)

'Best intentions' foods that you haven't used for six months to a year. That canned octopus and those ingredients for Thai cooking seemed like such good ideas at the time, but if you're never going to serve exotic seafood snacks or concoct an elaborate meal with coconut milk, curry paste and fish sauce, it's time to find them a new home

Step 2 RESTOCK YOUR CUPBOARDS

Keep these items – or put them on your next shopping list.

Canned beans: pinto, black, red kidney and haricot beans, and chickpeas

Canned chopped tomatoes, tomato paste and tomato sauce (lower-sodium versions are best)

Canned fruit in natural juices with no added sugar

Canned vegetables

Dried fruits, including single-serving boxes of raisins

Nuts: unsalted, unflavoured almonds, walnuts, pecans etc. (store extras in the freezer to keep them fresh for longer)

Brown rice: standard and quick-cooking varieties

Other whole grains, such as pearl barley, bulgur and quinoa (store in the freezer to retain freshness)

Old-fashioned oats

Whole-grain breakfast cereals that list a whole grain as the first ingredient and have at least 4g of fibre per 40g and not too much fat or sugar

Low-sodium, low-fat canned soups

Wholewheat pastry flour (store in the freezer for a longer shelf life)

Salt-free seasoning blends and individual herbs and spices

Whole-grain pastas and noodles

Water-packed canned light tuna

Canned salmon

Extra-virgin olive oil

Balsamic vinegar to be used in flavoursome dressings and cooking

Low-sodium vegetable juice

Sparkling water (delicious mixed with a little fruit juice)

Popcorn if you have an air popper, or no-salt, low-fat microwaveable popcorn if you don't

Fresh garlic

Small onions

Sweet potatoes

Step 3 PURGE YOUR FRIDGE

These fridge and freezer items also belong in the discard pile – or they can be used up then replaced with healthier choices:

Fizzy drinks, fruit punch, sweetened commercial tea and other sugar-laden drinks

Full-fat milk, cream, cheese, cream cheese, cottage cheese and/or yoghurt

High-sodium processed cheese spreads and slices, and processed meats

Margarine with trans fats

Full-fat mayonnaise

High-sodium condiments

Fatty minced beef, cuts of beef with visible streaks or margins of fat, fatty pork, bacon and sausage

Full-fat and premium ice cream as well as high-sugar sorbet and ice lollies

Frozen dinners and side dishes that contain trans fats or more than 25 per cent of the Recommended Daily Intake of saturated fat and/or sodium

Step 4 RESTOCK YOUR FRIDGE

Organise your shelving to best hold the following items:

Skimmed milk, low-fat cheese, yoghurt, cream cheese and cottage cheese

Low-fat mayonnaise

Boneless, skinless chicken breasts and thighs, turkey breast, minced skinless chicken or lean beef

Eggs high in omega-3 fatty acids

Jars of chopped garlic

100% orange juice, pomegranate juice or purple/red grape juice

Seasonal fruits such as berries, cherries, oranges, tangerines, peaches, grapefruit, grapes, kiwi fruit, plums, peaches and watermelon or other melons

Seasonal vegetables such as spinach, broccoli, cauliflower, aubergine, cucumbers, romaine lettuce, mushrooms, radishes, mangetouts, sugar snap peas, cabbage, carrots, green beans, asparagus or tomatoes

'Convenience' fruits and veg: presliced carrots, pineapple or salad bar fruit; shredded cabbage; prechopped broccoli and/or cauliflower florets; red and green pepper slices from the salad bar; boxes of cherry tomatoes; single-serving bags of baby carrots; prewashed salad greens; precut green beans

Bags of frozen unsweetened fruits such as blueberries, cherries, peaches, raspberries or strawberries

Bags of plain frozen vegetables such as spinach, broccoli, courgettes, carrots, corn, green beans, peas or mixed vegetables

Healthy frozen dinners for occasional quick meals – look for brands with fewer than 400 calories, no trans fats and less than 25 per cent of the Recommended Daily Intake of saturated fat and/or sodium

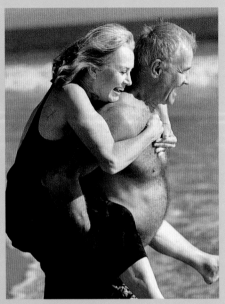
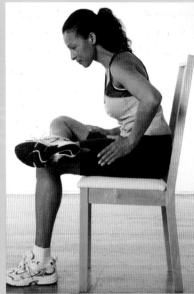
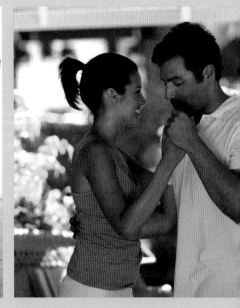

... improved memory and cognition
... better stress management
... stronger immunity

Move to feel good

In the summer of 1966, five healthy 20-year-old men went to bed for three weeks. They weren't tired; they were participating in what would become known as the Dallas Bed Rest and Training Study, a landmark study on the effects of exercise (and the lack thereof) on our bodies.

After three weeks of complete inactivity – the men even used wheelchairs to get to the bathroom – their muscle function deteriorated to the point where they could barely stand. As researchers later noted, 'Those three weeks of bed rest had a greater effect on their aerobic fitness than 30 years of ageing.'

After the bed rest part of the study, the men completed eight weeks of intensive exercise training, including treadmill work-outs and long-distance running. The results? They completely reversed the damage from the bed rest, proving conclusively the amazing power of physical activity.

What's more, studies since then have shown that immobilisation either in hospital or during space flight also causes loss of bone mass. But scientists have now found that this too can be recovered by exercise. Researchers from Manchester Metropolitan University and the Charité University Medicine Berlin persuaded 25 healthy young men to stay in bed for 90 days, then measured their bone mineral content (BMC). They lost an average of 3.5 per cent BMC, with the worst-affected man registering a staggering 15.6 per cent decline. Recovery took time, but 360 days later the volunteers' BMCs were virtually back to normal, and those men who had lost the largest amounts during the bed rest had made the larger gains – in fact, in the most extreme case, one man gained bone mass at a faster rate than during the growth spurt at puberty. So no matter how inactive you've been, it's never too late to compensate.

Fitness at all ages

Fast-forward 30 years. Researchers contacted the original five men from the Dallas study, now aged 50, for a follow-up study. All had become sedentary, gaining an average of 23kg (50lb) and doubling their overall body fat. They had also lost significant cardiovascular fitness. Not all of that loss was related to the natural effects of ageing; about 40 per cent was due to inactivity.

But here's the thing: after walking, jogging or cycling for 5 hours a week for six months, the men *again* completely reversed their age-related drop in cardiovascular fitness. Their resting heart rates, blood pressure levels and hearts' maximum pumping ability, or aerobic power, returned to the levels of 30 years earlier. The message? It's never too late to begin exercising.

You don't believe us? Well, how about this one, then: when 50 men and women with an average age of 87 worked out with weights for ten weeks, they more than doubled their muscle strength and improved their walking speed – even though they weren't doing any walking exercises.

The bottom line: your physical strength, heart health and breathing ability aren't bottoming out just because you're getting older. If they've declined, it's most likely because you've been sitting around instead of working your muscles regularly.

'Muscle mass seems to be very important to longevity,' says Mark Davis, a research associate at the Centre for Sport, Exercise and Health at the University of Bristol.

That's because the amount of muscle you have affects nearly every function in your body. If you maintain good muscle tone, you'll probably gain less weight, have a lower percentage of body fat and prevent insulin resistance. Your LDL cholesterol and blood sugar levels will be lower, and your HDL cholesterol levels higher. You'll also avoid constipation, keep your blood thin and moving smoothly through your veins and arteries, improve your sleep and reduce your risk of depression and memory lapses.

It doesn't take much to reap these benefits. Just a few weeks of regular, moderate to high-intensity physical activity each day, and almost every health measure is likely to improve – no matter *what* your age.

Of course, the benefits are greater if you've maintained an exercise programme throughout your life. One study, for instance, found that people who took long swims three to five times a week delayed their natural physical decline by decades. In other words, while the swimmers might be 60 years old, they had the medical measurements of 40 year olds.

Just as the human body needs food for life, so must we all have exercise to survive

But even if The Beatles were still touring the last time you put on a pair of plimsolls, it's not too late to see dramatic changes in your health and quality of life if you start exercising *today*. Consider this: one study found that men between the ages of 60 and 75 could increase their strength at the same rate as men in their 20s by performing basic weight-training exercises twice a week for 16 weeks. By the end of the study, these older men were raising about 270kg (600lb) on a leg-press machine, compared with the 170kg (375lb) they pressed when they began. They also had lower LDL and higher HDL cholesterol levels. All in just four months.

And a study of 1,020 healthy people ranging in age from 54 to 100 (average age 80) found that for every extra hour a week spent being active, their risk of becoming disabled dropped by 7 per cent. By 'disabled', we mean having joint pain, being depressed and/or overweight, and even being unable to walk – the problems that lead to the type of old age you're trying to avoid.

you've gained three extra years, but those extra years were spent doing the exercise,' notes Jere Mitchell, MD, professor of internal medicine and physiology at the University of Texas and one of the original investigators for the Dallas Bed Rest Study. What exercise does, however, is add *life* to your years. 'There's a big difference in the quality of life if you drop dead playing tennis at 90 or if you've been in a nursing home since age 60,' Dr Mitchell says.

Yet despite our lip service to an active life, most working adults spend little to none of their time exerting their bodies. The problem is particularly bad in the UK. More than half of all adults do no moderate-intensity physical activity in a typical week – not even *10 minutes a week* of vigorous leisure-time physical activity, such as brisk walking, bike riding or swimming. Even young adults (aged 16 to 24) are pretty inactive – 42 per cent of men and 63 per cent of women fail to achieve recommended activity levels – but the proportions rise to a staggering 93 per cent of men and 96 per cent of women aged 65 and over.

The more energy you expend today, the more energised you will be tomorrow

Plus, the more time the older participants spent being active, the lower their risk of dying. Those who spent 2¼ hours a week being physically active were nearly a quarter less likely to die during the 2½ year study than their couch-potato peers. When the physical activity was upped to 7 hours a week, their risk of dying during the study plummeted by 57 per cent. And remember – these were all healthy people to begin with.

It's not that exercise significantly extends your life. 'If you start exercising four times a week at the age of 20, by the end of your life,

That's one reason why the current generation of older adults is shaping up to be the first in modern history that will be *less* healthy in their older years than the generation before.

Don't let yourself be lumped into this generational deficiency. Push yourself out of that easy chair and vow that the rest of your life begins today. You won't go it alone, we promise. In the pages ahead you'll learn about the health-related benefits of exercise and, as a bonus, we've included three work-out routines of varying difficulty that you can pick up easily. ■

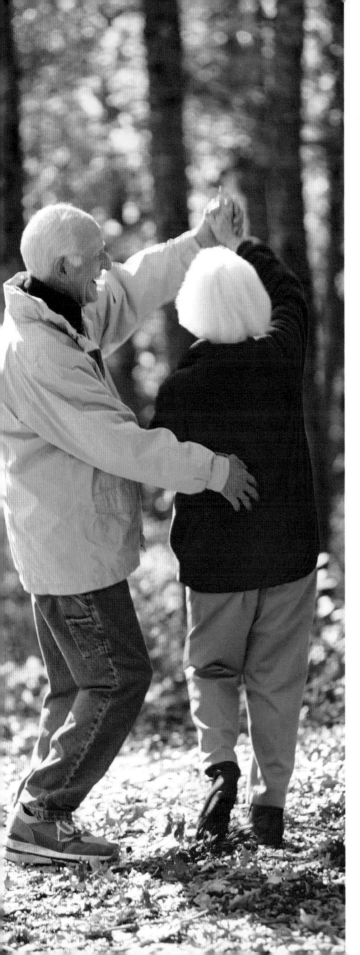

The benefits of exercise

Here are several ways that moderate physical activity – the equivalent of walking at a 5km/h (3mph) pace – can help your health.

Cardiovascular health
- Improves cholesterol levels
- Improves endurance
- Improves blood pressure
- Improves the ability of the heart to contract and expand

Body composition
- Reduces abdominal fat
- Increases muscle mass

Metabolism
- Increases the number of calories you burn, even at rest
- Reduces LDL cholesterol
- Reduces very low density cholesterol (vLDL), the type most likely to stick to the artery walls
- Reduces triglycerides
- Increases glucose tolerance and decreases insulin resistance

Bone health
- Slows decline in bone mineral density
- Increases total levels of bone-building calcium and nitrogen

Psychological well-being
- Improves perceived well-being and happiness
- Reduces levels of stress-related hormones
- Improves attention span
- Improves sleep

Muscle strength and function
- Reduces the risk of muscle or bone-related disability
- Improves strength and flexibility
- Reduces the risk of falls
- Improves balance

10 reasons to move

Ask non-exercisers why they don't get up and move, and you're likely to hear many similar stories. They don't have time. They're not in shape. They have too many aches and pains. And most tellingly, it's just too late to bother.

We hope we've convinced you that it's *never* too late to start exercising. But if your brain needs more evidence, here are ten major health improvements you're likely to see in as little as six months if you begin exercising regularly.

1 Improved memory and cognition

When you work out, whether it's walking through a forest or lifting weights in a gym, you're doing more than just strengthening the muscles. You're also stimulating numerous areas in your brain and central nervous system, each of which controls one tiny portion of the movement. Plus, you're stimulating the release of a variety of chemicals, including human growth hormone (HGH). Yes, this is the same hormone given to children with growth problems; the same one that certain 'anti-ageing' doctors give to patients at their clinics, even though it's generally illegal to use it for that reason.

Among its youth-promoting benefits, HGH triggers a hormonal and biochemical cascade that releases brain-derived neurotrophic factor (BDNF), a hormone that helps your brain to sprout new synapses, or connections between the neurons. One study of 59 healthy but sedentary people aged 60 to 79 found that working out aerobically for six months (and we're not talking about marathon training) increased their brain volume, an improvement missing in a control group that didn't work out. It's probably why several studies find that regular physical activity significantly slows mental decline in people who already have Alzheimer's or other forms of dementia.

It's also why the more BDNF you have circulating in your brain, the greater your ability to learn and remember. The less BDNF, the less any learning sticks. Another benefit: high levels of BDNF control appetite and reduce the risk of obesity. They also stimulate the release of neurotransmitters in the brain, such as serotonin and dopamine, which control mood and play a role in depression. Scientists suspect that these exercise-induced BDNF boosts may partially explain the benefits of exercise on people with depression.

Upping your BDNF levels doesn't take much; for rats, a week of running on a wheel is enough. In people, a single high-intensity work-out triggers results. Of course, the increase is short term, which is why regular physical activity is so important.

In fact, some researchers suggest that what we think of as 'age-related' mental decline – such as memory loss or some slowing of our thinking – is actually 'revenge of the sit'. We've fallen away from our genetic tendency to be physically active nearly 100 per cent of the day, and the resulting loss of BDNF and the neurotransmitters it affects, including serotonin, contributes to our current high rates of obesity, forgetfulness, dementia and depression.

We're not suggesting that you buy yourself a human-sized hamster wheel or begin testing your blood levels of BDNF every time you jog round the block. Just focus on the visible benefits. Simply walking briskly for 45 minutes three days a week for six months can make a huge difference to the kind of mental acuity that allows you to be more attuned to the world around you.

So stick with an exercise programme for three months and see what kind of memory, learning and decision-making benefits *you* get.

2 Lower risk of Alzheimer's disease

Exercise has other brain benefits beyond improved memory and reasoning. A long-term study that followed nearly 1,500 people for an average of 21 years found that just two sessions of physical leisure-time activity each week cut their risk of Alzheimer's in half. You can get benefits in an even shorter amount of time; exercising just three or more times a week during a six year period, one study found, reduced the risk of dementia by a third in older people compared with those who exercised less.

Some of this risk reduction is thought to be related to changes in the hippocampus, the part of the brain that controls higher thought and the part first affected by the physical changes that lead to Alzheimer's. The bottom line is that physically active people have healthier hippocampuses. So do rats. When rats specially bred to develop Alzheimer's get steady exercise over several months, they show a remarkable reduction in the plaques and other brain changes that signal the development of the disease.

3 Fewer hot flushes

If you're on the younger end of the ageing spectrum and the menopause is near, you have yet another reason to lace up your trainers: a Spanish study at the University of Granada found that 3 hours of exercise a week could significantly reduce severe hot flushes and other menopausal symptoms, increasing a woman's overall quality of life. While half of the exercising group had severe symptoms when they began working out, after a year, just 37 per cent did. Meanwhile, the percentage of women with severe menopausal symptoms in a control group that *didn't* exercise during that time rose from 58 to 67 per cent.

The real-life fitness test

There are many scientific ways to measure fitness. But for most of us, the signs of being fit are measured daily in what we can or can't do. For a person over the age of 45, you are probably in reasonable physical shape if you can:

- Dance to a fast beat for more than 10 minutes without feeling winded.
- Walk for 30 minutes straight without getting tired.
- Feel energised 14 hours after you woke up (so if you got up at 7am, you should still be awake and active at 9pm).
- Carry large containers of milk or water in each hand without feeling any strain.
- Load your luggage into the storage rack above your plane or train seat without it being too difficult.
- Jump up and down ten times without causing your heart to race.
- Carry a large basket of clothing up or down two staircases without struggling.
- Trim your toenails without any discomfort from the bending.
- Easily sit down on the floor and then stand up.
- Raise your foot as high as your hip when kicking.
- Twist and look behind you without moving your feet.

4 Improved self-esteem

We talk a lot about self-esteem in our children, but what about our own? Self-esteem can play a major role in your health and quality of life. If you feel good about yourself, you're more likely to live a healthier lifestyle, to remain active, to interact socially and to participate in community activities. All this works in a kind of circular way to keep you healthier. And now we know that exercise also helps to maintain or improve self-esteem in older people.

For instance, one study measured changes in self-esteem in overweight women aged 60 to 75 who participated in either a stretching-and-toning exercise programme or a brisk walking regimen for six months. Both programmes enhanced the women's self-esteem, although the stretching-and-toning group showed greater improvement. All the women felt better about their body images and their strength. The message? You don't have to up your heart rate to achieve a better feeling via exercise.

5 Better stress management

There's a reason we counsel people to take a walk when they need to 'let off steam'. All that steam – or stress – triggers a chemical cascade designed to prepare you to run. Your heart beats faster and harder, your lungs take in more oxygen, your liver releases glucose to provide energy for the muscles, and your immune system revs up in preparation for injury.

If all you do is sit there, all that physiological energy has nowhere to go, which damages key body systems over time. It suppresses the immune system; contributes to bone loss, muscle weakness and atherosclerosis; and increases insulin levels (you need more insulin to get all that glucose into cells), leading to higher levels of dangerous abdominal fat.

Enter exercise. Just 20 minutes jogging or stair-climbing does more to soothe stress-induced anxiety than sitting still in a quiet room for 20 minutes. Not only does physical activity reduce anxiety, but being physically fit acts as a buffer against the damaging effects of stress, such as high blood pressure. We're not talking about a lifetime of physical activity, either; just six months. This can do more to reduce stress-related high blood pressure than changing diet.

6 Stronger immunity

Ever noticed that people who work out a lot tend to get fewer colds and bouts of flu than those who avoid the gym like the plague? There's a reason for that. Every time you exercise, it puts stress on your entire body, stimulating the release of certain immune system hormones and chemicals. If you exercise too much, this has a negative effect, increasing inflammation and eventually *suppressing* the immune system. But if you exercise moderately on a regular basis, you're able to maintain a higher level of immune activity without triggering that suppression response.

Again, this does not require a lifetime of exercise. The response of your immune system to a single physical work-out is intense enough to supercharge the effects of a pneumonia or flu vaccine, particularly in older people, who tend to have weaker immune systems. Exercise regularly, and those vaccines are more likely to work. (It's a little-known fact that flu vaccines simply don't work in many, particularly older, people.) With or without a vaccine, physical activity reduces significantly the risk of developing an infection, studies find. When researchers examined the risk of hospitalisation for infectious disease in 1,365 women aged 55 to 80, they found that the inactive ones were more than three times as likely to be hospitalised for infections. ▶

the new exercise classes

For more than two decades, most fitness centres have offered classes that provide a limited range of aerobic options.

Some add in stepping exercises, some integrate martial arts moves, and others use stationary bicycles, but the basic class – loud music, a high-intensity instructor and even higher-intensity work-outs – hasn't changed much. Until recently. Happily, most recreation centres and fitness clubs today also offer a plethora of programmes; these may hark back to ancient Chinese traditions, borrow from professional ballerinas or even pull in techniques from the boxing ring. Some are quite intense and not for beginners, others are perfectly suited to an older or out-of-shape exerciser. Here we look at a few very different options.

TAI CHI CHUAN The name of this ancient Chinese martial art form (called tai chi for short) loosely translates to 'the supreme ultimate boxing system'. It involves slow, steady movements that incorporate both the physicality of the body through the motions and the mental strength of the mind through meditation. Most of the movements are performed in a standing position, with inner calm being a key component.

Numerous studies attest to tai chi's benefits in improving balance, flexibility and cardiovascular health in people of all ages, but particularly in older people with or without chronic conditions. It can reduce pain and disability from arthritis, significantly reduce the risk of falls, lower the blood pressure, relieve stress and improve aerobic capacity.

PILATES Pilates was created by the German fitness instructor Joseph Pilates in the early 1900s both as a way to rehabilitate from injury and to strengthen the body to reduce future injuries. It utilises a series of low-impact, controlled, precise movements that are designed to improve balance, flexibility and core strength, accompanied by slow, steady breathing. Programmes sometimes involve certain machines that Pilates invented.

Like tai chi, there are hundreds of research studies documenting the benefits of Pilates-type exercises for preventing injury, managing pain and core muscle training. So far, they've found Pilates can relieve lower-back pain better than standard medical treatments and improve flexibility. Best of all, the risk of injury is low with a properly trained teacher. Look for an instructor certified by a recognised UK Pilates association, who has had months, not a couple of weekends, of training.

BALL CLASSES You've probably seen those oversized rubber balls in shops or at fitness club. They're great tools for strengthening your abdomen and back, and improving your balance. But what do you do with them? Try lying across a ball on your back to do sit-ups. The combination of the abdominal exercise and the added effort required to balance on the ball supercharges the motion. Or simply sit on the ball with your feet hip-width apart and lift one foot at a time. Can you keep your balance? Classes that integrate balls offer a low-impact option for improving muscle strength and flexibility.

KICKBOXING You might call kickboxing the high-impact aerobics of the 21st century. This is the class for you if you're already fairly fit and strong, and you're looking for a great endurance exercise with strength-training thrown in. You'll even get a bit of stretching for improved flexibility. Moves include kicks, punches and squats, for a full-body work-out. Come to class prepared to work hard.

KETTLEBELLS Coming soon to a gym near you, kettlebells is a high-intensity Russian fitness routine – not for exercise beginners – that incorporates solid cast-iron weights that look like bowling balls with handles. Like Pilates and yoga, routines focus on strengthening core muscles; unlike those two programmes, you also get an aerobic work-out by working several muscles at a time.

Other studies find a much lower risk of upper respiratory tract infections such as colds and bronchitis, as well as pneumonia, among physically active older people. Again, we're not talking about training for a marathon. Something as gentle as tai chi can boost your immune system enough that it can better fight off the virus that causes shingles, a painful nerve disease more common in those over 50.

7 A better sex life

Just 30 minutes a day of vigorous exercise is enough to slash a man's risk of erectile dysfunction by between 37 and 58 per cent, depending on the intensity of the physical activity. Sexual frequency, enjoyment and satisfaction in older people is also directly linked to their fitness levels; the fitter you are, the more often you're having sex!

8 Less abdominal fat

Here's another good reason to be active: exercise is critical in reducing the size of fat cells around your abdomen, the so-called visceral fat. This is the fat that gives men their beer bellies and women an apple shape. It's also the type of fat that accumulates within your abdominal organs and liver, contributing to inflammation, insulin resistance and diabetes. Plus, it's associated with metabolic syndrome, a cluster of health markers that significantly increases your risk of heart disease as well as diabetes.

We now know that the *size* of these fat cells, as well as the number, is directly related to your risk of developing diabetes, regardless of your weight. Simply cutting calories may do little to shrink belly fat cells unless you exercise. That's what one team of researchers found when they studied three groups of women. All cut out 2,800 calories a week, either through dieting alone or a combination of dieting and exercise.

The two exercise groups burned 400 calories a week through walking and shrank their visceral fat cell size by 18 per cent; the dieters, who reduced their body fat, weight and waist and hip measurements exactly as much as the diet-and-exercisers, saw no change in the size of those fat cells. So it seems that exercise may be the key factor in controlling distribution of fat cells. A similar study found that while diet alone and diet-plus-exercise reduced total and abdominal fat in overweight women to the same degree, *only* exercise reduced blood levels of chronic inflammation markers such as C-reactive protein (CRP) and interleukin-6.

9 Relief of depression

Researchers took 156 people aged 50–77 who had been diagnosed with major depression and randomly assigned them to one of three groups: either exercise (30 minutes of bike riding, walking or jogging three times a week), medication (the prescription drug sertraline) or a combination of the two. After 16 weeks, all three groups showed similar improvements in depression, but only the exercise groups also improved their cognitive abilities. Plus, when researchers checked on the participants six months after the study ended, they found much lower relapse rates in the exercisers than in the medication group.

10 More muscle strength

Sometimes it's easy to overlook the obvious – in this case, that exercise makes you stronger. Exercise your arms, and carrying groceries becomes easy. Exercise your legs, and stairs won't be a problem. As little as two to four weeks of weight-training can create the kind of microscopic molecular changes in your body's production of hormones – including growth hormone and other chemicals, as well as proteins related to muscle growth – that contribute to muscle repair and strengthening. Researchers have even seen significant improvements in as few as four work-outs.

This is critical, according to Dr Mitchell, because the more muscle you have, the better your cells use insulin and take in glucose. Those two factors play a major role in inflammation, obesity, heart disease and diabetes, and are behind many of the health-related benefits of exercise and its ability to keep you feeling young. Yet he notes, 'There's no magic pill you can take to train your muscles.' He's not just touting the company line; Dr Mitchell, 79, walks an hour a day most days and works out with weights two or three times a week.

Slow or fast?

Is it better to walk slow or fast? Researchers at the University of Michigan in Ann Arbor in the USA wondered the same thing, so they tracked nine overweight, sedentary women aged 50 to 65. The women walked 5km (3 miles) a day, a total of 25km (15 miles) a week, for eight months. At the end of the study, those keeping a modest pace – covering 1.6km (1 mile) in roughly 20 minutes – increased their insulin sensitivity and thus reduced their risk of diabetes, although the improvement tapered off as their speed increased. The slower walkers also lost more body fat than the faster walkers.

On the other hand, faster walkers (who averaged a 15 minute a mile pace) secreted more growth hormone, while growth hormone levels in the slower walkers actually declined.

The message Just get out there and walk. Mix it up a bit – perhaps try walking fast uphill or slower coming down, or vice versa.

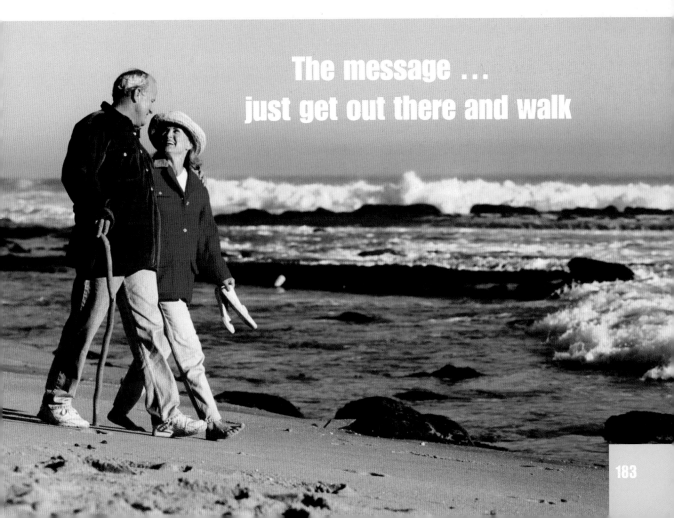

The message ...
just get out there and walk

Understanding exercise

Put simply, exercise is any activity that exerts your body beyond the point reached in normal daily activities. Sometimes we forget the simplicity of the definition. We get so caught up with shoes, gyms, programmes, stopwatches, science, clothing and fads with funny names such as 'yogilates' and 'super power sets' that we give up on the whole idea of exercise.

Throw all those complicated notions aside. Exercise is nothing more than moving your body for good health. Of course, some exercise is better than others, and different types of movement do affect your body in different ways. But understanding the different types is easy – and so is doing it – if you don't let trainers or overblown health magazines complicate things.

Here's what we suggest: throw out all you think you know about exercise and start over again, beginning right now. In the following pages, we'll give a concise explanation of the four essential types of fitness – ENDURANCE, STRENGTH, FLEXIBILITY and BALANCE. Then we'll tell you precisely which ones *you* need to focus on for optimal health today and tomorrow.

Finally, we'll provide specific exercise sequences for you to consider doing most mornings or evenings that deliver the best results for the minimum investment of time and effort.

fitness type 1
Endurance

Endurance activities are those that challenge large groups of muscles, such as those in your legs or arms and shoulders, for at least ten consecutive minutes. The most obvious examples are walking, cycling and swimming, but endurance activities also include lifestyle actions such as washing windows, vacuuming, sweeping, mopping, gardening, mowing the lawn, raking and pruning. A round of golf – without a cart – also counts.

These activities provide the biggest returns when it comes to protecting against the effects of chronic diseases associated with ageing, such as heart disease, diabetes and osteoporosis. One major reason: endurance exercises strengthen not only the muscle groups being used but also your heart, lungs and circulatory system. That's why endurance exercise is also called aerobic exercise: the word *aerobic* basically means it involves oxygen, which is what your heart, lungs and circulatory system are all about.

Endurance exercise is also the most straightforward. To build endurance, you just do your preferred activity at a high rate of intensity for as long as you are comfortable. Come ▶

great advice

Endurance exercise provides the best defence against most chronic diseases

10 ways to exercise naturally

Here are ten ways to get a moderate level of activity without setting foot in a formal exercise environment. Each burns up to seven calories a minute; your goal is to get at least 10 minutes of sustained activity at a time.

1 **Take a daily fitness walk** This is in addition to any other walking you do as part of your day. Commit to a pace slightly faster than your normal gait. Walking the dog is perfect. Don't let weather stop you – light snow or misty rain is no excuse to stay at home. If the weather is too bad for an outdoor walk, go to the shopping centre – but no window-shopping. Walk from one end to the other, but avoid food shops. You'll find that your daily walk not only strengthens your body but is also a great way to relax, think and socialise.

2 **Take up table tennis** An intense game of table tennis gets your heart rate up, increases the amount of oxygen going to your lungs and brain, and provides all the other amazing benefits of physical aerobic activity.

3 **Coach a children's team** Got extra time on your hands? Why not volunteer to help to coach a youth club football team? In addition to the fun you'll have and the appreciation you'll earn, you'll also get an unexpected work-out at least twice a week (more if you arrange more practices).

4 **Clean the old-fashioned way** For a cleaner house and a healthier you, get down on your hands and knees to scrub the floor, hang laundry out on a clothes line and wash the windows

yourself instead of calling someone to do it. All will provide a good, moderate work-out with a bonus at the end: a sparkling house.

5 **Play with the children or grandchildren** Try throwing a Frisbee or teaching them how to play badminton. Or even dance around the living room with them for 10 minutes.

6 **Go canoeing** Many parks offer canoes or rowing boats for hire, and rowing at a moderate pace of less than 6km/h (4mph) provides a moderate work-out.

7 **Sign up for dance classes** Ballroom dancing, line dancing, folk dancing, ballet and even disco or other forms of modern dance are great endurance exercises.

8 **Ride a horse** We're not talking about a gallop, although that's certainly something to build up to. But even a gentle trot or canter helps; you get an extra physical boost if you learn how to groom and saddle the horse.

9 **Audition for a musical** Most communities have local theatre groups that rely on volunteers for their talent. Singing while moving, as in walking across the stage, provides a moderate level of activity.

10 **Join a sports team** Maybe you're beyond the over-40s football team, but what about a doubles tennis club or other sociable activity group? Even joining a bowling group will provide a decent-enough work-out once or twice a week.

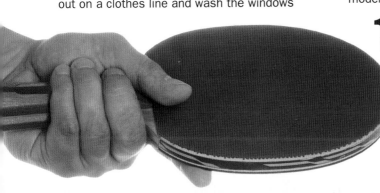

back to it in the next day or two, and you'll be able to do it a little longer. And so it goes on.

So what is a high-enough rate of intensity? It's simple: work hard enough to make yourself breathe harder than usual. Want us to be more specific? There are measurements you can take to gauge your ongoing exertion more objectively, but they often involve buying equipment such as a heart rate monitor. Instead, just measure your own rate of perceived exertion (RPE). This simply means your innate sense of how hard you're working, and is a guide to your work rate.

In determining your RPE, ten is the highest level of intensity; it essentially means you can't catch your breath and are about to fall over from exertion. Zero is the lowest level of intensity; it means you've probably been lying comfortably on your sofa for the past hour. When you're engaged in endurance activities, aim for somewhere between five, which is moderate, and seven, which is strong.

Another way to know that you're working hard enough is that you'll be sweating and slightly out of breath but still able to talk. Increase the intensity, and you may find yourself only able to gasp out 'yes' or 'no'. Any higher, and you need to bring it down a level.

Next question: how long should you exercise? Answer: ideally, up to 30 minutes of consecutive exertion. For now, though, start with 10 minutes. That's the minimum length of time in which you can get the respiratory and cardiovascular benefits you seek.

Ten minutes doesn't sound like much, but if you've been inactive for several years – or even a few months – start slowly. This is not the time to head out for a 30 minute hill climb. Instead, start with a 10 minute walk. Every day, add another 5 minutes and increase your speed until you're doing 30 minutes at the 'breathing-hard-but-can-still-talk' level. Interval training may be recommended for those who are very out of shape. This involves working at a slightly higher rate for a short period, then increasing the intensity for a short period. As you get into shape, you'll find your work-out gets easier. Then you can either choose to up the intensity or settle at a healthy fitness plateau.

Even better, start to diversify your endurance activities. If walking comes easily, then perhaps it's time to take up swimming or tennis or to get out your bicycle and take to the road. One great thing about endurance activities is that they tend to be done outdoors, making them much more natural and fun than being in a gym.

fitness type 2
Strength

Strength exercises increase the power of a specific muscle by challenging it with some form of resistance. That could be weights, exercise bands or even your own body weight. The usual method is careful, slow lifting and

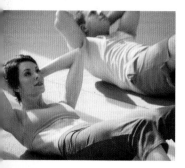

great advice

Forget measurements at first: you know when you're exerting yourself, and when you've had enough lowering of a weight to target a specific muscle or muscle group.

If you think this form of exercise is best left to the young ones, think again. This is probably the most important form of exercise when it comes to preventing the frailty and disability associated with ageing.

Why? Without muscle strength, your ability to walk, sit, stand and bend gradually fades. When you observe older people struggling to stand or walk, it's for one reason only – their muscle strength has gone. Yes, injury or disease may have curtailed their capacity for activity, but, in fact, it's still weak muscles that limit their mobility. And only healthier muscles – achieved through strengthening exercises – can return that mobility.

Strength-training has other important benefits. It reduces the risk and symptoms of osteoporosis, heart disease, arthritis and type 2 diabetes. It helps to improve your sleep and reduces your risk of depression. At least one study also found that it improves balance – even in middle-aged people whom you wouldn't think would have balance problems.

Think strength-training is too hard or too awkward for you? Think again. The fact is, strength-training is often *less* tiring than endurance work-outs. It can be done in limited space and with limited time. You need minimal gear – often just a few dumbbells – though technique is crucial. Best of all, you'll see the results in as little as a few weeks. Plus, strengthening exercises can boost your metabolism by as much as 15 per cent, which is a bonus when it comes to losing weight. Maybe that's why more than ever, people aged 65 and older are taking up strength-training.

One important thing to remember if you're taking up exercise in the hope of shaping up: volume for volume, muscle weighs more than fat. That's because it's denser. As you start ▶

Time to move up?

How do you know if you need to move to a lighter or heavier weight? Here's what the experts say.

Reduce the weight if:

- You can't complete two sets of ten repetitions in a stable position.

Keep the weight the same if:

- You need to rest after ten reps because the weight is too heavy to complete more reps in a stable position.

Increase the weight if:

- You could have done a few more reps in a stable position without a break. At your next work-out, do the first set of reps with your current weight and the second with the next-highest weight. For example, if you're currently using ½kg (1lb) dumbbells, use 1 or 1½kg (2 or 3lb) dumbbells for your second set.
- You could do all 20 repetitions at once without a break. At your next session, use heavier dumbbells for both sets.

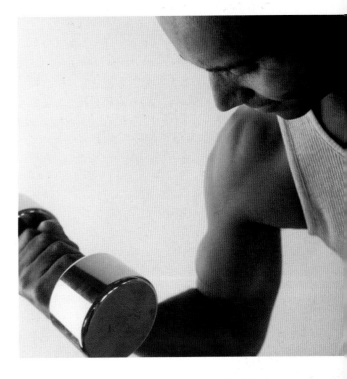

get back in the swing

I am a 58-year-old former athlete. I used to play football pretty seriously and was in good shape until I hit 40. But everyday life today is busy, and in my free time, I just want to sit and relax. How can I reclaim my body and strength?

answer: **Congratulations on your decision** to reclaim your body. It is never too late. Listed below are eight steps to getting you back on the 'active, healthy and fit' track.

1 If you've been inactive for a while, or you have any bone or joint problems, ongoing illnesses or risk factors such as high blood pressure, check with your doctor before starting an exercise routine.

2 Once cleared for training, address any previous injuries or musculoskeletal issues that could present problems when training. Ex-football players typically have chronic knee pain. Any chronic muscle or joint pain should be looked at before you start training to get to the root of the problem. Don't cover it up with medication. If you have chronic pain or lingering injuries that might affect exercise, contact a physical therapist, who can evaluate you and recommend corrective exercises.

3 If your eating and drinking patterns are an absolute disaster, book a few sessions with a registered dietitian or enrol in a weight-management programme. It is very important to steer clear of programmes that promise a quick fix.

4 Buy some decent work-out kit, especially footwear. But you don't need any track suits, heavy sweatshirts or other athletic paraphernalia.

5 Bury your old training methods and avoid saving all your exercise for the weekend. Plans, patterns and progressions (the three Ps) are the keys to permanent lifestyle changes.

6 Establish short and long-term goals. Be realistic and specific as to what you would like to achieve through regular training and lifestyle modifications. These might include:

● I don't want to end up like my father, sitting in a chair all day long. I want to be a healthy and fit 80 year old.

● I want to be able to carry my golf bag for 18 holes and not have to take a buggy.

● On my next hill-walking holiday, I would like to be able to climb something higher than I've climbed before.

● I need to slim down so I can move quicker on the tennis court.

● I just want more energy, and by getting fitter, leaner and stronger, I know I will have it.

7 Cardio, strength and mobility training are all integral components of a well-rounded training programme, regardless of your goals. The frequency, intensity, mode and rate of progress should be based on whether you're training for health, fitness, performance and/or fat loss.

8 To get started ...

● Gradually build up to 30–60 minutes of brisk walking five or six times a week (30 minutes for sedentary people, 60 for more active people).

● Stretch after you walk.

● For basic strength, complete two sets of 10–12 chair squats and desk push-ups every other day. Make sure your technique is correct.

● When you're ready for more, work with a certified personal trainer or join a good sports centre with qualified staff. Educate yourself through a variety of resources.

to exercise, you build muscle and lose fat, so you may lose flab without losing weight. That's why you can be working out and seeing your measurements change, but your weight remains the same. The same weight is simply taking up less space. In fact, some experts estimate that the space used by a pound of muscle is 22 per cent less than the space used by a pound of fat.

In general, there are just a handful of exercises you'll ever need to master. We'll show them to you in our routines beginning on page 201. In terms of what else you need to know, strength-training has a very simple process and vocabulary.

A repetition, or 'rep' is lifting, then returning a weight to its starting position once (or if you are using rubber bands, stretching then releasing the band). In general, you want to lift carefully and steadily, completing the lift in a slow count of two. Pause for a second at the peak of the lift, then return at half the speed of the lift (that is, to a count of four) until you are at the starting position. A rep should take 8–10 seconds. Typically, you exhale during the most difficult part of the movement – in most exercises, that's the lift – and inhale during the easier part. Whatever you do, *don't* hold your breath. That could increase blood pressure to dangerous levels. Again, technique is the most important factor.

A set is 8–12 reps in a row. A set should take anywhere from 1 to 2 minutes. When you complete a full set, pause for a minute or two to rest, then repeat the same exercise for a second set. If you really want to push yourself hard, pause again, then do one final set. Doing two sets of the same exercise takes between 4 and 8 minutes and is the perfect amount for everyday strength-training. Weightlifters and athletes may add a third set because they need particular muscles to be strong and have extra endurance.

If you pick a work-out that includes six exercises, it would take about 30 minutes in total to do the routine properly and safely. Think about it: you can complete a full strengthening work-out in the span of a typical TV comedy show – and you can even watch the programme while you're doing it.

As to how heavy the weight should be, that's simple: the amount you can just handle for two full sets. Those last few reps should be challenging but not painful or exhausting.

Over time, strengthening exercises get easier. When you get to the point where two sets of an exercise doesn't provide much of a challenge, move up to the next weight level. Simple. ▶

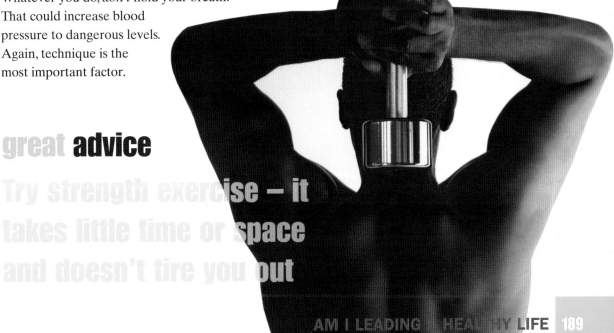

great advice

Try strength exercise – it takes little time or space and doesn't tire you out

Nordic walking

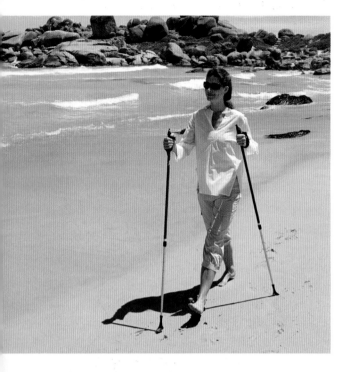

If you're interested in getting a full-body work-out while taking a walk, consider Nordic walking, which uses poles similar to ski poles. A relatively new sport, it was born in the late 1990s as a way to train Finnish cross-country skiers in summer. Using the poles is simple: you plant one pole in the ground and 'push off' against it with the foot on the same side. So if you're about to step with your left leg, you plant the pole on the right and use your right foot to push off.

Studies find that pole walking can burn up to 50 per cent more calories than regular brisk walking, as well as work out up to 90 per cent of your body's muscles, thanks to the abdominal and upper-body strength required to plant the poles and push off. A bonus for people with achy knees or hips is that some of the force of walking is transferred to the poles instead of your joints.

You can buy a pair of walking poles at some sporting goods shops or online for about £50.

New to all this? Consider not even using weights at first – just going through the motions with your hands closed in fists. You'll find that two sets of 12 movements without a weight can be strenuous enough, but use a dumbbell as soon as this starts to feel relatively easy.

Here are some other important things to remember for strengthening exercises.

Build in recovery time Always give yourself a day off between strength activities to give your muscles time to rebuild and recover. It's this recovery period that leads to stronger muscles.

Emphasise legs over arms When you think of weight-training, you tend to think of lifts involving arms and shoulders. That's not quite appropriate. Although you should incorporate both upper and lower-body strength-training exercises into your routine, strengthening the lower-body muscles around your hips, knees and ankles is particularly important for healthy ageing and mobility. Be sure that at least half of your exercises target legs, hips and lower back.

Posture matters Whether you're lifting a small dumbbell over your head or doing a leg lift, how you hold your body determines whether you get the most out of the movement. Stand or sit erect with your back straight, your hips aligned, your shoulders pulled down and your neck stretched high. Most important, as you exercise, try to move just the target muscles. Don't swing your whole body to help to lift a dumbbell. If the exercise is for your arms, for instance, only your arms should move.

Don't rush You'll get twice as much benefit if you take your time returning the weight to its starting position. For instance, once you lift that weight over your head, count to four as you slowly bring your arm down.

Keep your joints loose Locking your knee and elbow joints can result in pain and injury since you put all the stress of the weight on the joint instead of the muscle, where it belongs.

fitness type 3
Flexibility

The first two fitness types – endurance and strength – focus mostly on the capabilities of your major muscle groups. Flexibility, however, is in large part about your joints.

The definition of flexibility is simple: it's the range of motion your body can go through. With age, your range of motion naturally decreases. The goal of stretching and other flexibility exercises is to keep your range as wide as possible. 'You have to maintain a certain range of flexibility and mobility,' says Mark Davis of the University of Bristol, because without that, you start restricting your activities. That creates a vicious cycle in which you engage in less activity, further reducing not only your flexibility and mobility but also your strength and endurance. Before you know it, you're grunting just trying to get out of a chair and saying no to invitations to walk or shop because it's just too challenging to bother.

Flexibility exercises strive to do a few things. They wash the key parts of your joints – the bones, tendons, ligaments and cushion-like substances between them – with nutrients and blood. They also keep the tendons and ligaments strong and stretchable. And, just as important, they keep the muscles attached to your joints loose and flexible. After all, that's the key function of a muscle: to move your body through constant stretching and compressing.

Stretching, in other words, does a lot of important things. However, it's also one of the easiest and most pleasurable types of exercise there is. And it requires no gear whatsoever.

To stretch a muscle and its related tendons and ligaments properly, you want to get into the extended position slowly, then hold it for up to 2 minutes. This is much different from what many people do, however. Too often, people jerk and pull their muscles, holding the stretch for just a few seconds, if at all. Be patient! By slowly stretching a muscle then holding the stretch for the suggested time, you are maximising the benefits and minimising the chances of injury.

Aim to do flexibility exercises at least twice a week. These include basic stretching, reaching and bending. Activities such as yoga, tai chi and ▶

Get stretching – it's one of the easiest and most pleasurable exercises you can do

great **advice**

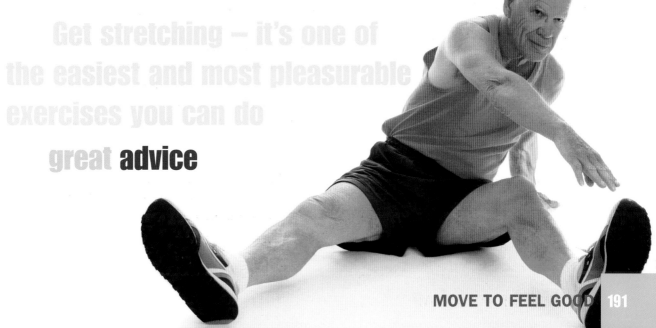

exercise gear worth buying

The beauty of exercise is that you need only good shoes and socks to do it. But if you want to go a step further, consider investing in one or more of the following.

A HIGH-QUALITY PEDOMETER This little gadget tracks the steps and miles you walk throughout the day (10,000 steps equals 8km/ 5 miles). Numerous studies find that wearing one is a great motivation to increase your steps. Don't buy the cheapest pedometer; research shows they're not so accurate. You should be able to find a good one for about £20. Health experts are so convinced that a pedometer encourages walking that in many areas the NHS will lend you one as part of the National Step-O-Meter Programme. Ask your GP, practice nurse or health visitor.

A HEART RATE MONITOR The key to aerobic or endurance activities is to get your heart rate up to a certain level and keep it there for 10 minutes or more. Using the breathing-heavy-but-can-still-talk approach generally gets you to the right pace. But if you want a more precise measurement, first determine your maximum heart rate by subtracting your age from 220. Your target heart rate is between 50 and 75 per cent of that. So if you're 50, your target heart rate is between 85 and 130 beats a minute. To monitor their heart rate continuously, athletes and serious exercisers use a heart rate monitor. The typical unit includes a band you wrap around your chest and a wristband or armband that picks up the signals from the chest monitor. It's an easy way to see if you need to increase the intensity – which becomes more important as you get fitter.

DUMBBELLS Exercise experts have a saying: 'dumbbells are smart'. That's because they make it difficult to push yourself too hard, thus avoiding injury. They're also flexible and can be used at any time and nearly anywhere.

Increasing the weight as you get stronger is as simple as picking up another set of dumbbells. You can even buy some that allow you to change the weight by turning a knob, but for durability, choose fixed-weight dumbbells. A popular type is hex dumbbells. The ends resemble hexagons so they don't roll when you lay them down. For travel, you can buy hollow weights that can be filled with water when you're ready to work-out.

AN INFLATABLE EXERCISE BALL As described on page 181, these exercise balls are terrific when it comes to strengthening core muscles and improving balance. Even just sitting on one when you're at the computer can provide some benefits. Size is important: buy one large enough so your feet are flat on the floor when you sit on it. If you're under 1m 65cm (5ft 5in), try a 55cm (22in) ball; if you're over 1m 89cm (5ft 11in), aim for a 75cm (30in) ball. Everyone else should do fine with a 65cm (26in) ball. Don't inflate it completely; a little give helps with stability.

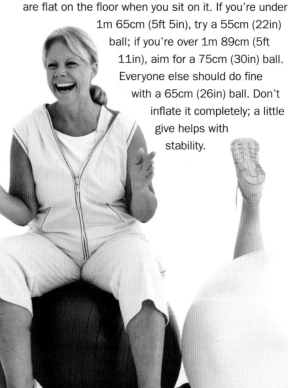

Pilates provide excellent opportunities for improving your flexibility. The beauty of these is that you can do them anywhere – even when sitting on a plane. But many of your daily activities also provide a good chance to stretch, including:

Waking Stand up and slowly reach for the ceiling. Hold for 20 to 30 seconds. First thing in the morning is a perfect time to do a little stretching. In fact, it's perfectly natural. Think of how many animals stretch themselves out after a nap or a night's rest.

Vacuuming As you vacuum, you reach forward, then back. You bend to move things and stretch to reach the corner or under the sofa. You're cleaning, but you're also stretching. Do you have a house full of hard-surfaced floors? You can get the same benefits from mopping them.

Cleaning windows The up-and-down motion of cleaning the windows and the stretching as you stand on your tiptoes to reach the higher parts provide a good flexibility work-out.

Bowling Every time you bend and stretch to bowl the ball or wood, you're extending muscles beyond their usual range. Take advantage of that by completing a few extra stretches while you wait to see how you've done.

Golf Reaching down to pick up your ball, swinging your arms and twisting your body as you move the club head to meet the ball are movements that can help to keep you flexible.

For the best health, you should also do a stretching routine. You can stretch all the major joints with a few simple movements. Hold each stretch for 30 seconds, and in 5 minutes you can do a whole body-stretching sequence, with enormous benefits. As part of 'The full-life fitness routines' that start on page 200, you'll see that we ask you to do four stretches a day, focused on a single body area.

fitness type 4
Balance

Balance activities are particularly important for people as they age because good balance helps to prevents falls. Yet each year in Britain one in three people over 65 and half of those over 80 sustain a fall – sometimes more than one.

Falls in later life, when bones are more brittle, risk a fracture, particularly of the hip. Ninety per cent of all hip fractures are due to falling, and athough fewer than one in ten falls results in a fracture, given the number of falls, that's a lot of broken bones. And hip fractures are a major cause of disability and loss of freedom – around 40 per cent of all care home admissions result from a fall. Worse, falls are the leading cause of death due to injury in people aged 75 and older in the UK.

There are two types of balance: static and dynamic. Static balance involves the ability to maintain your balance without moving, such as standing on one foot. Dynamic balance is the ability to maintain your balance while moving.

The good news is that many forms of exercise already challenge and improve your sense of balance. Examples include tai chi, yoga, dance and even strength-training. If you're an avid exerciser, it's unlikely that you need to do additional balancing exercises – but try some anyway. This is one area of fitness in which there isn't a lot of science or precision. Just do things that force you to stay up on your feet in awkward situations. Here are some ideas.

Do basic balance challenges each day at home For instance, stand on one leg and lift the other, or walk in a straight line heel to toe. If you're just starting, hold on to something when you try these. Eventually, the goal is to be able to perform these for longer times without holding on to anything, or with your eyes shut.

Dance Balance is about being light on your feet and having a good sense of your body and its movements. What teaches you that more than dancing? For the most benefits, sign up for ballroom dancing classes. You'll get the physical benefits of the dancing and the emotional and life-enhancing benefits of the social interaction.

Get off the beaten path Taking walks on an unpaved nature trail forces you to step over or around roots, boulders and other obstructions. It's the perfect activity to improve your balance.

Do more side-to-side activities Sports such as badminton and football force players to move forward, backwards and sideways, making them great for helping you to develop balance and a sense of assuredness on their feet. If you are relatively fit and have a willingness to play and laugh about it, consider a gentle game of these sports with your children or spouse.

Take up tai chi One study of 256 physically inactive people aged 70 to 92 found that taking part in this Chinese martial art for six months reduced falls by half compared with a similar group who did stretching exercises for six months. Plus, those in the tai chi group who did fall had far less serious incidents – just 7 per cent resulted in injuries versus 18 per cent of the stretchers.

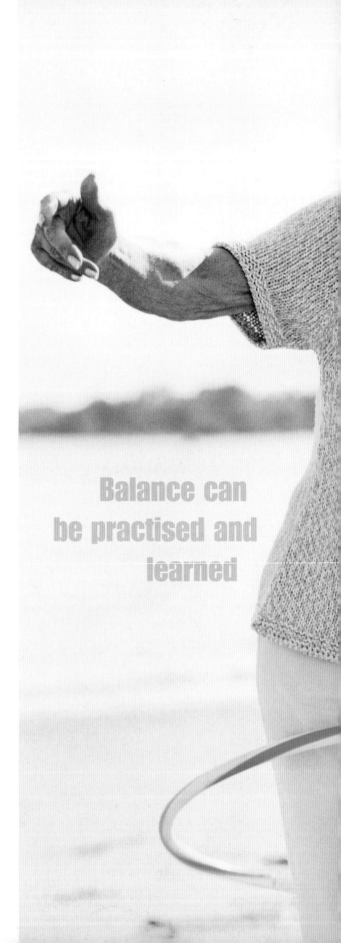

Balance can be practised and learned

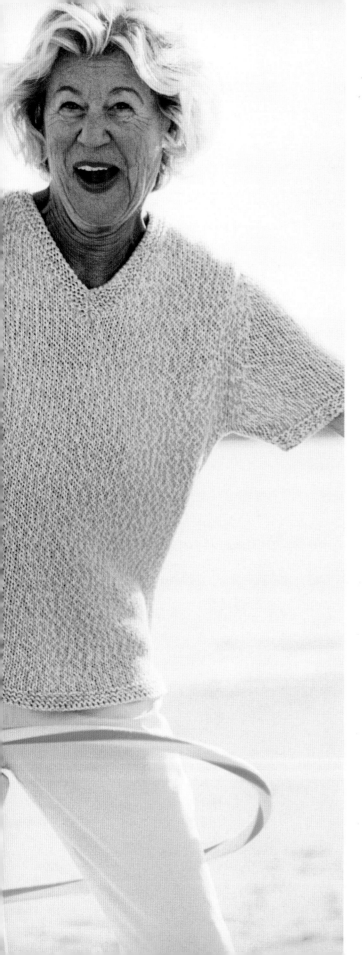

When *not* to exercise

You want to do some form of physical activity every day, if possible. However, if you have any of the following conditions or symptoms, either take a day off or check with your doctor first.

- A cold, the flu or an infection with a fever
- More fatigue than usual
- A swollen or painful muscle or joint
- A new or undiagnosed symptom
- Chest pain or an irregular, rapid or fluttery heartbeat
- Shortness of breath
- A hernia with symptoms

If you do only one thing ... garden

Gardening is one of those rare multiple-benefit activities, providing endurance, strength and flexibility activities all in one. How? Picture an early spring day when you're preparing your vegetable garden for the first planting. Digging the soil builds muscle strength as well as endurance. So does loading shovels of compost and topsoil into the wheelbarrow, wheeling it over to the garden, dumping it and turning the earth over as you work it in. When the time comes to plant the flower or vegetables seedlings, you bend and stretch to get them in the ground.

Other benefits of gardening?

- Cutting the grass with a walking mower (preferably manual) provides a great endurance work-out.
- Raking leaves provides flexibility and endurance benefits.
- Hauling compost, dirt and weeds is a good strength-building work-out.
- Pulling weeds is a wonderful way to stretch muscles stiff from too much sitting.

The best fitness of all: daily living

If you follow what trainers and experts tell you, a well-rounded fitness regimen would have you actively engaged in some type of formal exercise for an hour a day six or seven days a week. A lot of effort, a lot of time but not unreasonable if you want to be truly fit for a long life. But what of the other 15 hours a day that you're awake?

When you think about it, it's thoroughly illogical to believe that the optimal fitness schedule is '1 hour on, 15 hours off.' The truth is, fitness is best seen as a lifestyle, not as a task.

Every moment of your day, every task you do, is an opportunity to move in ways that help your health. When you think of fitness as a lifestyle, it means you walk a little faster, stand a little taller, stay outside a little longer, do tasks a little more intensely. It means you bypass the easy or lazy options and instead take the stairs, fetch the item from the garage yourself and take care of that fallen branch or broken step right now, by yourself.

When fitness becomes a lifestyle, it means that you are naturally walking more each day, so you don't have to schedule it formally, get dressed for it and recover from it. It means that you are naturally stretching your muscles, using your strength and challenging your sense of balance. It means that not half an hour goes by

So how do you start living a fitter lifestyle? Again, it's all in the choices. Here are some simple life rules to start.

- Always take the steps if you are going up or down two or fewer flights of stairs.
- Always stand when talking on the phone.
- Always get up and move when TV commercials come on.
- Always get the post, take out the rubbish, walk the dog and pick up the newspaper yourself rather than having it delivered.
- Always strive to be outdoors as much as possible (it's virtually impossible not to be more active outside than inside).
- Always get up and move after 30 minutes of sitting.

These are all easy to do, and the benefits will be enormous. Can you add to the list?

Does living the fit lifestyle mean you can stop thinking about exercise? No. Active living will do a great job of keeping you slim and maintaining your body's current physical condition. But remember the definition of exercise – using your body in ways that go *beyond* normal exertion levels. Only by mixing in a some formal exercise can you improve your strength, endurance, flexibility and balance.

To help to put all this in perspective, we've created the 'full-life fitness pyramid' (see opposite). This is a general guide to the range

Active living – the best exercise of all

when you haven't done some small thing with a little more exertion as a matter of habit.

And does this kind of living pay off! More energised living burns calories, strengthens muscles, builds endurance, improves your mood and makes you sleep more deeply. Science proves it, and living it quickly reveals it.

of exercise you should strive for in a week and in what amounts. Follow this plan and you are moving towards greater strength and better health. Make a copy of the fitness pyramid and put it by your desk or stick it on your fridge. Refer to it and you'll have an instant understanding of your fitness needs.

full-life
fitness pyramid

The comprehensive approach to building up a strong, healthy body through a combination of exercises and activities

Balance exercise
frequency: a few minutes a day
Examples: agility games and challenges, tai chi

Flexibility exercise
frequency: at least twice a week
Examples: stretching, yoga, Pilates

Strength exercise
frequency: each main muscle group exercised twice a week
Examples: weight-training, exercise bands, calisthenics

Endurance/aerobic exercise
frequency: 30 minute sessions at least three times a week
Examples: fast walking, cycling, aerobics, rowing

Hobbies and passions
frequency: seek a daily dose
Examples: sports, fishing, knitting, gardening, birdwatching

Active daily living
frequency: all waking hours
Examples: taking the stairs, getting outdoors, living energetically

Find your inner motivation

So you're going to get out there and become more physically active. But what if a week from now you're slumped back on the sofa watching television? Don't feel bad. Half of all people who begin exercise programmes drop out within the first six months. So how do you motivate yourself day in and day out?

Re-read this chapter It turns out that women who *believe* in the health benefits of exercise tend to work out more often and more intensely or for longer periods than those with negative thoughts about working out. It will also help to re-evalute your goals when you start to lapse.

Don't watch yourself Stop looking at the mirror and don't think about the movements, just *do* them. One study found that women who concentrated on their movements during exercise tended to exercise less often, less intensely and/or for less time than women who didn't.

Switch from negative to positive thinking For instance, if you hate sweating during exercise, turn it into a positive such as, 'Sweating clears toxins from my body and makes my skin look better', or 'The more I sweat, the more my muscles are working'. If you get out of breath when you exercise and perceive it as harmful, you'll stop, but what if you viewed it as an indication that you're building endurance? You'd be more likely to continue exercising.

Track your progress Use our fitness test (page 179) to track your work-outs and benefits. Research finds that you're more likely to stick with a physical activity if you can see or quantify the progress. (A food diary is also an excellent way to track your healthy-eating progress.)

Join a class The social aspects of an exercise class serve as a powerful motivator for anyone of any age. As one woman told researchers trying to learn what motivates older people to exercise, 'Most of us live alone, so it's better to come and exercise in a group. I do not do too well at home, as I cheat a little. When I am in the class, I've got to keep up. You do not want to cheat with the instructor.'

Set rewards for yourself Maybe tell yourself that every week in which you complete at least four 30 minute exercise sessions, you'll treat yourself to a massage or, if you have a hobby, such as woodworking, you'll buy a new tool.

Find a caring, motivating instructor or personal trainer Having someone who cares about your progress provides a powerful incentive. 'We need supervision!' one woman explained when addressing issues of motivation with researchers. 'We need the instructor to help us to keep it up, or else we do not do it. At least once a week, we need that external boost. It's not easy to do the exercise on your own.'

Sign a health contract This is a written agreement to accomplish a health goal. In your case, to walk 30 minutes a day five days a week. Or to spend 45 minutes two days a week doing

The toughest exercise is convincing yourself to stick with it. Don't just rely on will-power

resistance training. Or to sign up for a tai chi class or a gym spinning class. The contract should include a calendar for you to track your progress and to reinforce your commitment.

Tell everyone you know It turns out that social support for your exercise programme keeps you motivated – so call your children and email the grandchildren. Let your next-door neighbour and your best friend know that you're starting a new physical fitness programme. They'll keep asking how you're doing, and to avoid the embarrassment of telling them you gave up, you'll keep at it.

Sign up for a 5K walk or run that's two months away Having a goal you're working towards is one of the best motivators. You can get help training for the event from the internet, books or your local gym.

Have we convinced you of the age-defying benefits of physical activity yet? Are you ready to take up a sport, lift a weight, try to touch your toes? We hope so. The simple truth is this: there's no better prescription for living a long, healthy life than exercise. To borrow from one of the leaders in the field: just do it! ■

Matching goals to exercises

If you want to ...

Lose weight

● Walk slowly but for longer distances. A study at Colorado University in Boulder, USA, found that obese people who walk at a leisurely pace burn more calories than if they cover the same distance at their normal pace. And there's a bonus: the slower pace puts less stress on your knee joints. Another approach is to tackle your cardio work-out before breakfast, forcing your body to break into fat reserves for fuel.

Prevent diabetes

● Add strength-training to your life. By building muscle, you increase the ability of your cells to take in glucose, reducing insulin resistance and your risk of diabetes.

Prevent falls

● Do 10 minutes of balance training four or five days a week.

Prevent heart disease

● Participate in some kind of endurance activity several times a week for at least 30 minutes.

Prevent osteoporosis

● Get some form of weight-bearing exercise that forces you to work against gravity. This could be endurance or resistance. It includes activities such as walking, running, dancing, climbing stairs, weightlifting and calisthenics. And don't forget gardening. One study found that gardening was second only to weight-training when it came to reducing the risk of osteoporosis in 3,310 women aged 50 plus.

Rid yourself of back pain

● Try a programme that focuses on your core, such as Pilates, yoga or tai chi. These disciplines stretch and strengthen all the muscles in your trunk, including the back, abdomen and shoulders, which can relieve an aching lower back.

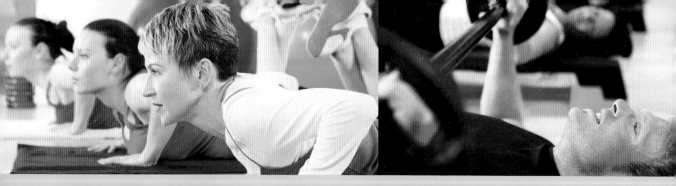

Full-life fitness routines

Can you spare half an hour to rejuvenate your health, spark your energy and improve your mood? We've come up with three fitness routines that combine simple moves into an any time, any place, 30 to 45 minute session. They are:

routine 1 Easy does it

routine 2 Antidote to ageing

routine 3 Spread stopper

While these routines vary in their intensity and requisite skill and strength levels, they are all structured the same.

- Four strength exercises and four stretches a day.
- Each day focuses on one of three body regions – upper (arms, shoulders and neck), core (chest, back and abs), or lower (hips, legs and feet).

Many of the exercises identify which muscles are being targeted. However, for the exercises targeted at your body's core section, we've skipped the list since so many small muscles in the back and abs area are simultaneously challenged by these moves.

THE PLAN

Each routine is made up of three 30-minute stretching and strengthening sequences, each focused on a different part of your body. Do the three sequences on consecutive days, then take the fourth day off. If you want to vary routines, you can ask a qualified fitness instructor to write an individual programme for you.

THE PROCESS

- Do strength exercises first, then stretches.
- Do the indicated number of sets and reps of each strength exercise, as noted.
- Take no more than two minutes of rest between sets.
- Take no more than two minutes of rest between exercises.
- To improve endurance, shorten rests to under 30 seconds.
- Hold each stretch for the times noted – never more than 30 seconds.
- Concentrate on what you are doing and feeling. Music is good, TV isn't.
- Focus on deep, long breathing throughout.
- No eating during the exercise sequence. Sips of water are OK as it's important that you are well-hydrated before and after exercise.

routine 1 Easy does it

A routine for **beginners** or people recovering from illness or injury.

rating Easy

Perfect for people who:
- Have not exercised for two years or more
- Are overweight or have limited movement
- Are recovering from prolonged injury or illness
- Are new to formal fitness plans

What's needed:
- Light dumbbells
- Towel
- Mat, bed or daybed
- Supportive chair
- Wall space

routine 2 Antidote to ageing

A medium-challenge routine for healthy, **active people** who currently lack any formal exercise in their lives.

rating Medium

Perfect for people who:
- Are middle-aged with busy lives
- Are sedentary but in good health
- Are active, healthy and older
- Have noticed a recent decline in energy

What's needed:
- Light to medium dumbbells
- Towel
- Pillow
- Supportive chair and a mat
- Wall space

routine 3 Spread stopper

A more difficult fitness routine for **fit people** that delivers a leaner body and stronger muscles.

rating Hard

Perfect for people who:
- Are seeking to tone their abs, back and legs
- Are active at weekends
- Used to play sports but now lack the time
- Are seeking to lose weight
- Have experience of working out

What's needed:
- Medium to heavy dumbbells
- Towel
- Supportive chair and a mat
- Stairs

THE PROMISE: If you live in a higher-energy way, pursue an active hobby and add one of these routines, you will achieve a level of healthy, comfortable fitness that could have a huge positive impact on all parts of your life. Get started!

DAY 1 Strength exercises
Easy

SHRUG Tones upper back, mid back and shoulders

1 Stand with your feet hip-width apart. Hold a dumbbell in each hand and let your arms hang straight down so your hands rest by the sides of your thighs, palms facing in.

2 Keeping your arms straight, slowly raise your shoulders towards your ears as if you were shrugging. Roll your shoulders back as far as is comfortably possible, then return to start.

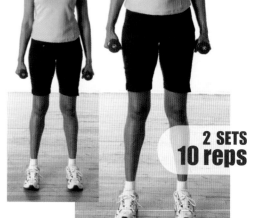

**2 SETS
10 reps**

WATER JUG RAISE
Tones shoulders

1 Stand with your feet hip to shoulder-width apart and hold a dumbbell in each hand. Bend your elbows, keeping them close to your body, so your forearms are straight out in front of you and form 90 degree angles, with the palms facing each other.

2 Keeping your hands in front of you, raise your upper arms and elbows to the side. Don't raise your shoulders. Keep your elbows below shoulder height. The weights should rotate towards each other as if you were pouring water out in front of you. Pause, then return to start.

**2 SETS
10 reps**

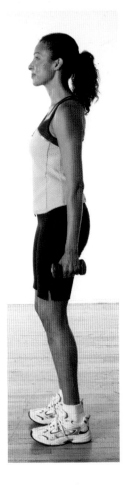
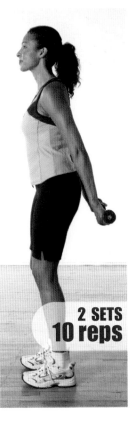

REVERSE RAISE
Tones triceps

1 Stand with your feet about hip-width apart with your knees slightly bent. Hold a dumbbell in each hand, allowing your arms to hang naturally by your sides, palms facing in.

2 Keeping your arms straight, slowly raise them behind you as high as is comfortably possible, rotating your palms so they face the ceiling. Pause, then slowly lower back to start.

2 SETS
10 reps

PULLOVER

Tones chest and back

1 Lie on a mat on the floor with your knees bent and your feet flat on the mat (if this is uncomfortable, you can do this exercise on a bed). Grasp a dumbbell by the ends with both hands and raise it above your chest.

2 Keeping your elbows straight, lower your arms back and over your head as far as is comfortably possible (don't arch your back). Pause, then return to start.

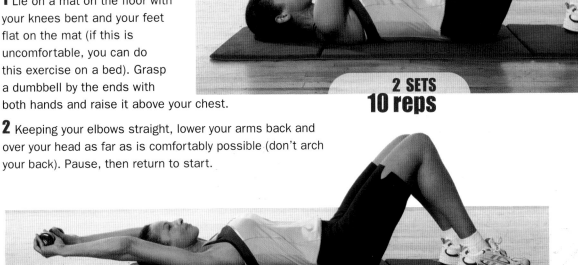

2 SETS
10 reps

DAY 1 Stretches
Easy

WALL TWIST

Stretches chest and shoulders

Stand with your left side at a rightangle to a wall, then reach out with your right arm and place your hand against the wall. Gently turn your torso towards the left, away from your arm, as far as is comfortably possible. Hold, then switch sides.

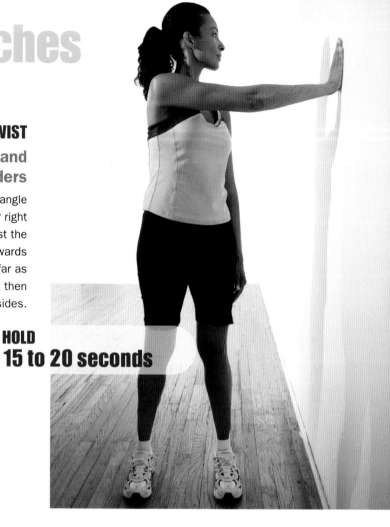

HOLD
15 to 20 seconds

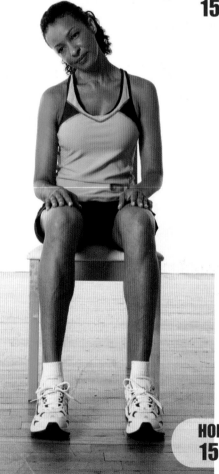

NECK STRETCH

Stretches neck and upper back

Sit up straight in a supportive chair and drop your chin towards your chest. Slowly drop your head towards your right shoulder, trying to touch your ear to your shoulder as you let your shoulders drop. Hold, return to centre, then switch sides. Put your right hand over to your left ear to help with the stretch.

HOLD
15 to 20 seconds

HAND PULL

Stretches hands, wrists and forearms

Sit up straight in a chair and extend your right arm with your wrist flexed and your fingers pointed towards the ceiling. Using your left hand, pull your right fingertips back towards your body as far as is comfortably possible. Hold, then switch sides.

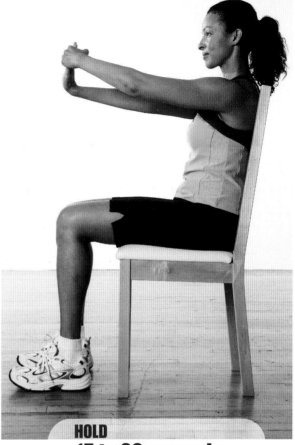

HOLD
15 to 20 seconds

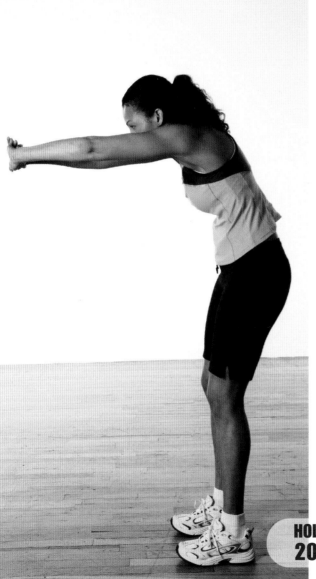

BACK STRETCH

Stretches upper back

Stand with your feet hip to shoulder-width apart. Extend both arms straight in front of you and lace your fingertips together, turning your hands so your palms face outwards. Press your palms away from you, straightening your arms and rounding your back as far as is comfortably possible.

HOLD
20 to 30 seconds

DAY 2 Strength exercises
Easy

SEATED LEG EXTENSION Strengthens quadriceps

Sit on a chair with your feet flat on the floor and hold onto the sides of the seat for support. Slowly lift your left leg until it's straight in front of you. Pause for 1 or 2 seconds, then slowly lower your leg. Repeat with the opposite leg. Alternate ten times for one set.

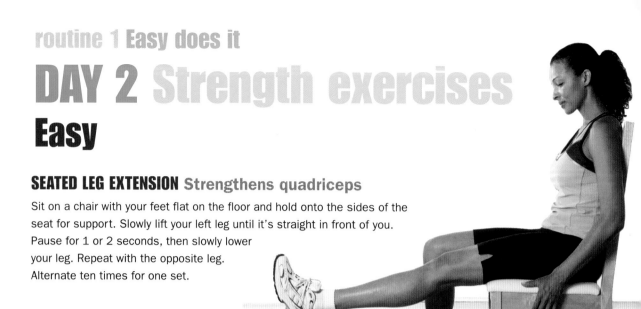

2 SETS
10 reps EACH LEG

STANDING LEG CURL
Strengthens hamstrings

Stand facing a wall with your feet about hip-width apart and place your hands against the wall for support. Keeping your back straight, slowly bend your right leg at the knee, raising your heel towards your bottom until your shin is parallel to the floor. Pause for 2 seconds, then return to start. Complete a full set with one leg before switching to the other.

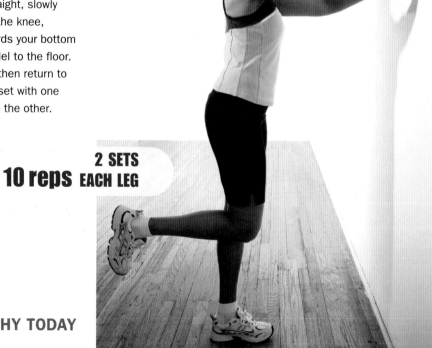

2 SETS
10 reps EACH LEG

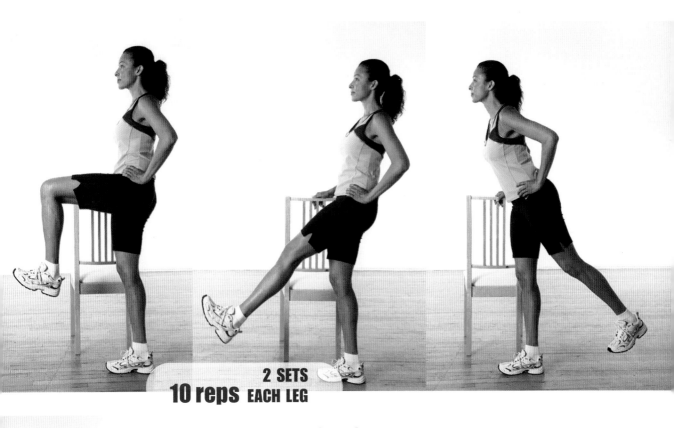

2 SETS
10 reps EACH LEG

MARCH AND SWING Strengthens legs, bottom and back

1 Stand with your left hand on your hip and the other on a chair back or tabletop for support. Raise your left knee until the thigh is parallel to the floor, with the foot flexed.

2 Straighten your left leg, pressing the heel forward and towards the floor as you lean your torso slightly backwards.

3 Return to the knee-lifted position, then straighten your left leg behind you, leaning forward with your torso. Complete a full set with one leg before switching to the other.

TIP-TOES Strengthens calves

1 Stand behind a chair with your feet hip-width apart and one hand planted on the chair for support.

2 Using your calf muscles, slowly rise onto your toes as high as is comfortably possible. Pause, then slowly lower your heels back to the floor.

2 SETS
10 reps

DAY 2 Stretches
Easy

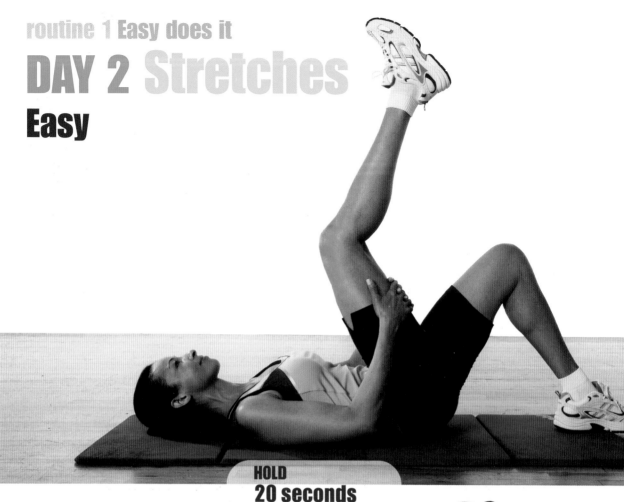

HOLD
20 seconds

HAMSTRING STRETCH
Stretches hamstrings

Lie on your back with your knees bent and both feet flat on the floor. Raise your right leg towards the ceiling, then clasp your hands round the back of your right thigh and gently pull it towards your chest (use a towel if you can't reach). Hold, then switch legs.

SEATED FIGURE 4 Stretches glutes, lower back and hips

Sit on a chair with your feet flat on the floor. Cross your right ankle over your left knee so your calf is parallel to the floor and your right knee is pointing to the right. Keeping your back straight, lean forward from the hips until you feel a stretch deep in your right glute muscle. Hold, then switch legs.

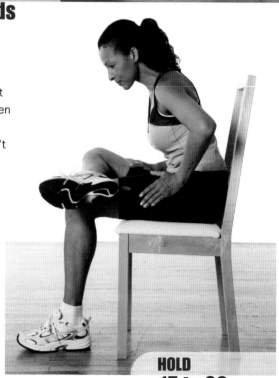

HOLD
15 to 20 secon

SEATED CALF STRETCH
Stretches calves

Sit on the edge of a chair with your left foot flat on the floor and your right leg extended with the foot flexed. Loop a towel around the ball of your right foot and, keeping your back straight, gently pull your foot towards you as far as is comfortably possible. Hold, then switch legs.

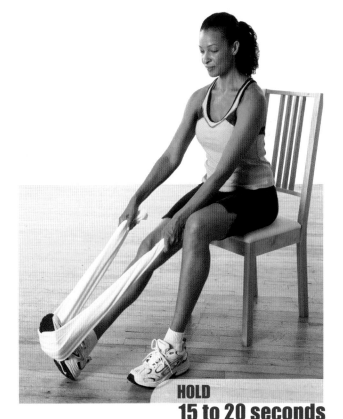

HOLD
15 to 20 seconds

KNEE DROP Stretches groin and inner thigh

Lie on a mat on the floor (or, if more comfortable, on a bed) with your knees bent and your feet flat. Place your hands on the inside of your legs and gently let your knees fall out and down towards the floor or bed. Then gently press down to deepen the stretch as far as is comfortably possible. Hold, relax, then repeat.

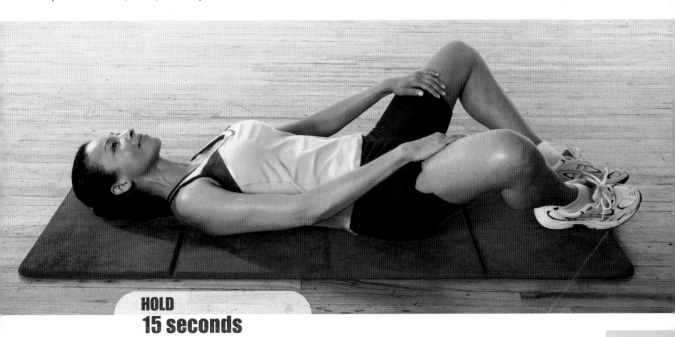

HOLD
15 seconds

DAY 3 Strength exercises
Easy

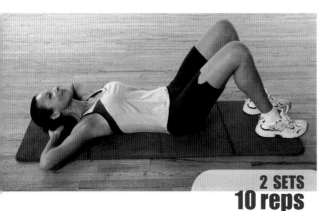

2 SETS
10 reps

PELVIC TILT

1 Lie flat on your back with your knees bent, your hands behind your head, and your elbows extended to the sides.

2 Lift your pelvis up and towards your ribcage, tightening your lower abdominal muscles and gently 'pushing' back into the floor. Hold for 2 seconds, then relax and let your pelvis rotate back to its normal position. Repeat the exercise in a slow, controlled manner.

STANDING TWIST

1 Stand straight with your legs hip to shoulder-width apart. Hold a dumbbell with two hands and extend your arms straight in front of you, keeping your elbows soft. Keep your shoulders low and your hand below shoulder height.

2 Keeping your arms extended, contract your abdominal muscles and turn your torso to the right as far as is comfortably possible. Pause, then return to start. Repeat on the opposite side. Continue alternating for a full set of reps on each side.

2 SETS
10 reps EACH SIDE

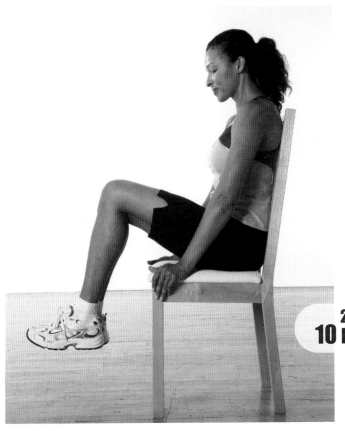

SEATED TOE LIFT

Sit straight all the way back in a chair and place your hands on the sides of the seat in front of your hips or on the chair arms. Contract your abdominal muscles and slowly lift your feet off the floor as far as is comfortably possible. Pause, then lower your feet back to the floor.

2 SETS
10 reps

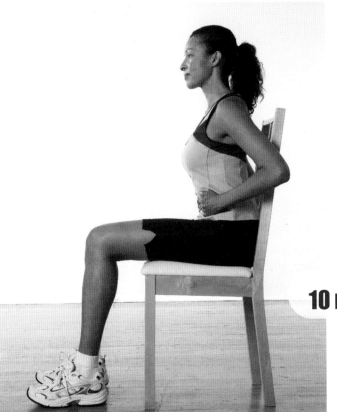

NAVEL PULL

Sit in a chair with your hands on your stomach. Contract your abdominal muscles and pull your navel in towards your spine. Keeping your abs tight, slowly inhale for 4 or 5 seconds and exhale for 8 to 10 seconds. Relax and repeat.

1 SET
10 reps

DAY 3 Stretches
Easy

MORNING STRETCH

Lie on a mat on the floor (or, if more comfortable, on a bed), raise your arms overhead, and extend your legs so your body forms a straight line from your heels to your head. Imagine that strings are pulling your arms and feet in opposite directions and try to extend your limbs as far as you can. Keep your feet flexed. Hold for 10 seconds, then relax.

REPEAT 3 times

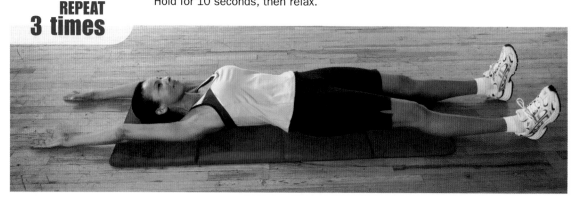

LYING ROTATION

Lie on a mat on the floor (or, if more comfortable, on a bed) on your right side with your right arm bent and right hand under your head. Bend both legs (you can put a pillow between your knees for added comfort). Extend your left arm straight in front of you. Then slowly rotate it up towards your head and all the way round (your torso will naturally roll back and your palm will flip so it's facing up; but keep your lower body stable) past your head, behind your back, and over your hips until it's back to the starting position. Switch sides.

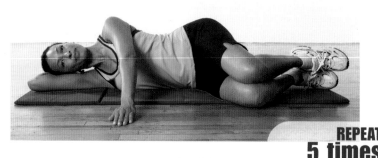

REPEAT 5 times

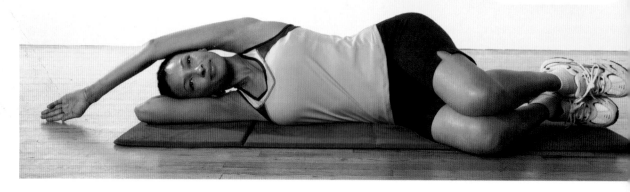

REACH AND BEND

Stand straight with your feet about shoulder-width apart. Gently lean to the left as you raise your right arm towards the ceiling, curving it slightly overhead, palm facing down. Hold, then repeat on the other side.

SIDE STRETCH

Sit in a chair (preferably one without arms) and grasp the back of the seat beside your left buttock with your left hand, palm facing your body. Hold on as you gently lean forward and drop your right ear towards your right shoulder. Hold, then repeat on the other side.

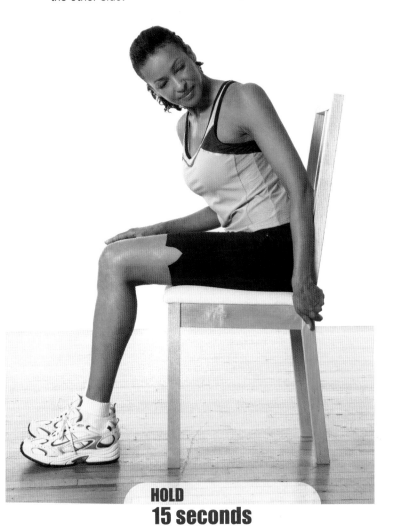

HOLD
15 seconds

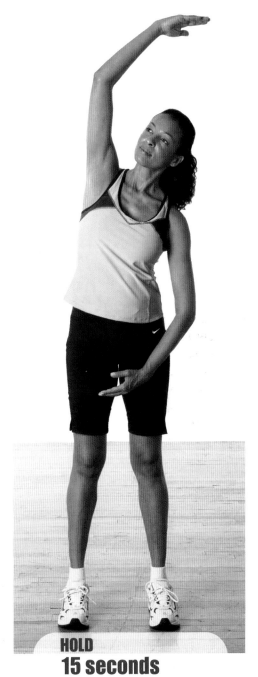

HOLD
15 seconds

DAY 1 Strength exercises

Medium

CHEST SQUEEZE
Tones chest and shoulders

1 Stand holding a light dumbbell in each hand. Bend your arms at a 90 degree angle and extend them to the sides so your upper arms are parallel to the floor, palms facing forward. Keep your shoulders down (do not shrug them).

2 Squeezing your chest muscles, bring your elbows towards each other until they are about shoulder-width apart. Return to start.

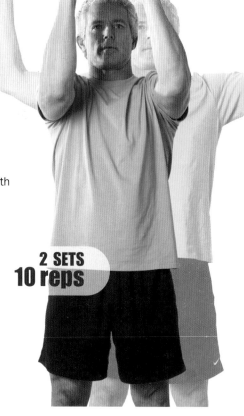

2 SETS
10 reps

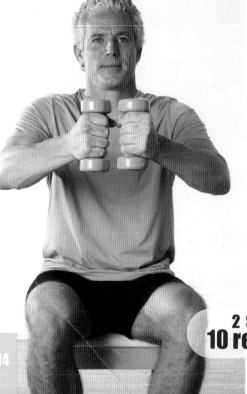

BACK FLY Tones upper back and shoulders

1 Sit in a chair with your feet flat on the floor about hip-width apart. Hold a dumbbell in each hand with the weights at about chest level and about 30cm (12in) from your body, palms facing each other and elbows slightly bent (imagine you're hugging a beach ball). Keep your elbows below shoulder height.

2 Bend forward from the hips (don't hunch your back) about 7–12cm (3–5in). Keeping your back straight, squeeze your shoulder blades together and pull your elbows back as far as is comfortably possible. Pause, then return to start.

2 SETS
10 reps

JAB Tones shoulders and upper and mid back

1 Stand with your feet hip-width apart with your left foot about a stride's length in front of your right foot, keeping your knees slightly bent. Raise your arms in front of you as though sparring. Your elbows should be bent, with your left hand in front of your face and your right hand just below your chin.

2 Punch straight out in front of you with your left arm (don't fully extend or lock the elbow), then bring it back to start. Repeat, then switch sides.

REPEAT FOR
30 seconds

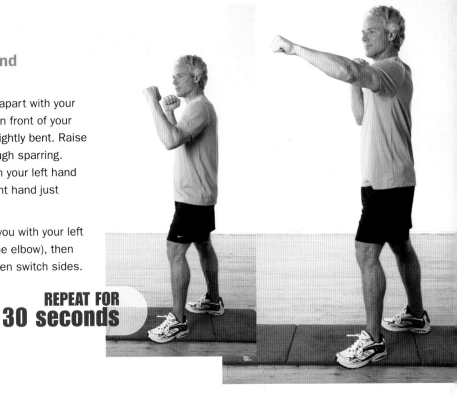

BICEP CURL Tones biceps

1 Stand with your knees slightly bent and your feet hip-width apart and hold a pair of dumbbells down at your sides with your arms rotated so that your palms are facing out as far as is comfortably possible.

2 Keeping your back straight and your elbows tucked close to your sides, slowly curl the weights up towards the outsides of your shoulders. Pause, then return to start.

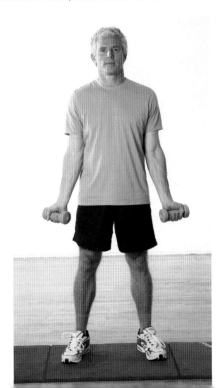

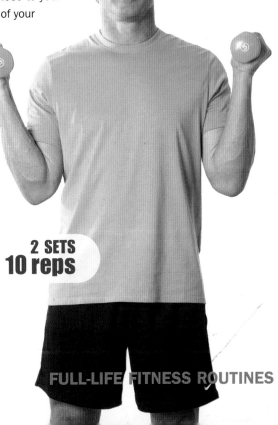

2 SETS
10 reps

DAY 1 Stretches
Medium

LIFT AND ARCH
Stretches chest, shoulders and abs

Sit on the floor with your legs crossed and hold a towel overhead with both hands so that your arms form a V. Keeping your lower back in the neutral position (don't arch it), lift your chest and arch your upper back slightly as you gently pull on the ends of the towel. Keep your shoulders down and make sure your arms go up and behind your back.

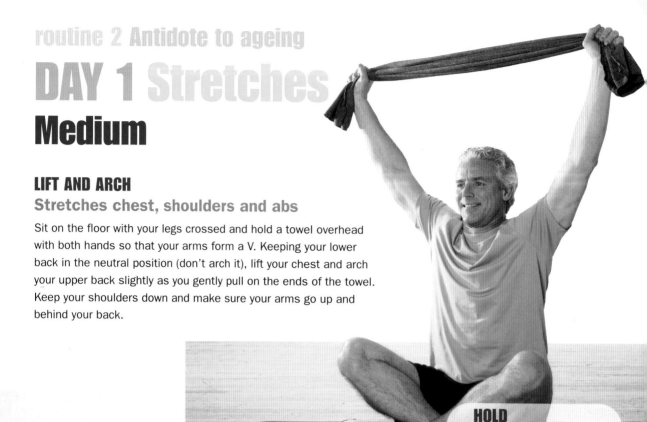

HOLD 20 seconds

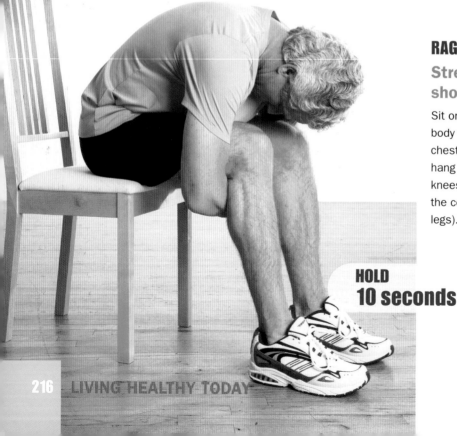

HOLD 10 seconds

RAG DOLL
Stretches back and shoulders

Sit on the edge of a chair and slump your body forward over your legs so your chest rests on your knees and your arms hang down. Wrap your arms under your knees and press your back up towards the ceiling (your chest will rise off your legs). Hold, then repeat three times.

DE-HUNCH STRETCH
Stretches chest, shoulders and upper back

Sit on the edge of a chair with your legs open and your pelvis tilted slightly forward. Lift your chest and squeeze your shoulder blades together and down away from your ears. Extend your arms at 45 degree angles from your body and then slightly behind you, palms facing forward. Hold, then repeat three times.

**HOLD
10 seconds**

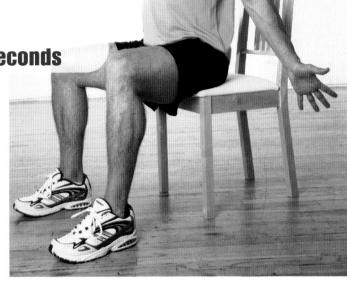

SIT AND REACH
Stretches back, shoulders and sides

Sit straight in a chair with your feet flat on the floor and place your left hand on your right upper arm. Twist to the left and grasp the back of the chair on the left with your right hand, bringing your chin over your left shoulder as you turn. Hold, then switch sides.

**HOLD
15 seconds**

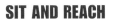

DAY 2 Strength exercises
Medium

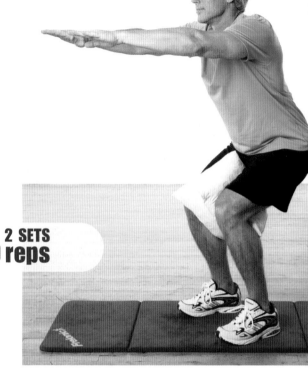

PILLOW SQUAT
Tones inner thighs and glutes

1 Stand with your feet hip or shoulder-width apart. Place a pillow between your legs just above your knees.

2 Keeping the pillow in place, extend your arms straight in front of you and simultaneously lower your bottom as if to sit in a chair. Your legs should be bent at about 45 degrees. Pause, then return to start.

2 SETS
10 reps

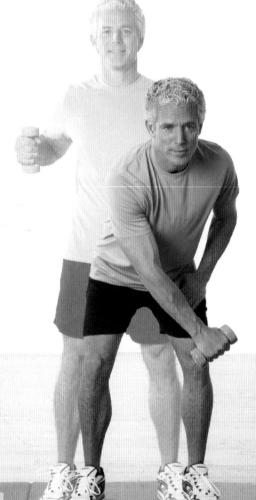

LAWNMOWER PULL Tones glutes and thighs

1 Stand with your feet hip-width apart and hold a light dumbbell in your right hand. Squat slightly until your legs are bent at about 45 degrees and place your left hand on your left thigh for support. Reach across your body with your right arm, placing the hand with the dumbbell directly in front of your left knee.

2 In one smooth motion, pull your right arm back across your body (as though pulling a lawnmower cord) and stand up slightly, though not fully. Complete a full set on one side before switching to the other.

2 SETS
5 reps EACH SIDE

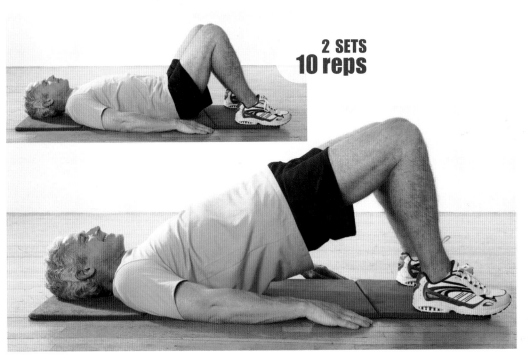

2 SETS
10 reps

BRIDGE Tones hips and glutes

1 Lie on your back with your legs bent and your feet flat on the floor. Rest your arms at your sides, palms facing down.

2 Contract your buttocks and raise your hips towards the ceiling until your body forms a straight line from your knees to your shoulders with your knees aligned with your hips. Pause, then return to start.

CHAIR TAP
Tones thighs, hips and glutes

1 Stand tall facing a chair with your feet about hip-width apart and your hands on your hips. (You can also place one hand on a wall for balance if you need to.)

2 Keeping your abdominal muscles tensed for back support, raise your left foot and tap the seat of the chair with your toes. Return to start. Complete a full set with one leg before switching to the other. Don't step fully onto the chair during this exercise.

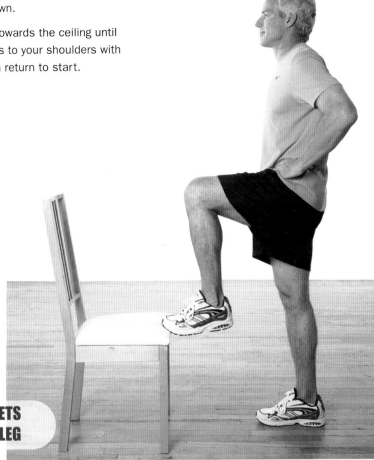

2 SETS
10 reps EACH LEG

DAY 2 Stretches
Medium

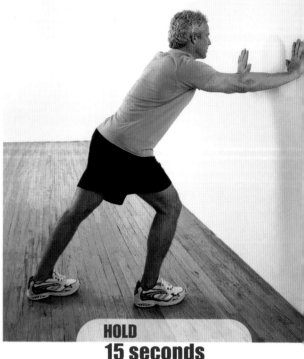

STANDING CALF STRETCH
Stretches calves

Stand at arm's length from a wall and place your palms flat against the wall. Extend your left leg 60–90cm (2–3ft) behind you and press your left heel to the floor. Make sure your back stays straight. (Your right knee will bend naturally as you extend your left leg.) Keeping both heels flat on the floor, press against the wall until you feel a nice stretch in your calf. Hold, then repeat with the other leg.

HOLD
15 seconds

CROSS AND PULL Stretches glutes and lower back

Lie on your back and cross your right leg over the left. Lightly grasp your right knee with your left hand and your left knee with your right hand. Gently pull your knee towards your chest as far as is comfortably possible. Hold, then release and repeat on the opposite side.

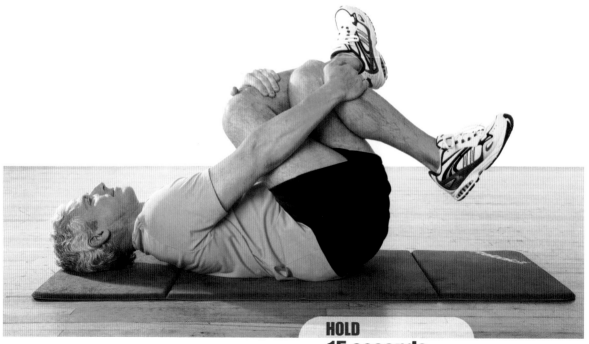

HOLD
15 seconds

FLAMINGO Stretches quadriceps and hips

Stand (with your right hand resting on a wall for support, if needed) and bend your left leg behind you. Grasp the top of your left foot with your left hand, keeping your back straight. Slowly pull your heel towards your bottom, stopping when you feel tension in your quads (the front of your thigh). Keep your hips and knees in alignment and tilt your pelvis slightly forward to deepen the stretch. Hold, then switch sides.

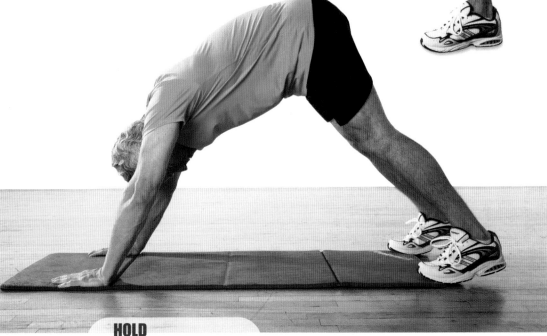

HOLD
20 to 30 seconds

DOWNWARD DOG

Stretches hamstrings, glutes and calves

Kneel on all fours with your feet flexed. Press your hands and feet into the floor, raising your hips towards the ceiling (your body should look like an upside-down V). Keep lifting your tailbone towards the ceiling as you lower your heels to the floor as far as is comfortably possible.

HOLD
15 seconds

DAY 3 Strength exercises
Medium

BIRD DOG

1 Kneel on all fours with your hands directly below your shoulders and your knees directly below your hips. Keep your head in line with your back (don't tilt it up or down).

2 Slowly extend your right arm and left leg so they're in line with or slightly above your back, pointing the toes of your left foot. (Don't arch your back while doing this exercise.) Pause, then return to start. Repeat on the opposite side.

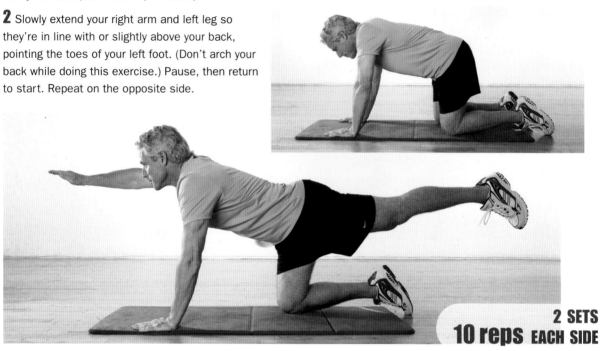

2 SETS
10 reps EACH SIDE

HOVER

Lie face down on the floor with your upper body propped on your forearms and your elbows directly beneath your shoulders. Lift your torso off the floor so your body is in a straight line, supported by your forearms and toes. Your back and pelvis should not arch or droop. Hold, relax, then repeat three times.

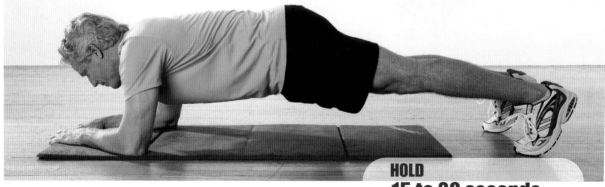

HOLD
15 to 20 seconds

MODIFIED 100

1 Lie on your back with your knees bent at a 90 degree angle and your calves parallel to the floor. Keep your arms straight at your sides.

2 Contract your stomach muscles, pulling your navel towards your spine, and press your lower back into the floor. Roll your head and shoulder blades off the floor, sliding your fingertips forward along the floor as you do so. Hold for five breaths, inhaling and exhaling forcefully, then roll back down to the floor.

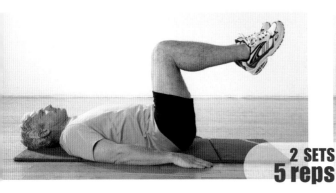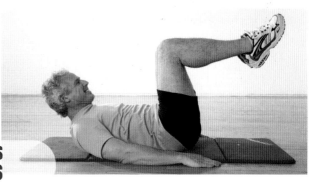

**2 SETS
5 reps**

TOWEL CRISS-CROSS

1 Lie on the floor with your knees bent and aligned over your hips, then raise your calves so they're parallel to the floor. Hold a small towel outstretched in both hands with your arms extended so the towel is by your knees.

2 Roll your head and shoulder blades off the floor. Extend your left leg and simultaneously move the outstretched towel to the outside of your right knee. Next, extend your right leg and bend your left knee, moving the towel to the outside of your left knee, keeping your shoulders off the floor. Your neck should stay in a neutral position. Alternate ten times for one set.

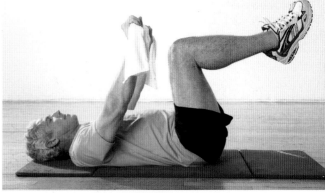

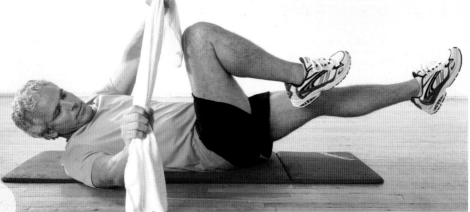

**2 SETS
10 reps**

DAY 3 Stretches
Medium

BACK CURL

Lie on your back with your feet off the floor and your knees bent towards your chest. Wrap a towel round the backs of your legs just below your knees, then grasp one end of the towel with each hand and pull your knees towards your chest until your lower back rolls off the floor slightly (or as far as is comfortably possible).

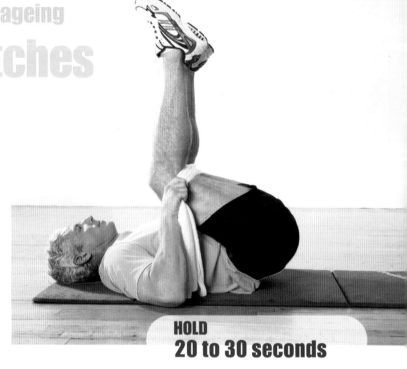

**HOLD
20 to 30 seconds**

SHIRT PULL

Stand straight with your feet hip-width apart and your arms crossed at your wrists in front of your body, as though preparing to pull off a shirt. Tilt your chin upwards and pull your crossed arms up, raising them and uncrossing them until they are fully extended overhead. Stretch your fingertips towards the ceiling as high as possible. Hold, then relax and return to start. Repeat five times.

**HOLD
5 to 10 seconds**

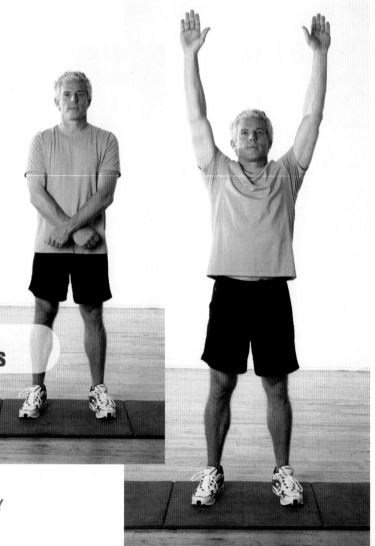

CHILD'S POSE

Kneel with the tops of your feet on the floor and your toes pointed behind you. Sit back on your heels and lower your chest to your thighs. Reach out with your arms and rest your palms on the floor. You may get a better stretch by having your knees and feet slightly apart.

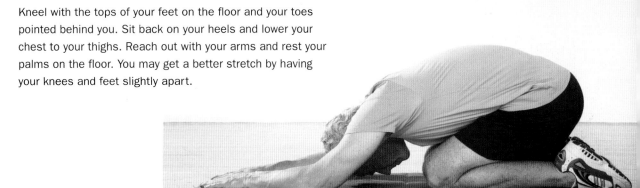

**HOLD
15 seconds**

TRIANGLE

Stand with your feet wide apart in a straddle stance with your left toes pointed forward and right toes pointed to the side; extend your arms straight to the sides. Keeping your arms outstretched, bend your torso gradually to the right and run your right hand slowly down the shin of your right leg as far as is comfortably possible. Reach towards the ceiling with your left fingertips and look up towards your left hand. Hold, then release and switch sides. It's important to do this stretch slowly.

**HOLD
20 to 30 seconds**

DAY 1 Strength exercises
Hard

STANDING ROW Tones back and shoulders

1 Holding a dumbbell in your left hand, stand with your right leg a wide step in front of your left with your left heel lifted off the floor. Rest your right hand on your right thigh for support and lean forward slightly.

2 Bend your left arm at a 90 degree angle in front of you, palm facing in. Pull your left arm up until your elbow is even with your shoulder. Pause, then return to start. Complete a full set with one arm before switching to the other.

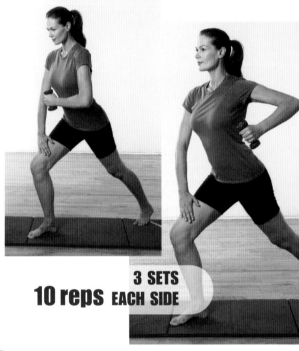

3 SETS
10 reps EACH SIDE

3 SETS
10 reps

CURL AND PRESS
Tones biceps and shoulders

1 Sit on a chair (preferably one without arms) with your feet flat on the floor. Hold a dumbbell in each hand with your arms down by your sides, palms facing out.

2 Keeping your upper body stable, bend your elbows and curl the weights up to your shoulders. Rotate your wrists so your palms are facing away from you and lift the weights overhead. Pause, then reverse the move, lowering your arms to return to the starting position.

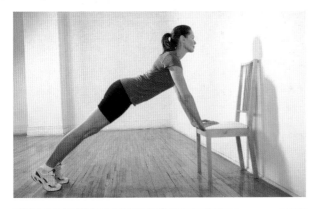

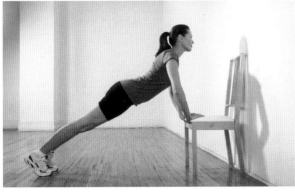

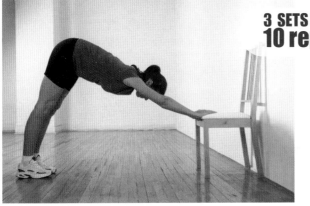

CHAIR PRESS-UP
Tones chest, triceps and shoulders

1 Place a chair against the wall and assume a push-up position with your hands as if on the third step of a flight of stairs (this exercise works with stairs or a chair). Your arms should be extended with your hands directly below your shoulders, and your body should form a straight diagonal line from your head to your heels.

2 Bend your elbows, keeping your arms close to your body as you lower yourself towards the chair (or step).

3 Straighten your arms and press your hips back and up towards the ceiling so you're in an inverted V position, dropping your heels towards the floor. Return to start.

It is very important to monitor your technique here, to avoid putting strain on your lower back.

3 SETS
10 reps

CHAIR DIP Tones triceps, shoulders and upper back

1 Have a chair pushed up against the wall. Sit on the edge of the chair with your hands grasping the seat on either side of your bottom, and your feet flat on the floor. Slide your bottom off the chair and walk your feet forward slightly, keeping your legs at a 90 degree angle.

2 Keeping your shoulders down, slowly bend your elbows, lowering your hips towards the floor until your upper arms are nearly parallel to the floor. Pause, then push up to return to start.

3 SETS
10 reps

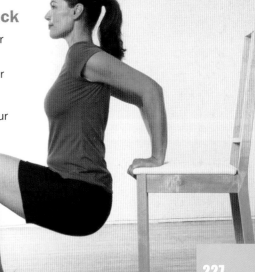

227

DAY 1 Stretches
Hard

OVERHEAD GRASP AND BEND
Stretches triceps and sides

Stand with your feet about shoulder-width apart. Extend your left arm overhead, bend the elbow, and reach down the middle of your back with your left hand, pointing your elbow towards the ceiling. Keep your shoulders down as you gently grasp your left elbow with your right hand and push it as far as is comfortably possible into a deeper stretch. Hold, then switch sides.

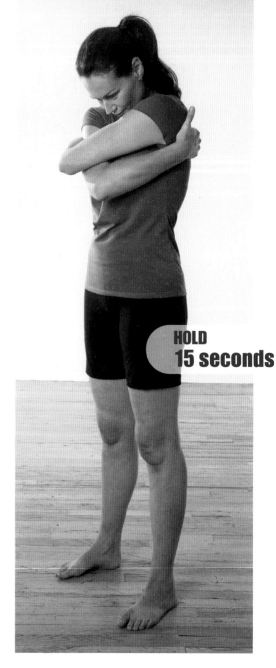

HOLD
15 seconds

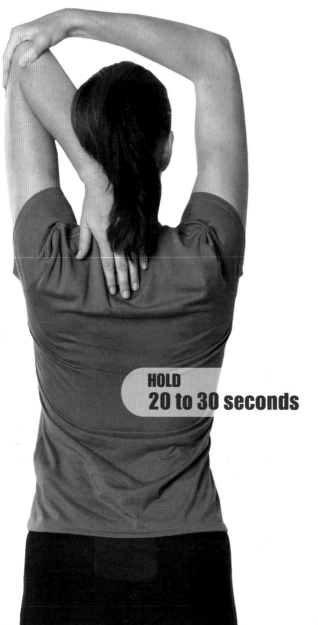

HOLD
20 to 30 seconds

SELF-HUG
Stretches upper back

Stand with your feet hip-width apart and your knees slightly bent. Wrap your arms around the front of your body as if you were giving yourself a hug, grasping the backs of your shoulders with your hands. Keeping your torso steady, relax your upper back and shoulders and let your head hang forward as far as is comfortably possible.

WALL STRETCH
Stretches chest and shoulders

Stand next to a wall and raise your left arm, pressing your hand and forearm against it. Slowly rotate your body towards the opposite shoulder until you feel a stretch across your chest and in your shoulder. Hold, then repeat on the other side.

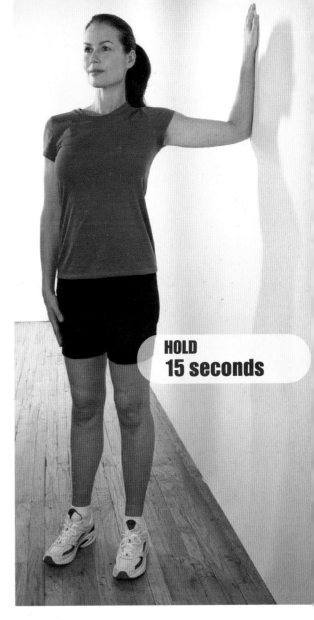

HOLD
15 seconds

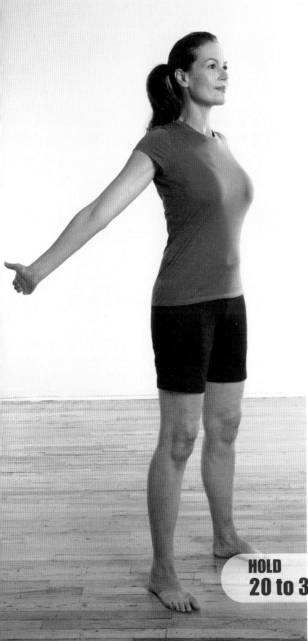

OPEN ARMS
Stretches biceps, forearms and chest

Stand with your feet hip-width apart and your knees slightly bent. Slowly raise your arms out to the sides until they reach shoulder level. Then, with your palms facing forward, gently stretch your arms behind you, keeping them just slightly below shoulder level. When you've pulled back as far as is comfortably possible, bend your wrists back until you feel a stretch in the fronts of your arms.

HOLD
20 to 30 seconds

DAY 2 Strength exercises
Hard

3 SETS
3 reps

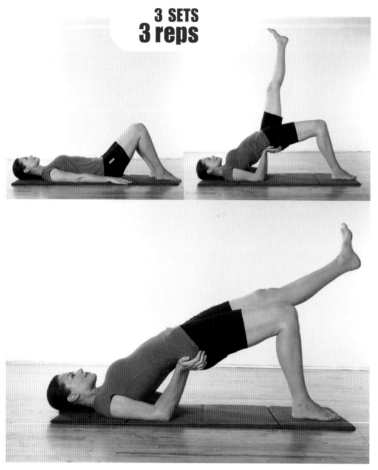

SINGLE BRIDGE
Tones glutes and thighs

1 Lie on your back with knees bent and your feet flat on the floor about hip-width apart. Contract your buttocks and lift your bottom so your body forms a straight line from your knees to your shoulders. Support your hips with your hands, keeping your elbows and upper arms planted on the floor.

2 If you can, straighten your left leg towards the ceiling, pointing the toe, then flex your foot.

3 Lower your leg until your knees line up, then raise the leg again. Repeat three times, then switch sides. (If this is too difficult, skip step 2 and just raise your leg so your knees are in line with one another. If it's too easy, take your hands off your hips.)

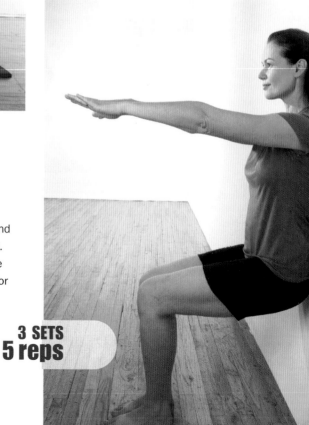

WALL SQUAT
Tones glutes and thighs

1 Stand with your back against a wall, your legs straight and your feet about 60cm (2ft) from the wall and slightly apart. Raise your arms straight in front of you and slide down the wall until your thighs are nearly parallel to the floor. Hold for three to five counts, then slide back up to the starting position, lowering your arms as you stand.

3 SETS
5 reps

STEP-UP
Tones thighs and glutes

1 Stand facing a step and hold dumbbells at your sides, palms facing in.

2 Place your left foot on the step, then press up so your right foot is also on the step. Next, step down with your left foot, followed by the right. Repeat, starting with your right leg. Alternate ten times for one set. (If you are older or have balance problems, use a single step to avoid tripping.)

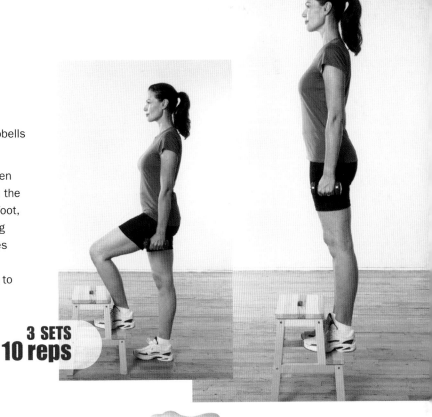

3 SETS
10 reps

L-LIFT Tones hips and glutes

1 Lie on your right side with both legs extended straight in front of you so your body forms an L shape. (If you have tight hamstrings or back, angle your legs at 45 degrees.) Extend your right arm overhead, resting your head on your upper arm, and place your left hand on the floor in front of you for support.

2 Keeping your feet flexed and your abdominal muscles tensed for back support, lift your left leg towards the ceiling as high as is comfortable. Pause, then return to start. Complete a full set with one leg before switching to the other (if it's too difficult, bend your knees).

3 SETS
10 reps EACH LEG

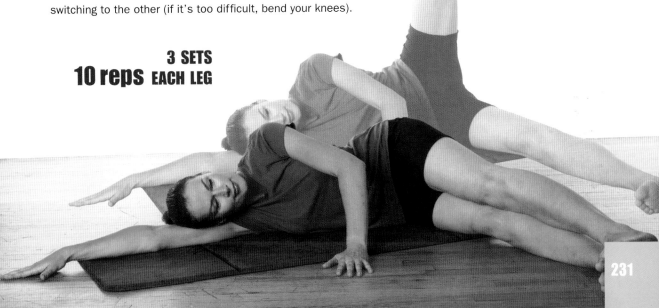

DAY 2 Stretches
Hard

CROSS-BODY LEG STRETCH
Stretches glutes and outer leg

Lie on your back with a towel or tie looped around the arch of your right foot. Pull the leg off the floor as high as is comfortably possible (you can bend your knee slightly if you need to). Then place your right arm on the floor and, using your left hand, pull the leg slowly across your body as far as you comfortably can, keeping your hips on the floor. Hold, then switch sides.

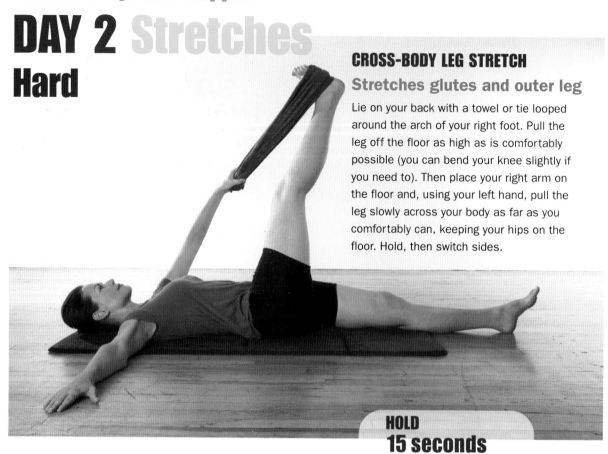

HOLD
15 seconds

LYING ROPE STRETCH
Stretches hamstrings

Lie on your back with a towel or tie looped around the arch of your left foot. Contract your left quadriceps (front of thigh) and pull the towel back, lifting your left leg as far as is comfortably possible. Keep your right leg straight, or bend it slightly if your back or hamstring is very tight. Hold, then switch legs.

HOLD
15 seconds

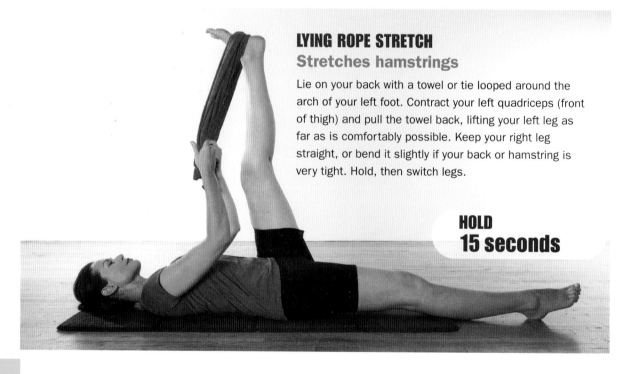

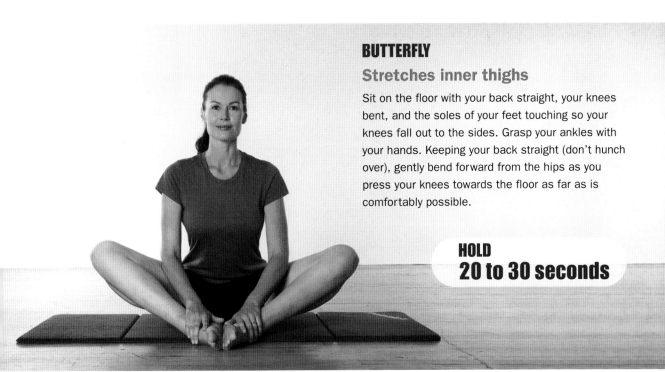

BUTTERFLY
Stretches inner thighs

Sit on the floor with your back straight, your knees bent, and the soles of your feet touching so your knees fall out to the sides. Grasp your ankles with your hands. Keeping your back straight (don't hunch over), gently bend forward from the hips as you press your knees towards the floor as far as is comfortably possible.

HOLD
20 to 30 seconds

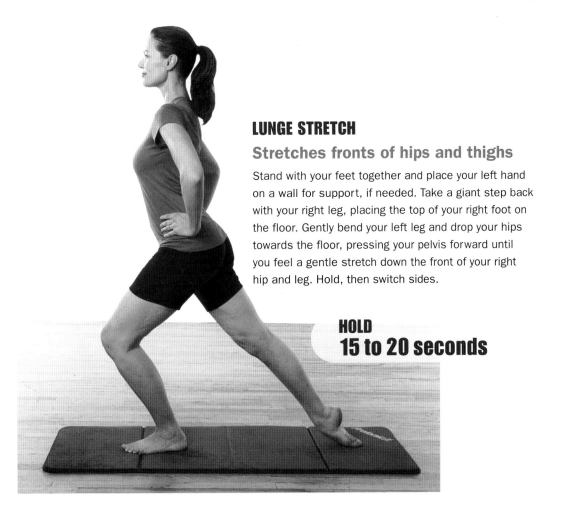

LUNGE STRETCH
Stretches fronts of hips and thighs

Stand with your feet together and place your left hand on a wall for support, if needed. Take a giant step back with your right leg, placing the top of your right foot on the floor. Gently bend your left leg and drop your hips towards the floor, pressing your pelvis forward until you feel a gentle stretch down the front of your right hip and leg. Hold, then switch sides.

HOLD
15 to 20 seconds

DAY 3 Strength exercises
Hard

SINGLE LEG STRETCH

1 Lie on your back with your legs straight. Bring your left knee into your chest. Grasp your left ankle with your left hand and put your right hand on your knee.

2 Keeping your abdominals tight, curl your head and shoulders up off the floor, pull your left knee into your chest, and lift and stretch your right leg straight out, with your heel a few inches off the floor. Pause, then return to start. Alternate ten times for one set.

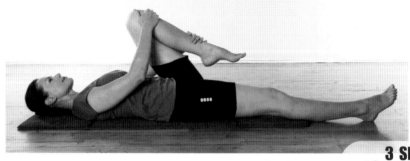

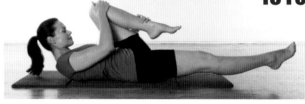

**3 SETS
10 reps**

PLANK TORSO TWIST

1 Assume a push-up position with your arms extended, your hands directly below your shoulders, and your legs extended and supported on the balls of your feet. Your body should form a straight line from your head to your heels.

2 Keeping your upper body stable, bend your left knee towards your right shoulder, twisting your hips slightly to the right. Pause, then return to start. Repeat with your right leg. Alternate ten times for one set.

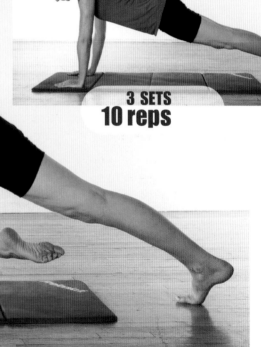

**3 SETS
10 reps**

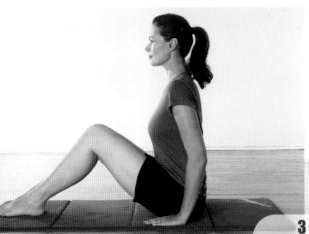

3 SETS
5 reps

BOAT

1 Sit on the floor with your back straight, your knees bent and your feet flat on the floor.

2 Keeping your back straight, contract your abdominal muscles, lean back and extend your legs so your body forms a right-angle. Extend your arms straight out on either side of your knees. Hold for 3 to 5 seconds, then return to start.

This exercise is one of the hardest and requires some practice. You should tackle it only if you're confident that you're fit enough and have sufficient balance.

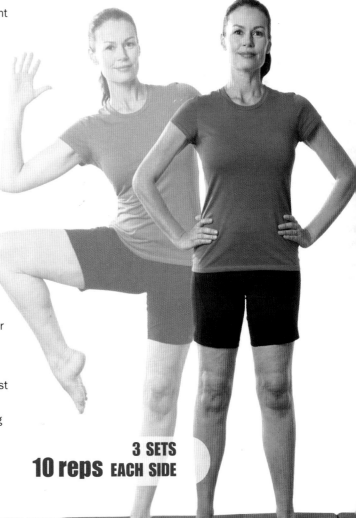

STANDING SIDE CRUNCH

1 Stand with your feet hip-width apart. Slightly point your right toes out to the side. Place your left hand on your hip and extend your right arm straight overhead.

2 Raise your right knee out to the side, raising it to waist height as you bring your right elbow down to meet your knee. Complete a full set with one side before switching to the other.

Don't be surprised if you fall over when you first try this exercise! It will become easier with practice.

3 SETS
10 reps EACH SIDE

DAY 3 Stretches
Hard

COBRA

Lie face down with your feet together, your toes pointed, and your hands on the floor, palms down, just in front of your shoulders. Lift your chin and gently extend your arms, raising your upper body off the floor as far as is comfortably possible. (If you feel any strain in your back, keep your elbows bent and your forearms on the floor.)

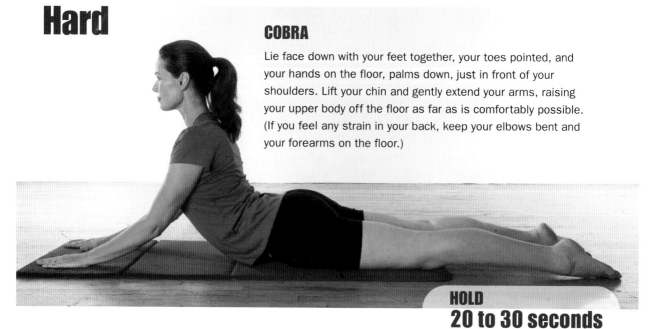

HOLD
20 to 30 seconds

CAT STRETCH

1 Kneel on all fours with your hands directly below your shoulders and your knees directly below your hips. Pull your abdominal muscles in, drop your head, and press your back up, rounding it up towards the ceiling. Hold.

2 Then raise your head and drop your belly towards the floor, arching your back in the opposite direction. Hold.

HOLD
15 seconds

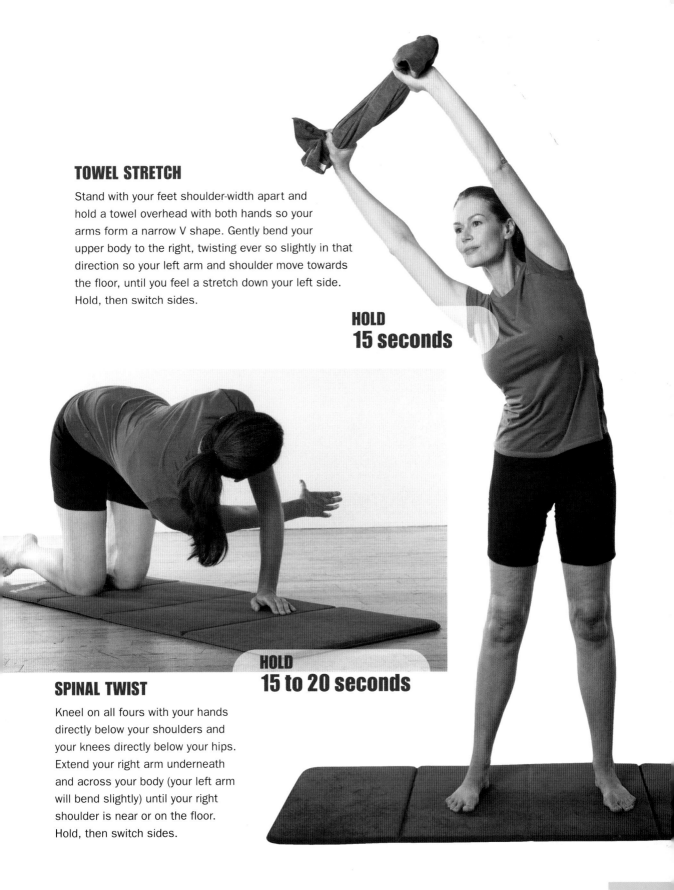

TOWEL STRETCH

Stand with your feet shoulder-width apart and hold a towel overhead with both hands so your arms form a narrow V shape. Gently bend your upper body to the right, twisting ever so slightly in that direction so your left arm and shoulder move towards the floor, until you feel a stretch down your left side. Hold, then switch sides.

**HOLD
15 seconds**

**HOLD
15 to 20 seconds**

SPINAL TWIST

Kneel on all fours with your hands directly below your shoulders and your knees directly below your hips. Extend your right arm underneath and across your body (your left arm will bend slightly) until your right shoulder is near or on the floor. Hold, then switch sides.

… managing depression

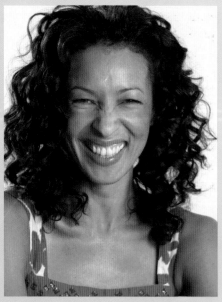
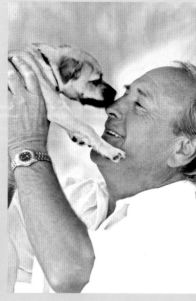
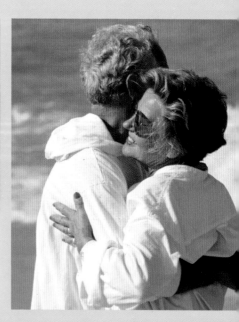

… happiness – what is it anyway?

… resisting stress

Live to feel good

What does it take to age successfully? It's a question researchers have only begun to explore in earnest in the past 20 years, ever since it became clear that our understanding of ageing was no longer sufficient in a world increasingly filled with active adults in their 80s, 90s and beyond.

What those researchers have found is thoroughly fascinating. Yes, nutrition and exercise are key elements of a healthy, disease-resistant body. But what matters as much as, if not more than, the daily details of food and fitness are the attitudes and mind-sets that guide our lives. As it turns out, good health may or may not make us happy, but happiness without question contributes enormously to good health.

This is an important point. For too long now, the medical community has scoffed at the notion of a 'mind-body connection', as have many people. But the research is in, and it is irrefutable: your thoughts and emotions greatly affect your physical well-being. Put simply, there is no cheaper and easier way to improve your health than to smile regularly. ■

Optimism, resilience, social activities and faith

Happiness –
what is it, anyway?

On any given day, we all tend to be a bundle of emotions and moods, from angry to ecstatic, from bored to bubbly. It's naive to think that we should be constantly smiling. Concepts such as joy, purpose and self-worth are far too complicated to reduce to a simple 'Are you happy?' If only there were some type of measuring machine, like a blood pressure kit, that could tell us our happiness levels on a numbered scale. Now that would be useful!

Surprise. Researchers haven't created such a machine, but they have come up with the next best thing: they've identified the specific attitudes, lifestyle choices and personal traits that best contribute to both long life and long health. We call them the:

Fabulous 5 traits

TRAIT 1 Resilience in response to life's changes and challenges

TRAIT 2 A healthy, active social life

TRAIT 3 The ability to prevent or manage depression

TRAIT 4 Embracing some form of spirituality or higher purpose

TRAIT 5 The skill to defuse the stresses of daily life

Research definitively shows that people who exercise these five traits are far less susceptible to the diseases and breakdowns of ageing. Better still, they actually do seem to be more joyous, more purposeful and more active.

It's no surprise that these positive psychological traits are deeply enmeshed in the cultures of long-lived people. On the Japanese island of Okinawa, home to the world's largest concentration of healthy, happy people over the age of 100, people embrace a 'don't worry, be happy' philosophy of life called *taygay* that minimises stress and protects people's emotions from life's slings and arrows.

Okinawans also practise a deep, meditative spirituality that links them with their ancestors, their gods and the universe. They stay connected with friends, family and neighbours. Okinawan village life is based on the value of *yuimaru*, or mutual assistance. Friends, work colleagues or neighbours meet regularly in groups called *moais*, where everyone puts a little money into a pot, and whoever needs it most takes it home. Elder Okinawans are proud of their status and revered by their communities – something Western cultures would do well to imitate. For them, there's no word for 'retirement', and most older people do not feel lonely.

The benefits of positive attitudes and practices like these don't manifest themselves in the distant future. Optimism, resilience, social activities and faith make *today* better. And, as revealed in Okinawa, they also make you more likely to enjoy life many years from now.

The bottom line: if you think that living a healthy lifestyle is just about food and exercise, you are badly mistaken. Everyday attitudes are as important to your health, short *and* long term, as anything else you can do.

So read on. We'll explore each of the Fabulous 5 attributes in detail and show you specific, easy ways to embrace them. Remember: making a change is easier than you think, if you go about it one small step at a time. You can improve your mind-set, your social life and your direction. The first step is merely gathering enough courage and conviction to *take* a first step. The second one will follow much more easily. ■

make today better – and add years to your life

TRAIT 1 Resilience

When Dutch researchers asked 600 people aged 85 and over to identify the key components of successful ageing, they came up with one that surprised even the experts: psychological health. But rather than defining psychological health as the lack of depression or other mental-health conditions, they told researchers it meant being able to adjust to circumstances, focus on gains rather than losses and appreciate your blessings. We have another word for it: *resilience*.

Resilience is why certain children who grow up surrounded by poverty or cruelty still manage to get into top universities and become successful. It's why some people rebuild after storms and flooding, despite the challenges and hardships. It's why you say of someone who's just been diagnosed with cancer or who has just lost a husband or whose business has just failed: 'I can't believe how well she's handling this'. We like to think of a resilient person as a human rubber band – able to be stretched almost to breaking point and still snap back.

Resilience isn't 'positive psychology' or 'always looking on the bright side'. It's about accepting that life will always present challenges and being able to focus on dealing with them successfully. One measure of resilience is what psychologists call 'sense of coherence', meaning having the ability to define life events as less stressful, the motivation to cope and the capacity to mobilise resources to deal with stresses encountered. A strong sense of coherence is associated with both physical and mental health, and may even enhance survival. In one major European study of more than 20,000 people aged 41–80, it was linked with a 24 per cent reduction in the risk of stroke over a seven-year follow-up period, after taking account of age, risk factors, social class, educational level and the number of adverse events that had occurred in someone's life. In another study of nearly 6,000 Finnish men, a strong sense of coherence almost halved their risk of developing diabetes over the following two decades.

Everyone has some measure of resilience. Older adults, who have had decades of coping with challenging situations, may even be best placed to create and maintain a resilient attitude. If you're faced with financial trouble, for instance, you can think back to another similar time and draw strength from the fact that you managed the situation then, so you can manage it now.

Resilience really comes into play when you're confronted with stress. If you're resilient, studies find, you recover from stress faster, reducing the damaging impact it can have and readying yourself more quickly for the next challenge.

Researchers have identified certain common traits of resilient people. How many apply to you? Resilient people:

- Adapt to change easily
- Feel in control of their lives
- Are able to bounce back after difficult times
- Have close, dependable relationships
- Remain optimistic and have a sense of humour, even in the face of challenges
- Can function well under pressure
- Have a sense of confidence and strength in themselves as individuals

Have you laughed

- Believe things happen for a reason
- Can handle uncertainty or unpleasantness
- Know where to turn for help
- Like challenges
- Enjoy taking the lead
- Have hobbies and enjoy other activities.

Even if you're on the low end of the resilience scale, you can take steps today to build your inner resilience. While the following tips provide a start, every other tip throughout this chapter will also add to your resilience.

Laugh at least five times a day Humour and resilience are actually quite similar. After all, what is humour but the ability to make light of real life? Laughter keeps you optimistic, helps you to cope, reduces stress and reminds you of what's important in life. If you don't have a sense of humour, now is the time to work on one. Start with the professionals: watch comedies on TV, rent funny films, read funny books. Be less stern and more playful with your family. Have animated conversations about unimportant subjects with friends. Learn the art of the gentle tease – and be open to teasing in return. Come bedtime, look back on your day and think about whether you laughed enough. Then vow to laugh more tomorrow. Just one warning: avoid sarcasm, mockery and any other forms of humour that degrade or hurt others. Humour, when twisted improperly, can be more bitter than sweet.

Choose laughter over anger Let's be honest: there's no shortage of people and things that can make us angry, be it the government, a rude shop assistant, your spouse's insensitive

comment, the mess in the living room, the inconsiderate driver in front of you, your boss and so on. In every case, you have a choice: become angry, or don't. We recommend choosing the latter. Anger *solves* nothing. But it does accomplish something: it ruins your mood, hurts your health and gets in the way of constructive responses. Resilient people avoid anger. Rather, if they can control the situation, they work to improve it – and if they can't control it directly, they find ways to cope with it. So the next time anger starts to sweep over you, shut it down, smile at the absurdity and frustrations of life and get busy fixing things.

Have empathy This is closely related to the tip on controlling anger. Most people do what they do by choice. People who take the time to ponder the other side's perspective

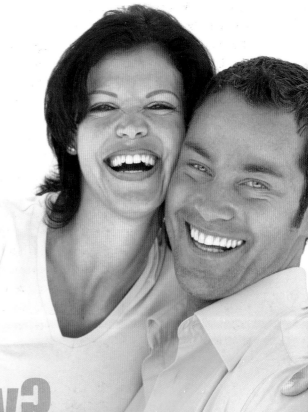

enough today?

LIVE TO FEEL GOOD **241**

almost always sidestep anger and respond constructively. Rather than just getting angry at your boss, for example, take a moment to think through why he or she said or did what bothered you (more often than not, your boss will be acting in response to someone else's unreasonable demands). The ability to see situations from multiple viewpoints is extremely handy for building a more resilient personality.

List your strengths. This could be everything from your ability to interact with anyone at any time to your talent for baking. Don't do this on your own; ask people who know you well to contribute to the list. Knowing your strengths, becoming *aware* of your strengths, is like putting money into the resilience bank. When it's time for a withdrawal, you'll know just how much you have to use.

Write down your blessings It may sound corny, but recognising the many things you have to be thankful for is a sign of resilience. Don't leave anything out. If you're blessed because you moved into a house with the master bedroom on the ground floor and you don't have to climb stairs, add it to the list. Make copies of the list and put one in your bedroom, the kitchen and the glove compartment of your car. Whenever you're tempted to have a moan, pull out the list and remind yourself how lucky you really are.

Don't panic When adversity hits, take a deep breath, think about the situation, then list five things you can do without falling apart. Say to yourself, 'In the near future, this will already be worked out, and things will be getting better.'

Ask the right questions People often let situations control them instead of *them* controlling the situation. Many times, this occurs because they haven't bothered to get the information they need. When problems occur, ask questions. Lots of questions. This provides you with enough information to develop alternative responses, at least one of which will enable you to bounce back from the situation.

Identify one positive thing in every situation No matter how bleak a situation is, there's always something positive to be found. Even for one couple whose house burned down on Christmas Eve, just two days after they'd moved in, when the husband tried to light a fire in the fireplace. They lost everything they had accumulated over their 40 year marriage. But they still had each other. And, they said, starting over was actually a positive experience.

Manage your expectations If you expect everything to go perfectly when you travel, you're setting yourself up for a disappointment. Instead, anticipate long delays and lost luggage by taking extra reading material or playing cards and not putting anything you can't live without in your checked-in bags. Then, when disaster *doesn't* strike, you're three steps ahead. This kind of thinking also works well for family reunions, house renovations and medical appointments.

Set daily goals You need a sense of accomplishment every day to strengthen your own belief in yourself. These goals could be small, such as calling on a housebound elderly neighbour every week, or designed to add up

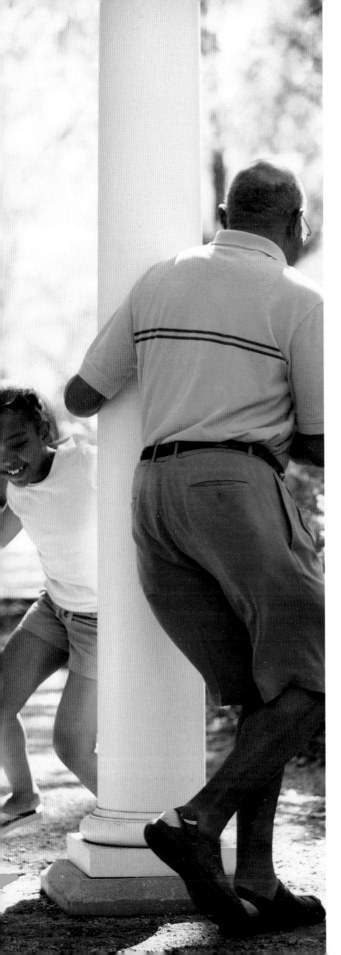

to a larger achievement, such as getting another degree or building a gazebo.

Compare yourself only to yourself Just because Mary lost her job and had to declare bankruptcy doesn't mean you will. Just because your neighbour Sam had lots more good fortune this past year than you did doesn't mean you're a failure. Focus on your situation in the context of your life, not that of anyone else around you.

Recognise what you can and cannot control If you have diabetes, for instance, and you're following a healthy diet, taking your medication and exercising regularly, but you still have fluctuating blood sugar, recognise that you're doing all you can to control the situation, and that you may need to put the rest of the problem in your doctor's hands.

Change one thing every day With age, we move in smaller circles, becoming so entrenched in our routines that we don't even notice them any longer. Then, when something happens to change that routine, we lack the flexibility to cope with it. To prevent this from happening, aim to change one thing about your routine every day. You might brush your teeth with your left hand, take a different route while riding your bike to work, or sleep in a different bedroom in the house. ■

toxic thinking about ... ageing

If you think ageing means pain, disability or poor health, **you're living in the past.** A landmark study published in 2002 found that people who perceive ageing negatively live an average of seven and a half years less than people who view ageing in a positive light.

Since then, other studies have found numerous connections between the perception of ageing and overall health and well-being. For instance, one found that people who viewed ageing positively were more likely to remain physically active, a key component of ageing well. Those who thought negatively about ageing, however, were less likely to remain physically active and more likely to age 'unsuccessfully'. Other studies found that views about ageing affect memory, well-being, the will to live and overall satisfaction with life.

Your expectations about ageing also affect how your body reacts to stress, particularly when it comes to the effect of stress on your heart. View ageing as all downhill, and your heart goes mad when you're under stress; view ageing as a well-deserved benefit of a well-lived life, and your heart reacts to stress as a minor blip in the scheme of things.

Your perceptions about ageing also affect how you live your life. For instance, if you believe that brain function inevitably declines with age – a total falsehood – you might refuse to learn to use a computer, cutting yourself off from a valuable tool for learning, staying in touch with people and finding new activities and interests – all of which, as you now know, are keys to ageing well.

All this creates a vicious circle: if you think ageing means infirmity, and your health or memory deteriorates because of your belief, it only reinforces that mistaken belief and results in greater problems.

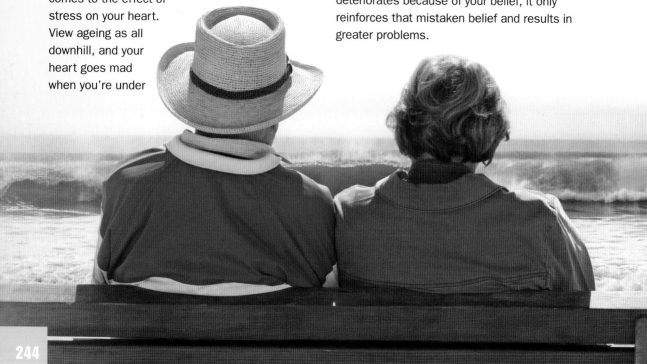

To readjust your perceptions of ageing ...

Increase your walking pace
One study of 47 healthy men and women with an average age of 70 found that those who received subliminally negative messages about ageing (senility, dependency and disease), and who then took a walk, travelled at the same speed as before they received the messages. Those who received positive messages about ageing (wisdom, astuteness, accomplishment) walked 9 per cent faster. It may seem a small change, but other studies found that walking speed is a good way of measuring your overall fitness and physical function. Studies also link walking speed to the risk of nursing-home admission and death in older people. Generally, your walking speed drops 9 to 30 per cent as you age, so any increase is a good thing.

Focus on other successful older people
Many of today's greatest authors, orchestra conductors, actors, commentators, teachers and visionaries are people over the age of 70. Role models abound for people seeking an active path for their later years.

Watch your language
Instead of chalking up forgetfulness to a 'senior moment', call it what it is: a brain hiccup, a sign that you're under too much stress, an indication that you didn't pay close-enough attention the first time.

When you were 20 and you forgot someone's name, you didn't refer to it as a senior moment, did you? This really works; one major study of 230 60 year olds found that those who chalked up their difficulty in completing certain tasks such as cutting their toenails or walking moderate distances to 'old age' were much more likely to have arthritis, heart disease and hearing loss than those who attributed their difficulties to other reasons.

Get the TV out of the bedroom and living room
In fact, turn it off altogether. It turns out that the more television older people watch, the worse their perceptions of ageing are. That's because older people are depicted so negatively on TV. In one study, participants aged between 60 and 90 who watched an average of 21 hours of TV a week found that older people were often the brunt of jokes or were left out altogether. As one 68-year-old participant wrote in her viewing diary: 'I feel like we've been ignored. I feel like we are non-existent.' Overall, the study found, less than 2 per cent of primetime television characters are 65 or older.

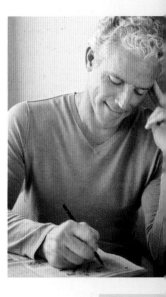

The bottom line
Your attitudes have the power to
programme your body to perform as
you think it should perform

TRAIT 2
Active social life

Are you lonely? Not 'alone', but lonely. There *is* a difference. For instance, you can be married with children at home and still feel lonely. Loneliness occurs not only when your social life is less active than you'd like but also when you don't get the level of intimacy you need from the relationships you *do* have.

Loneliness is not just a state of mind. Studies find that feeling lonely significantly increases your risk of heart disease and depression and that lonely people are more than twice as likely to develop Alzheimer's disease as those with stronger social connections. In fact, loneliness is as threatening to your overall health as obesity.

Researchers from University College London discovered one reason: in a study of 240 people aged 47–59, women with higher loneliness scores had significantly greater blood-pressure reactions to acute mental stress. And in response to stress, both men and women who were lonely had higher levels of fibrinogen, a protein involved in blood clotting. The more fibrinogen, the greater the risk of heart attack or stroke.

In another study, older adults who reported feelings of loneliness had higher blood pressure than those who didn't. Loneliness accounted for as much as a 30mmHg increase in systolic pressure (the top number), equivalent to the difference between normal and high blood pressure. The researchers suggest that reducing loneliness among older people could be as beneficial to health as losing excess weight or taking regular exercise.

The good news is that reaching out to make new social connections can indeed improve both feelings of loneliness and physical health. In a remarkable experiment in Sweden, half of the residents in an apartment building for elderly people were invited to participate in a programme of social activity involving interest groups in topics such as botany, art, history,

To have friends first takes the willingness to be a friend. Are you ready to give what it takes?

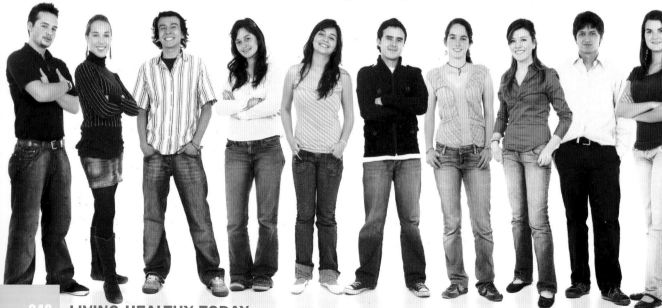

music, song and local interest, along with outings, picnics and visits to the theatre and opera.

Over six months, these residents increased their social activities threefold, both inside and outside the planned activities – they were also more likely to get together for coffee, walks and shopping – and were only a third as likely as the non-invited residents to report feeling that their days were monotonous and boring. Those in the social group were also significantly more inclined to protest when things went wrong.

What's more, these emotional changes were parallelled by improvements in hormonal and metabolic status that suggested a reduced risk of conditions such as diabetes and osteoporosis and indicated less stress and depression. Even more incredible, the sociable group actually showed a slight increase in average height, whereas the controls shrunk a little.

Now, we admit that as you get older, it can become more difficult to make friends, especially if you're retired or work from home. It wasn't always this way. Remember when your children were little? You made friends at the park and the school and through parents' groups, football teams and Boy Scout troops. Everywhere you turned, someone else was dealing with the same issues you were and was happy to get together for coffee to thrash through solutions.

Fast-forward to today. The children are gone or nearly gone, and chances are life is more solitary, with fewer external activities than 20 years ago. Even stranger is when you find you're in a neighbourhood filled with families living life at a different pace. All this can be overcome and, if you read on, we'll give you lots of ideas to add social connections to your life.

One thing is crucial to each of these ideas: the willingness to reach out. For some people, making that first phone call, enquiry or appearance is as tough a task as running a

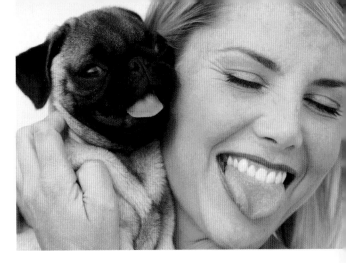

Adding dog years to your life

Talk about great companionship! Dogs worship the very ground you walk on. They don't care if you snap at them when you're in a bad mood or if you sit for hours saying nothing. But they do require that you get out of bed and walk them, at the very least. And that, studies find, is a very good thing for older people. When researchers looked at dog owners aged between 71 and 82, they found that those who walked their dogs were more likely to get 150 minutes of walking a week and to have faster walking speeds than those who didn't have dogs.

Other studies find significant health benefits in owning a dog (more so than owning a cat), including faster recovery from heart attacks, a greater ability to live independently and better overall well-being. If your living situation allows it, seriously consider adding a dog to your immediate family.

marathon. We understand, but there's no denying it: making new social connections requires reaching out. It takes courage, but when you acknowledge all your strengths, all your successes and all that you have to offer, it gets much easier. Do what it takes to confirm your sense of self-worth and venture forth.

When you reach out to people, you will be astounded at the results. Yes, a minority will be too fearful to accept, and you will ▶

Finding friends on the internet

Once, letter writing was common. Then it declined. Now it's back and better than ever in the form of emails and Internet bulletin boards.

With the rise of the internet over the past decade, all the modern rules of communication have changed. On any given day, billions of email messages are flying around among friends, families, business associates and hobbyists all over the world. Whether you live in a remote village in the Shetland Islands or in a city centre, there are people out there who share your passions. You just have to find them.

In the past few years, older people have been the fastest-growing group of internet users. In fact, a quarter of all British internet users are now over 50, and people over 65 are the most active users, spending an average of 42 hours online every month. So make the effort to get connected and join in, whether it's for news, shopping, information, hobbies, keeping in touch with friends and family or socialising. If you don't have a computer, pop into your local library, where you can get help learning to use one if necessary. The more time you spend using the internet, studies find, the greater your social network. Many older people find that their lives have been transformed by a few hours a day online.

For the perfect place to start your search for information and like-minded communities, try the groups section on http://uk.yahoo.com. Often, there's a 'groups' heading on a site's first page. Click there and enter your area of interest. Within minutes, you'll be off on an amazing journey through new communities and other similar websites. And so-called 'silver surfers' even have their own networking site, called Saga Zone, for people aged 50-plus (www.sagazone.co.uk).

Just as you would do at an airport or visiting a new major city, protect yourself when roaming online. Make sure your computer has protective software to prevent intruders. And never, *ever* publicly reveal personal information on the internet. Be constantly cautious and smart.

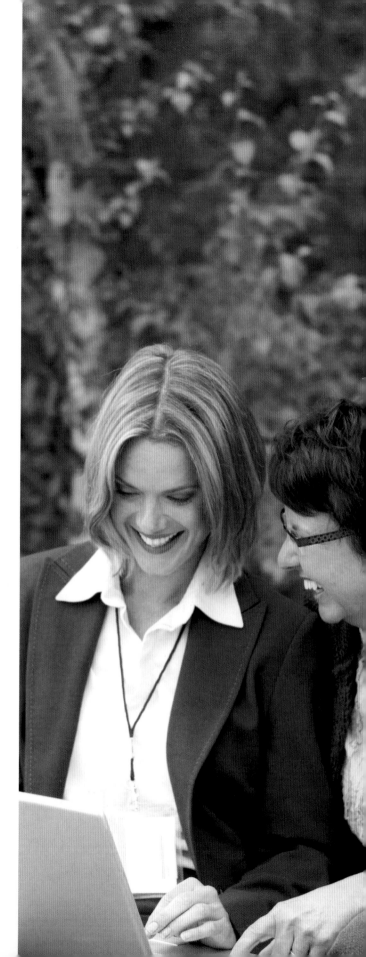

Fill your life with routines that involve friends and family

occasionally be rebuffed. But most people will be thrilled at your offer. A social invitation is a wonderful thing, whether you are a 6 year old being invited to a birthday party or a 68 year old being asked to join a bridge game. For a sense of personal satisfaction, there's little that can match bringing people together.

Here's how to get started.

Revive the dinner party ritual When was the last time you invited four people over for dinner? Once, dinner parties were a natural part of life. But over time, they've become less common. Change that. The fanciness of your cooking is not important. What's important is the opportunity to sit at a table together, not rushed by a waiter or intimidated by crowds or noise, and to talk freely over a glass of wine and a plate of food. Make a vow: two Sundays from now, you're having guests.

Be bold and take up a sport It may sound like a cliché, but try golf. With 3 to 6 hours spent on the course, you've got plenty of time for conversation and companionship. Plus, there are the required post-play refreshments at the 19th hole. If golf just isn't your thing, other good 'companion' sports include tennis and bowling.

Or take up a game Chess, poker, bridge, mah-jong, pool and darts are all great choices. Sitting around a table with friends and jovially playing a game for a few hours is one of the best things you can do for your health. (Beware, though, of all the snacks and alcohol.) Make it a twice-a-week ritual.

Or join a club Enjoy wine? Check with your local wine merchant. They'll have information on wine groups in your community. If not, put a leaflet up in the shop offering to start one. The key here is to take something you enjoy – tasting wine, solving puzzles, knitting, fishing, woodworking, gardening – and turn it from a solitary activity into a social one. The wine club formula works for nearly any hobby.

Meet your neighbours You may well know the postman better than you know the person you've lived next door to for six years. Why not throw a barbecue for a few neighbouring households, organise a street party or start a neighbourhood newsletter, in print or online, to get to know the people surrounding you.

Get a job Of course you've looked forward to retirement for 40 years. But studies find that people who aren't working are more likely to be lonely than those who work. You don't have to work full-time; some kind of part-time job that requires you to interact with your colleagues and the public is just the ticket. In other words, not a solitary desk job.

Register for college courses If you never went to college or university, or never had a chance to finish, now is the time. The more education you have, studies find, the more social connections you have as you age. Conversely, the less education you have, the more likely you are to become a loner because you don't trust others enough. A higher educational level means you're more likely to volunteer and, as the next tip shows, that's also a key quality in successful ageing.

Volunteer Nothing makes a person feel more wanted and appreciated than volunteering. We know this instinctively, but researchers around the world have reams of data proving it. When you help others, your own sense of control increases. And with a stronger sense of control, you're less likely to become depressed. It also makes you more likely to accept help from others, another key component of successful ageing. And you don't have to offer your services to other people if you don't want to – why not volunteer at a local animal sanctuary?

Visit the café every morning Instead of drinking your coffee or tea at home alone, have it in the company of the 'regulars' at your local café or coffee shop. Not only will you get a boost from the caffeine (which studies find reduces the risk of depression by more than 50 per cent), but you'll also get another boost from the social scene, and once you become one of the regular faces, you'll make new friends.

Commit to connections Instead of a vague, 'we must get together some time', whip out your diary and ask which day is best. That which we put off till tomorrow … well, you know what happens.

Weed out bad connections If you want to get the most from your relationships, quality is better than quantity. To find the time to focus on the best relationships, weed out the people who suck energy and joy from your life (like your friend who never stops whining about her sore back, her credit card bill and her 35-year-old son still living at home, and who never asks how you are). Next time she calls, gently extricate yourself from the conversation. After a couple of times, she'll get the message. If not, have the courage to say what you mean. Be kind but honest: 'I just don't think our relationship is working. I need to pull back for a while. I hope you understand.' The short-term pain will be worth the long-term gain.

Develop rituals with others We know of a couple who like to host an annual karaoke evening. Another family celebrates the first sighting of the spring daffodils with an open house, and a third has a summer barbecue that's a must on every calendar in the neighbourhood. Such activities keep you connected with people in your life, provide pleasurable activities to plan for, and ensure that you'll have regular opportunities for meeting new people (tell your old friends to bring a new friend).

Visit a nursing home It may sound depressing, but it's one of the best things you can do for yourself and the residents of the home. Ask the staff to recommend someone who doesn't get many, if any, visitors. Introduce yourself and start talking. Most important: listen. Ask the person about his or her family, former job and so on. If you don't click with one person, try another. You'll make a friend, and you'll be helping someone else even more than you're helping yourself. It also provides a powerful motivation to keep up with all the other advice in this book, to ensure that you maintain your own independence and physical strength. ■

Sometimes, an exchange of smiles is the best medicine in the world

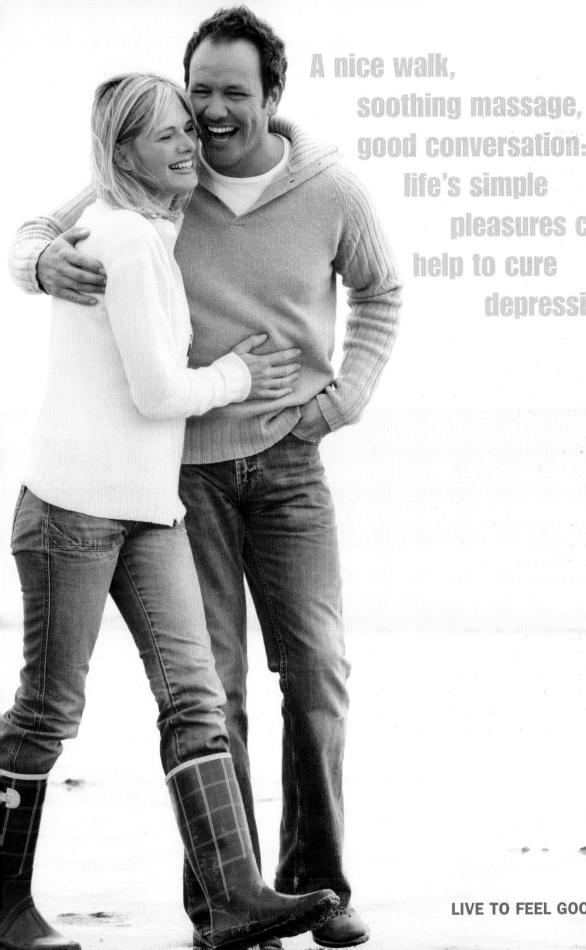

A nice walk,
soothing massage,
good conversation:
life's simple
pleasures can
help to cure
depression

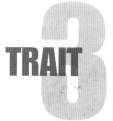

TRAIT 3 An ability to manage depression

When it comes to avoiding the frailty and disability of ageing, nothing beats preventing or treating depression. While we've known for years that depression significantly increases your risk of death from heart disease, a major Norwegian study has found it also increases the risk of death from stroke, pneumonia, influenza, Parkinson's disease and multiple sclerosis. One American study found that people with symptoms of depression were 42 per cent more likely to develop diabetes – the worse the depression, the higher the risk of diabetes. And a Dutch study showed that a history of depression raised the risk of Alzheimer's disease by 2.5 times.

Depression is far more than just a low mood. Feelings of sadness and a lack of enjoyment of normal activities occur for most of the day, almost every day, and persist for weeks without relief. Typically they are most intense at the start of the day. People affected lose motivation, may find it difficult to concentrate and may feel exhausted, irritable, guilty, hopeless or worthless. General aches and pains may develop along with headaches, palpitations and chest pain, and sleep patterns and appetite are disturbed.

This is a complicated condition with many interacting causes. Sometimes depression is set off by external events, such as bereavement, debt, major surgery or a diagnosis of serious illness, including cancer or a heart attack. And sometimes it just happens – so-called endogenous depression. People with a family history of depression seem to be more vulnerable, as do those who abuse alcohol or drugs. Even some prescribed medications may precipitate depression. People with sleep disorders, women with young children and unemployed people are all more likely to become depressed, as are people in unhappy marriages, whereas those with supportive relationships seem to be protected. Some diseases, such as an underactive thyroid gland, are directly linked with depression. And researchers from the Institute for the Health of the Elderly at the University of Newcastle upon Tyne have shown that depression in later life may be associated with narrowing and hardening of the arteries supplying the brain.

The link between depression, disease and death? Recently an outpouring of research has highlighted links with chronic inflammation – the state of heightened immune system activity that doctors now believe is the underlying cause of so many diseases. People who are depressed have overactive immune systems that produce inflammation-promoting chemicals such as cytokines, which are known to influence many conditions that become more common with age. And people with inflammatory diseases are more likely to become depressed. Those with

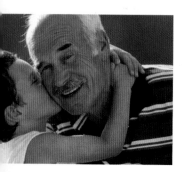

Depression is not a prolonged bad mood. It's a serious disease, connected to many major causes of death

rheumatoid arthritis, for example, are two or three times as likely to become depressed as the rest of the general population – and when they are depressed their arthritis tends to get worse. This suggests that there is 'cross-talk' between the brain and the immune system.

Stress increases the production of cytokines, which may explain why stressful events can precipitate depression. Both stress and depression increase the risk of infections, which in turn promotes a further output of cytokines. The same vicious circle occurs with sleep disorders. There is also some evidence that stress and depression may permanently alter immune responsiveness, so that cytokine production and an enhanced inflammatory response are more likely even with minor stress or trivial infections.

All of which may explain why sometimes depression is prolonged, hard to treat and recurrent, and why it is linked with many chronic diseases associated with ageing. The good news is that taking steps to reduce stress, depression or inflammation may all enhance health. According to psychiatrists at the University of Glasgow, antidepressant drugs have potential anti-inflammatory effects, and treatments that reduce inflammation may have antidepressant effects. By getting your depression under control, you can minimise its impact on your overall life expectancy. So get professional help if you need it, and meanwhile try these tactics to prevent depression, or reduce its effects if it does.

Pick a walkable neighbourhood to live in

Exercise triggers the release of a mood-enhancing brain chemical called serotonin. In one study, regular exercise was as effective as medication in improving symptoms of depression. More time spent outdoors has also been shown to reduce depression – light boosts serotonin production, too, and contact with nature reduces stress and depression.

A study of 740 older adults found that living in 'walkable' neighbourhoods protected older men from depression better than less walker-friendly areas. And it wasn't just the exercise that played a role, but something within the neighbourhood itself, possibly the sense of connection it provided.

Do something – anything – relaxing

Depression feeds on stress. Get practice in managing your stress levels before tension and anxiety become overwhelming. It doesn't really matter what you do, as long as it's effective. Take up yoga, learn to meditate, have a massage or try deep breathing exercises, guided imagery or progressive relaxation techniques – all easily learned at home from books or audiotapes.

Get help for a troubled relationship

Surprisingly perhaps, marriage seems to be quite good for depression – in one study, depressed people who got married scored much lower on a depression test than those who stayed single. But other studies suggest that unhappy marriages are linked with depression, and getting divorced even more so. So it's worth seeking help if you can (see the Resources section).

Eat more omega-3s
The good fats in oily fish and some vegetables are not just good for your physical health, they may also protect against depression. Countries with higher rates of fish consumption generally have lower rates of depression – so make sure you get your two portions of oily fish a week, and keep a container of flaxseeds in the fridge. The seed of the flax plant is one of the richest dietary sources of omega-3 fatty acids, and many studies find that this valuable fat significantly reduces the risk of depression. Sprinkle it over yoghurt and salads, mix into pasta sauce or blend into smoothies.

But consume less vegetable oil Just as important as adding omega-3s to your diet is cutting back on omega-6 fatty acids, found in vegetable oils used to make everything from margarine to cakes to crisps. One study found that people with major depression had nearly 18 times as many omega-6s as omega-3s in their blood, compared with about 13 times as many for subjects who weren't depressed.

Take a B-vitamin supplement A major Finnish study found that taking B supplements boosts the benefits of depression treatment. Other studies found low blood levels of vitamin B_{12} and folate (another B vitamin) in depressed people, with older women with vitamin B_{12} deficiencies having twice the risk of depression compared with women with normal blood levels of the vitamin. The benefit is probably related to the importance of B vitamins in brain health and their ability to reduce levels of homocysteine, a marker of inflammation that has also been linked to depression.

Touch your loved ones The bottom line – particularly for women – is that the more loved you feel, the less likely you are to become depressed. So, arrange a lunch date with a good friend; work on your relationship with your children; tell your partner 'I love you' every day; and light candles and get out the massage oil – this is the time to bring sex back into your life. What better way to feel loved than to make love?

Talk to your GP As mentioned, your depression may not be related to anything emotional but rather to something physical. And given all the links between depression and physical diseases, it's worth getting your general health checked. Most importantly, your GP can recognise and treat depression before it gets worse. Many people with depression delay talking to their doctor – but it's one of the most common problems that GPs deal with, and 90 per cent of people can be successfully treated by their GP alone.

Take a brisk 15 minute walk a day You probably know that exercise can help to prevent or treat mild depression. For years, though, researchers thought you needed a pretty high level for it to have any effect. But one study found that just 15 minutes at a brisk pace could help, bringing greater energy, less tiredness, more pleasurable emotions and a greater feeling of calmness. And in a survey from University College London, just 20 minutes of sustained activity each week – anything from jogging to housework, as long as it's enough to work up a bit of a sweat – had a positive effect on mood.

Mix up a bowl of guacamole Filled with healthy monounsaturated fat, the avocados in this tasty snack are also great sources of folate. A Finnish study found that people with the highest amounts of folate in their diets had the lowest risk of depression.

Walk outside in the sun, particularly during winter You need a daily dose of sunlight to keep seasonal affective disorder, or SAD, at bay. This form of depression is related to a lack of ultraviolet light. If the weather is too bad for walking, consider buying a full-spectrum light, which mimics natural sunlight (see our Resources section for retailers).

Visit public gardens once a week Walk around the gardens in all seasons and note what's new and how the winter landscape differs from that of spring and summer. The peacefulness of the place will help to reduce stress. ■

Are you depressed?

To determine if you might be depressed – or close to it – choose the best answer for the following questions, focusing on your emotions and thoughts of just the past week.

yes/no

1 Are you basically satisfied with your life? ☐ ○

2 Have you dropped many of your activities and interests? ○ ☐

3 Do you feel that your life is empty? ○ ☐

4 Do you often get bored? ○ ☐

5 Are you in good spirits most of the time? ☐ ○

6 Are you afraid that something bad is going to happen to you? ○ ☐

7 Do you feel happy most of the time? ☐ ○

8 Do you often feel helpless? ○ ☐

9 Do you prefer to stay at home rather than going out and doing new things? ○ ☐

10 Do you feel you have more problems with memory than most? ○ ☐

11 Do you think it is wonderful to be alive now? ☐ ○

12 Do you feel pretty worthless the way you are now? ○ ☐

13 Do you feel full of energy? ☐ ○

14 Do you feel that your situation is hopeless? ○ ☐

15 Do you think that most people are better off than you are? ○ ☐

Now count the number of circles you checked and find your score

0–4: Relax; you're doing well and have nothing to worry about in terms of depression. But retake this test every six months just to be sure.

5–8: You may have some mild depression. Now is the time to talk to a friend, spiritual adviser or therapist to make sure it doesn't become any worse and to identify steps you can take to improve it.

9–11: You may have moderate depression. You should make an appointment with your GP to discuss possible solutions, which could involve cognitive behaviour therapy or medication.

12–15: You are at risk of severe depression. Call your doctor immediately and ask for an urgent appointment. The sooner you get help, the better you will feel – and the less likely you are to damage your health.

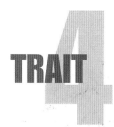

Spiritual engagement

TRAIT 4

Are you a spiritual person? Spirituality may become important when you start to ask 'why' about life, when you feel a sense of the mystery of it all or foster a belief that there is more to life than what we can see or fully understand. As one researcher noted, 'Spirituality is the ability to stand outside of ourselves and consider the meaning of our actions, the complexity of our motives and the impact we have on the world.' That could be religion – or not.

Spirituality is also strongly connected with resilience and successful ageing. For instance, a spiritual outlook on life enables you to focus beyond any physical disabilities because the spiritual perception views such functioning as just one aspect of living. It also helps you to answer and cope with the question of 'Why me?' when bad things happen because it helps you to view yourself as part of something bigger, not as the centre of the world.

A spiritual perspective also helps you to cope with situations that you can't control, which is a key component of stress. If you view the world as bigger than yourself and admit to the existence of some 'greater power', whether it's God or something else, it becomes easier to relinquish control.

Spirituality also focuses your mind on the present, emphasising mindfulness over the way we tend to rush and focus on the future so much in modern life. Finally, a spiritual perspective recognises the importance of social support, in terms of both giving and receiving. All have been found to improve overall health and well-being and to help people to age better, regardless of any physical or mental disabilities.

For instance, one study of 400 elderly Brazilians found that those who perceived their health to be good or very good were five times more likely to be 'ageing successfully' than those who perceived their health as bad. However, those who said their personal beliefs gave meaning to their lives were *ten times* more likely to be classified as ageing successfully.

Other studies of older adults find that attending religious services once a week significantly reduces levels of inflammatory markers in the blood and leads to lower death rates over a 12 year period regardless of a person's weight, diseases, social support network, depression levels or age.

Researchers from the University of Dundee found that people who had strong religious beliefs were less likely to be lonely in older age, while Canadian researchers found that older people who participated in church-related activities were much healthier overall over a six year period than those who didn't take part in such activities. In fact, other researchers found that once-a-week churchgoers had lower blood pressure, less abdominal fat, higher HDL cholesterol (the good kind) and lower levels of inflammatory stress hormones than people who skipped Sunday services.

For many, spirituality and organised religion are one and the same – but they needn't be. A passion for nature, a belief in healing energy, faith in science and the natural laws of existence or merely a strong sense of good versus evil can all provide purpose and direction in your life. What ultimately matters to your health isn't *what* you believe in but merely that you believe in *something* with your heart and soul.

Even if you aren't religious or spiritual today, you're likely to become more so as you age. Studies find that religion appears to increase with age as spirituality becomes more important.

Pause and give thanks – it enriches your

While we strongly believe in the power of spirituality to help people to live longer, healthier lives, we also acknowledge that this is particularly personal, fraught with emotions, traditions, history and even politics. That said, here are a few suggestions that you may find useful in growing your personal spirituality.

For health, focus on yourself As we all know, there is a difference between personal spirituality and organised religion. Spirituality is about one person – you. Organised religion can be a path to personal spirituality, but it also encompasses much more. Whatever path you choose, it's what happens in your *own* heart and soul that matters to your health.

Find a spiritual adviser This could be a vicar, rabbi, imam, yoga instructor, teacher, close friend or even someone from your church who is grappling with the same questions you are. The two of you should meet weekly for an hour to talk about your week and address larger issues. Spiritual growth is achieved more easily through shared experience and discussion than in isolation.

Take up music or art Both enable you to express yourself, allowing you to reflect the sense of something larger than yourself in your work. Not only that, but these new skills have added benefits in terms of keeping your memory sharp and your mind clear.

Devote time to the spiritual Whether it's going to a church, meditating, taking a nature walk, reading a spiritual guide or saying a nightly prayer, spending regular time cultivating your sense of the greater good is rewarding for your mind, heart and overall health. ■

Are you spiritual?

Answer the following true-or-false questions to assess your current level of spirituality. Be honest – no one but you will know your answers. Remember too that there are no right or wrong answers. However, 'true' answers reflect a greater level of spirituality than 'false' answers. Retake the quiz every six months to see if your spiritual attitudes are evolving.

- I believe in the existence of a higher power.
- I often experience a heartfelt connection to nature.
- During spiritual moments, such as when praying or meditating, I often feel a joy beyond ordinary happiness.
- I believe that things happen that have no rational, scientific explanation.
- My religion or spirituality is the main source of moral guidelines in my life.
- Overall, I'm at peace with the world around me.
- Sometimes I ask for the help of a higher spiritual power.
- I genuinely feel thankful for all that I have.
- It is important to me to help others.
- I accept others even when they do things I think are wrong.
- I take time out at least once a week to focus on my spiritual or religious needs.
- I belong to a spiritual community or organisation.

heart, and protects it, too

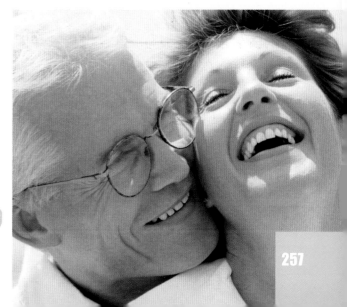

Resistance to stress

The word *stress* is so overused today that it has nearly lost its meaning. So, let's introduce some new words.

First, say hello to adrenaline, noradrenaline, cortisol, vasopressin and aldosterone. These are all hormones your body releases when a psychological or physical challenge suddenly confronts you. These chemicals play a major role in the inflammation we've talked about in this book. Recall that this inflammation damages cells, leading to a host of health problems. Every time you are scared, pressurised, angered or frustrated, your body releases chemicals that lead to inflammation, and this is one of the major problems caused by acute stress.

But there is fresh news in the world of stress. To understand it, you first need to know that there's a second type of stress that's much more problematic than the type caused when someone shouts an insult at you. *Chronic* psychological stress is when troubles gnaw at you persistently over time. Think of ongoing financial woes, out-of-control children, tough daily commutes, an underlying sense of insecurity and even deep resentments about neighbours. It turns out that chronic stress ages you cell by cell. It does so by shortening a part of the cell called a telomere.

Telomeres are caps on the ends of the cell's chromosomes that help to keep chromosomes stable, just as the cap on a pen prevents ink from leaking. Every time a chromosome unzips to make copies of its genetic material so the cell can divide, the telomere gets a tiny bit shorter. The shorter the telomere, the worse the cell functions. Studies link shrinking telomeres to numerous age-related conditions, including high blood pressure and cholesterol, insulin resistance and early death, primarily from infection and cardiovascular disease.

Telomeres get some help in maintaining their length from an enzyme called telomerase, which is released by immune system cells. Telomerase builds up telomeres after replication, keeping the cell alive longer and functioning better. Eventually, however, the telomere gets so short it disappears, and the cell self-destructs and dies.

The new discovery: chronic psychological stress can shrink telomeres the same way hot water shrinks a woolly jumper. It also seems to lower the amount of telomerase the immune cells release. And, in a vicious circle, the less telomerase you have, the greater your body's response to stress and the more inflammatory chemicals released.

These findings are important because they show how psychological issues such as stress have a harmful physical effect on our cells. The findings also provide crucial good news: it's how you *perceive* stress, rather than the actual cause of the stress, that leads to the harm.

If you can find ways to inoculate your body against overreacting to perceived stressors, you will halt the flow of inflammatory chemicals and stop unnatural damage to your cells' telomeres. One study found that people who practised transcendental meditation for 16 weeks had much better blood pressure, insulin resistance and heart-rate readings when exposed to stress compared with those who didn't meditate.

This all becomes even more important as you age, since studies find that your body's reaction to stress *increases* with age.

Along those lines, then, here's our advice for protecting yourself against the ageing effects of stress and changing your conscious perception of the stress you encounter. Add these tips to those in the sections above, and you will have all the information you need to live more calmly and happily and for a longer time. ▶

conquering clutter

There – in that pile of month-old post. There – in that stack of newspapers. There – in the collection of china scattered across the mantelpiece, in the overstuffed hall cupboard, in the junk under your bed. Clutter! The bane of a long-lived life.

Clutter means more than a messy living room. It takes away your sense of control ('I just don't know what to do with all this stuff.'). It isolates you ('I can't invite anyone over to the house until I get the clutter under control.'). Clutter can even be physically dangerous, leading to tripping accidents, increased allergens and insects and other vermin.

1 Make a list of cluttered spaces you wish to clear out. It could include drawers, cupboards or surfaces. Do not list an entire room, such as 'living room'.

2 Schedule 'clutter-control' mornings or evenings, giving yourself enough time to complete one item on your list.

3 Approach the cluttered area with three boxes labelled 'keep', 'donate' and 'rubbish'.

4 Pull every item out of or off the cluttered area. Don't put anything back without asking yourself the following questions.

- 'Have I used this in the past six months?'
- 'Will I need to use this in the coming six months?'
- 'Does this hold significant sentimental value?'

If the answer is **no** to all of these questions, put the item in the donation or rubbish box. If the

The key to controlling clutter is to start with a little at a time and maintain the clear space as you move towards the next cluttered area. Here, then, is our clutter-control prescription.

answer is **yes** to any of these questions, ask yourself one more:

- 'Does this need to be in this location, or is there a better place for it?'

Then put it in a more appropriate spot.

5 Once you've completed the decluttering, take a picture. Tape the picture to the bottom of the decluttered drawer, stick it on the inside of the door of the decluttered cupboard or tuck it under an item on the shelf/desk.

6 Make sure you give away your donations within a week of the clean-up. You may need to do some research about who accepts what and whether they will collect. Likewise, some rubbish – such as old cans of paint or glue – needs special treatment. Whatever you do, don't just transfer the clutter from one space to another. The job isn't done until the rubbish and donations are long gone.

Every week, look at a photo you took of your cleaned and organised room. It will motivate you like nothing else to keep it clutter-free

Just choose not to There's an old expression: 'don't take the bait'. It means that when given the opportunity to get angry or stressed, choose not to. Make this your mantra. The next time someone does something that would typically anger you or increase your stress, smile, let the hostile emotions pass right by and deal with things calmly. Over time, you can teach yourself an amazing amount of healthy self-restraint, even in the face of constant pressure.

Walk away Any time – and we mean *any time* – you can feel your heart rate rising due to stress or anger, excuse yourself from the situation and do what it takes to recover. Breathe deeply, think positive thoughts, go outside, have some cold water, force yourself to smile and remind yourself that you are in control. Re-enter the situation only when you know that you can handle it calmly and positively. You'll not only help your health but also prevent challenging situations from deteriorating further.

Practise mindfulness Mindfulness is a way of approaching life based on the concept that 'the present is the only time that any of us have to be alive – to know anything – to perceive – to learn – to act – to change – to heal,' according to its originator, Jon Kabat-Zinn. It's a technique shown to have multiple health benefits, and has successfully alleviated anxiety and depression in many people. The idea is to focus on your thoughts, so that when you ruminate on negatives you can redirect your attention elsewhere. For instance, you might redirect your musings about a big car repair bill to the day you spent last week with your grandson. When people practise this every day for about 30 minutes, their stress levels and feelings of being overwhelmed fall and their sense of coping increases.

A specific technique called Mindfulness-based Cognitive Therapy (MBCT), partly developed by Professor Mark Williams at the Centre for Mindfulness Research and Practice at Bangor University, has been shown in trials to help even relapsing depression resistant to ordinary treatments – so much so that the National Institute of Clinical Excellence (NICE) now recommends it for such patients on the NHS. You can learn this form of mindfulness meditation through classes, tapes or books.

Turn on Beethoven People who feel stressed are more likely to listen to music than they are to do anything else, including eating, crying or sleeping. Numerous studies find that listening to music during stressful situations, including surgery, reduces stress hormones. Our advice is to skip the heavy rock and stick with the classics. One study comparing Mozart with New Age music found that people listening to classical music relaxed more and reported greater levels of 'mental quiet', 'awe and wonder' and 'mystery', suggesting that the music provided a sense of spirituality as well.

Make yourself laugh Really. Start by smiling. Then say 'ha, ha, ha'. Then think about how ridiculous you look and let out a real laugh. Not working? Then try some of the ideas in our laughter advice for building resilience on page 241. Laughter helps to shut down your body's stress response, cutting off the release of harmful stress hormones. When researchers compared people who received an hour of quiet time with those who had an hour of humour and laughter, they found that the laughter group showed significant drops in the blood levels of several key stress hormones, while the group sitting quietly had no change.

Build bonding into your schedule We talked about social networks and friends earlier. This is so important to successful ageing that it's worth addressing again. Particularly for women, having close friends with whom to vent and bond makes more of a difference to chronic stress levels than the most luxuriant bubble bath.

Surround yourself with stress-relieving tools These include fresh flowers, peppermint or vanilla candles, pictures of people you love, photographs of a particularly good holiday, works of art and a sign that says 'Breathe'. All can reduce stress levels, studies find.

Stop multi-tasking All you're doing is increasing stress hormones on a regular basis, even when nothing really stressful is happening. Instead, do one thing at a time. When that one thing is particularly stressful, take a break before you move on to the next task. During that break time, practise your mindfulness meditation or deep breathing, or simply lie down with a cold cloth over your eyes and drift.

Clean a cupboard There is simply nothing that puts more control into your life than cleaning up a mess you encounter frequently.

Take up yoga Just one class is enough to reduce stress hormone levels, studies find.

Hold hands with your partner A good relationship is a great stress-buster. In fact, simply holding hands with someone you love reduces brain activity related to stress better than holding a stranger's hands. The better your relationship, the calmer the brain response.

Munch pistachios After four weeks of a heart-healthy diet containing 45–85g of pistachios daily, participants in one study had reduced stress responses, including lower blood pressure and greater artery relaxation.

Spend time in a garden Even if you live in a high-rise flat, try a container garden. The greenery has a tremendous effect when it comes to reducing stress. The best are 'healing gardens', which contain some form of water, green vegetation and flowers, in either an indoor or outdoor environment. Design it properly, though. The garden should be easily controlled and tended, offer social opportunities (with a bench or small table and chairs), allow for physical movement (an indoor or patio garden can do this with a variety of potted plants in different spaces and at different levels) and provide natural distractions (plants that attract butterflies are ideal). ▪

Stress isn't just in your mind. It is real, and affects your entire body in strong, measurable ways

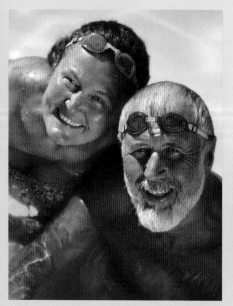

... dental problems   ... colds and flu

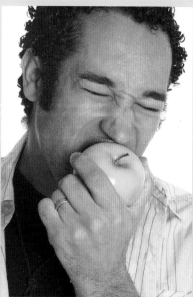

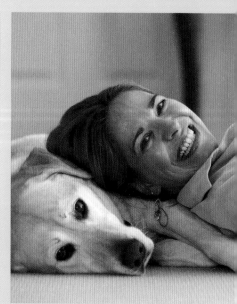

... balance   ... sleep problems

... joint and muscle pain

Take charge of
everyday health

Your body speaks to you all the time. But do you listen to what it's saying? Most people don't. Life is much easier if we ignore those little pains, that bad week of sleep, the occasional stomach ache, the recurrent colds. Most of the time the problem just goes away on its own, doesn't it?

And the truth is, a lot of people seem to get by just fine ignoring their symptoms and health problems. But that doesn't change this important fact: your body has told you that something is wrong, and you chose to ignore it. Perhaps your stomach pain was merely a reaction to a bad piece of fruit, or maybe it means that your stomach is beginning to have serious troubles. You just don't know.

Is this how you would treat a car that suddenly made odd noises, or what you would do if a wet spot started to appear on a ceiling at home? We hope not.

One of the great truisms of life is that a problem ignored is a problem that will soon grow worse. This holds true in relationships, the workplace, the government, your home and with your own body. Perhaps it's time to turn your ear inwards.

LISTENING AND REACTING

It's easy to categorise health into two parts. The first part is healthy everyday living and covers issues such as food, exercise, sleep, stress control and energy. Up until this point, we've focused

Your body constantly alerts you to potential health trouble ahead. Your job is to listen – and respond

entirely on just this – how to live every moment in a way that will extend and enrich your health and happiness for decades to come.

The second part of health is what you could call 'capital-letter' diseases: formally named health issues such as diabetes, arthritis, asthma, cancer and hundreds of other diagnosable chronic conditions. These are the age robbers, the killers, the conditions that researchers focus on, the ones all of us fear and each of us wants to avoid. These conditions are the focus of part 4 of this book, 'Preventing the diseases of ageing'; there we'll show you all the best ways to prevent these health traps of the future from catching you.

But there's a third part to health, and that's the focus of the next pages. It's the small health problems, the symptoms, the nagging little health issues that mean you fall between being healthy and having a serious chronic disease.

Starting from around the age of 45, most adults begin to experience more nagging symptoms than when they were younger. The main reason is simple – after four decades of life, natural wear-and-tear is beginning to catch up with you. Suddenly, your joints hurt more, your digestion isn't so reliable, your hearing is less sharp and your alertness is in decline come midafternoon.

More often than not, these health issues are small. But our message is big: by taking positive steps to remedy small health issues now, you are taking positive steps to lengthen your life and stay vibrant when you're older.

Why? Because symptoms are exactly that: the way an emerging problem reveals itself to you. The pain isn't the real problem, for example; it's the cause of the pain that often matters more. Or take a cold. You may be focused on stopping your runny nose, but that's not the most important task to consider – it's stopping the underlying virus from spreading. One doesn't have much to do with the other.

In the pages ahead, you'll discover clever ways to remedy several of the most common symptoms and simple health problems of people aged 40 and above. More importantly, you'll find these remedies also address the underyling health issues.

You'll probably recognise many of these problems – from sore gums to aching leg veins, common colds to after-dinner indigestion, these are the most regular everyday health complaints of adults. We also address a few more specialised issues, such as a decreasing sense of balance and skin problems, which if you handle them now, should have minimal impact on you later.

The big message: long-life living is more than just eating well, exercising and maintaining a great attitude. It also includes listening to your body, and responding quickly and thoughtfully to what it's telling you. With the quick-healing advice in the pages ahead, you'll find out what you need to get the healthy long life you want. ■

It happens to *everyone* at some time. You get lightheaded, or your foot catches on a loose rug or you don't spot that patch of ice. Suddenly, you're on the ground, hurt and embarrassed. If only we could all instantly bounce back up like six year olds. Unfortunately, as you age, falling becomes more than just a passing episode barely to be considered; instead, it becomes a serious risk to your health and independence.

People generally underestimate the impact of falling, and the potentially dire consequences, even at a relatively young age. A single fall can be even more debilitating than a heart attack. If you're over 65 and you fall and break a hip, for instance, you have a 33 per cent risk of dying the following year. If you consider that one out of every three people over 65 falls each year, the scope of the damage is pretty considerable.

Overall, falls are the leading cause of injury, death and disability among people aged 65 and older. Yes, that's right: you're more likely to die from falling in the bathroom than from being in a car accident. Yet by government estimates, half of all falls are preventable. That's why balance is part of the fitness pyramid on page 197.

We don't want you suddenly to become obsessed with falling, but a little mindfulness and some pre-emptive home adjustments could go a long way towards diminishing this concern now and for decades to come.

Evaluate your balance

It's simple enough. You need either a stopwatch or someone to help you who has a watch with a second hand. Wear flat shoes or have bare feet. Stand up straight with a countertop or chair back in front of you – to grab if you wobble. If you are frail, have osteoporosis or balance problems, stand in front of a bed as well, and have someone else around in case you fall.

When you're ready, fold your arms across your chest, shut your eyes and at the same time raise one leg, bending it at the knee as close to a right angle as you can. At the moment you raise your leg, start the stopwatch or have your partner note the position of the second hand. Stop timing as soon as you either uncross your arms or have to put your foot down. You can try this several times if you like – the sensation can take a bit of getting used to. Then take a break for a few minutes and repeat with the other leg.

Here are the average scores per age group:
- 20–49: 26 seconds
- 50–59: 21 seconds
- 60–69: 10 seconds
- 70–79: 4 seconds
- 80+: most people can't keep their foot off the floor for more than a second or two.

If your time is less than the average for your age, talk to your GP in case any health problems or medication are affecting your balance. If you managed less than 26 seconds – whatever your age – look at our suggestions for improving your balance. Then take the test again in a few weeks to see if your time has improved.

Improve your balance

Exercise, exercise, exercise No matter what you do – walking, strength-training or specific balance exercises – it will help your balance. One physical activity touted for improving balance is the ancient Chinese martial art of tai chi (see page 181). Yoga, dance, hiking and stretching also challenge your sense of balance, as do sports that emphasise side-to-side movement, such as badminton, tennis and football.

Try an exercise ball These giant balls are ideal for strengthening parts of your body to prevent falls, and they improve your overall balance. Sit on the ball with your feet about hip-width apart on the floor, then do the following exercises.

Hula Pretend you're balancing a glass of champagne on your head as you shift your hips in a circular motion from right to front and left to back, as if doing the hula. Try not to move your upper body at all. Repeat five times each way.

Foot lifts Slowly raise one foot, keeping the other on the floor. Try to maintain your balance and stability by tightening your core (abdomen, chest and back). Count to three, then gently return your foot to the floor and raise the other. Repeat ten times on each side. As you get better at balancing, increase the amount of time each foot is raised.

Knee lifts Tighten your core, then try raising your knees together without falling backwards. Initially, you might try lifting one knee at a time until your balance improves. Repeat five times with each knee, ten times if you're lifting both.

Get off the beaten path Take walks frequently on natural surfaces rather than paved walkways. A nature path, with its tree roots and rocks, presents a great challenge to your sense of balance. The same is true of a sandy beach.

Wear shoes that grip the ground Yes, life sometimes calls for high heels, dress shoes or, best of all, dance shoes. But for everyday life, wear shoes that have the best possible traction. Today, every style of shoe – from sleek work shoes to sandals – is available with rubber soles that are as ground-grabbing as hiking shoes.

Vibrating shoes?

In the not-too-distant future, you may put on a pair of vibrating shoes to prevent falls. A study published in the medical journal the *Lancet* found that these shoes, which include a pair of battery-operated insoles that randomly vibrate so slightly you can't even feel it, improved balance in older people. They help to boost the messages your nervous system sends to your brain when you walk and turn, enabling you to adjust your posture. The shoes aren't available yet, but their success in studies means you could see them soon.

Take a calcium/magnesium/vitamin D supplement daily While it won't build bone you've already lost, this mineral/vitamin combination can help to slow any future loss. The stronger your bones, the less likely you are to fall and, if you do fall, to seriously injure yourself. Vitamin D also contributes to neuromuscular strength. One analysis of five studies found that taking this vitamin reduced the risk of falls by more than 20 per cent.

Review your medication Get out all of the medication and vitamin, mineral, herb and other nutritional supplements you're taking – even if you take them only once a week or once a month – and list the names, dosages and when and how you take them. Then ask your GP if any individual medication or supplements (or combinations of them) could contribute to dizziness or balance problems.

Drink up If you spend most of your time at home, keep a large jug filled with iced water or diluted juice in your fridge and be sure to drink all of it – or more – every day. If you're on the road, carry a large refillable water bottle with you. Dehydration, which becomes more common as we age, can contribute to low blood pressure, dizziness and falls.

Consider hip protectors If your risk of falling is particularly high due to age or infirmity, wear padded cloths that either sit on the hip joint or are built into special underwear. If you do fall, these pads, available at many health supply shops or online, reduce the risk of hip fracture by shunting the energy away from the point of impact. In one study, frail women living in their homes who wore hip pads reduced their risk of hip fracture by nearly 80 per cent.

Reduce fall risk at home

Alarm your pets A cat weaving in and out of your legs or a dog sneaking up behind you is a fall waiting to happen. Add a bell or jangling tag to your pet's collar to avoid surprises.

Buy lots of double-sided carpet tape Use it to prevent rugs from slipping and sliding. Also put non-slip mats by the side of the bath and in front of the shower, and at bathroom and kitchen sinks.

Call an electrician Have sockets added in rooms where you have electrical cords attached to extension cords. The fewer cords, the less likely you are to trip over one. Also ask the electrician to install extra light fixtures in dark areas of your home, such as hallways, and make sure you have switches at the top *and* bottom of your stairs, and at both ends of corridors.

Measure your thresholds Doorway thresholds should be no more than 1.3cm (½in) high; otherwise, they're tripping hazards. Replace high thresholds with lower ones.

Evaluate your stairways Are the backs of your steps closed in? Are there handrails about waist height on both sides? Do the steps have non-slip surfaces? In addition to good lighting, these will reduce your risk of falling.

Visit the flooring shop If it's time to replace that carpet anyway, consider hard-surface flooring or Berber-style carpeting. Both are less likely to trip you up than most popular deep-pile carpets. Just make sure the flooring isn't slippery. There's even a special kind of hard-surface flooring that's been developed for nursing homes that you might consider for your kitchen or bathroom. It's designed to provide a firm walking surface, but if you do fall, it reduces the force of impact. It's similar to the type of flooring you might see in a dance or Pilates studio and can be ordered through commercial flooring distributors.

Add extra phones The closer the phone is, the less likely you are to run to answer it, reducing your risk of tripping and falling. Also make sure you have a phone extension by your bed.

Check outside lighting Make sure you have outside lights with high-wattage bulbs (75 watts or more) near all entrances and the garage. If you are likely to be out and about after dark, install lights with motion sensors that come on automatically as you approach. Put high-wattage bulbs (if appropriate for the fitting) in all the lamps and overhead lights indoors as well.

Forget about floor wax If you must use it, make sure it's the non-slip type.

Attach your reading glasses or bifocals to a cord or chain around your neck That way, when you walk upstairs – or anywhere else – you can take them off and let them hang. If you keep them on, they affect your distance vision, so you may misjudge a step; if you take them off and hold them in one hand, you're more likely to lose your balance and fall. ■

why we fall

No one forgets how to walk. But starting as early as our 40s, any number of physical factors make us more prone to falls. With time, many of these risks grow considerably. Be most mindful of the following.

LACK OF EXERCISE Leg weakness is the greatest cause of falls, increasing your fall risk more than fourfold. Weak muscles not only make you prone to falling but also make it less likely that you'll break your fall or regain your balance if you start to slip. If you have time for only one activity, make it walking or leg strength-training.

VISION PROBLEMS Eye conditions such as glaucoma, macular degeneration and cataracts become more common with age; because sight often deteriorates gradually, you may not notice at first. It's important to detect such conditions early. Don't just accept vision changes as part of ageing – there are usually effective treatments to preserve your sight from further damage. Have your eyes tested regularly by an optometrist (optician) – if you're over 60, you're entitled to free vision checks on the NHS.

MEDICATION Certain types of medication, including antidepressants, anti-arrhythmia drugs, digoxin and diuretics, significantly increase your risk of a fall. Plus, if you're taking three or more types of medication, you're also more likely to fall.

ENVIRONMENTAL HAZARDS Rugs, clutter and overcrowded rooms become minefields as you age. Even wall-to-wall carpeting can be a tripping risk if the sole of your shoe catches on it. Other potential problems in your home include low lighting, missing or loose handrails on stairs and lack of handrails in the shower/bath.

ARTHRITIS If you have arthritis, you're more than twice as likely to fall as someone without it. It's not the arthritis itself that increases the risk but the fact that people with it often stop exercising, so their muscles become weak. This doesn't have to happen. See page 349 for ways to maintain your strength even if you have arthritis.

DEPRESSION Depression doubles your risk of falling. Possible reasons include not paying attention to your surroundings, drinking more alcohol and eating less, or the side effects of medication.

AGE If you're over 80, your risk of falling is double that of someone younger.

PREVIOUS FALLS If you've fallen before, you're three times more likely to fall again than someone who has never fallen.

Colds and flu

How is it possible that you've seen men walk on the moon in your lifetime but no one's come up with a cure for the common cold? It's because getting to the moon is *easy* compared with curing colds. Space travel is just a matter of figuring out how to get from one point to another. When it comes to colds, however, researchers have to contend with more than 100 different cold-causing viruses, all of which are constantly changing.

The common cold has been around since the days of ancient Egypt; the Greek physician Hippocrates described colds as early as the 5th century BC. Today, adults typically get two to four colds a year. While primarily simply a nuisance in younger people, in older people colds can be the precursors of more serious diseases, such as bronchitis and viral pneumonia.

The flu isn't much easier to confront. Another illness that's been around for a long time (the first flu epidemic was recorded in AD 1173), it's also caused by wily viruses that change almost weekly.

Like colds, the flu is much more dangerous in older people than in younger folk. Most of the 36,000 yearly deaths from influenza that occur in the United States, for example, are in people aged over 65. Overall, those aged 75 and older have the greatest risk of dying from the flu, followed by children under the age of four.

Have you got into the habit of ignoring minor colds and flu? That could spell trouble as you get older. Take charge of colds and flu today so they won't become issues tomorrow.

To prevent colds and flu

Set a timer for 45 minutes, five days a week That's all the time you need to spend exercising over a year to reduce your risk of colds by more than threefold. And we're talking about moderate exercise, such as walking or cycling at an intensity level that still enables you to talk. As it turns out, moderate exercise is one of the best ways to prevent viral infections.

Don't worry; be happy And you'll have fewer colds – even if a researcher happens to squirt some cold virus in

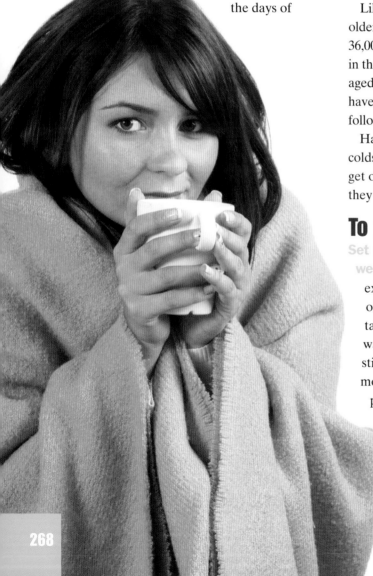

your nose. It seems people who are happy, relaxed and energetic are simply less likely to catch colds, even if they're infected with the virus. Researchers have yet to figure out the link between psychological states and the immune system, but studies confirm it exists.

Carry some hand cleaner If you think that coughs and sneezes are the most likely way to spread diseases, you're wrong. You're far more likely to catch someone's cold by shaking hands. In fact, you're more at risk of infection from a handshake than from kissing. That's why hospitals now encourage medical staff to use hand-sanitiser gel before touching patients, and why it's a good idea for you to carry a little bottle of it with you wherever you go. If you can't avoid shaking hands, rub yours well with the gel as soon as you can – and avoid touching your face in the meantime so germs don't transfer to your nose.

Wipe down your hotel room Start packing a disinfectant spray or mini-wipes to rid your room of the previous occupants' germs. When researchers infected volunteers with cold viruses and had them spend the night in a hotel room, they found afterwards that nearly everything in the room – from the telephone to the light switch, taps and TV remote control – was contaminated with the virus. Even though the room has been cleaned, it's a pretty good bet the cleaner didn't disinfect the phones, light switches and remote control.

Take some vitamin C There's a lot of controversy over the benefits of vitamin C when it comes to preventing or treating colds. One thing is quite clear, though: it doesn't make much difference in treating colds or reducing their severity or duration. A large Japanese study found, however, that people who took daily doses

The etiquette of sneezing

Don't cover your mouth with your hand when you cough or sneeze. Instead, do what your children and grandchildren may have been trained to do: sneeze or cough into the crook of your elbow. That way you don't touch your mouth, nose or eyes with your elbow, nor do you shake hands or smooth a child's hair with it, so you'll be less likely to pass on the germs.

of vitamin C over five years had many fewer colds than people who skipped the extra C. If you choose to take supplements, take 500mg a day. Participants taking this dosage were a third less likely to have three or more colds during the study than those taking just 50mg.

Swallow a garlic supplement daily It won't cure the common cold, but it may help to prevent it. That's what British researchers found when they gave 146 volunteers either daily garlic capsules or placebos from November through to February (the primary cold season). There were 24 colds in the garlic group versus 65 in the placebo group, a significant difference. Plus, the placebo group's colds lasted longer and were more severe than the garlic group's.

Get some sun Scientists now think that lack of vitamin D – correlated with the lack of sunshine in winter – helps to explain why winter is the peak season for colds and flu. In one study at the University of Tampere in Finland, young men with low levels of vitamin D were twice as likely to catch a cold over the winter season as those with higher levels. And several other studies have now shown that vitamin D, either produced by sunlight exposure or taken as a supplement, may protect against all kinds of respiratory infections. Why? Vitamin D is a key component in keeping the immune system ▶

a vaccine worth having

A flu jab doesn't just protect you against getting flu. More importantly, it may also protect you against complications of influenza, which can be serious in people who are elderly, frail or institutionalised, as well as in anyone who has multiple existing medical conditions.

Complications include a higher risk of hospitalisation for conditions such as pneumonia, heart failure and stroke, and a higher risk of dying as a result. Studies on the benefits of influenza vaccination among different groups have produced very varied results – possibly because of other differences between the people who are likely to get the vaccine and those who don't.

However, in general, although opinion differs on how well it may or may not protect elderly people, most studies do suggest significant benefits in terms of it lowering complication rates among vulnerable groups. That's why the NHS offers an annual flu vaccination to everyone over 65 and to anyone with chronic respiratory, heart, liver or kidney disease, diabetics and to people with compromised immune systems. The vaccine is also offered to people who live in nursing homes or other long-stay residential care, to carers of elderly or disabled people, and to health-care staff.

The vaccine has been proven to be safe and usually has no greater side effects than temporary mild soreness at the site of injection. It sometimes provokes flu-like symptoms such as mild fever or slight muscle aches for a day or two, as the body's immune system responds to the vaccine, but this does not lead to influenza itself – it can't, because live viruses are not used in the vaccine. Allergic or other reactions to the immunisation are extremely rare.

WHY YOU'LL NEED A JAB AGAIN NEXT YEAR

Should you get a flu jab each year? Yes – because the viruses that cause influenza change slightly from year to year, so a new vaccine has to be developed for each year's strains. It's important to get a flu jab annually if you're in any of the groups at risk of influenza complications.

WHEN IS THE JAB AVAILABLE?

As influenza occurs mostly in winter, with a peak between December and March, most GPs organise vaccination sessions in September and October, before the main flu season starts. It takes between 10 and 14 days for your immune system to respond fully to the jab by producing antibodies against influenza viruses.

WHAT ABOUT MERCURY IN THE VACCINE?

Some brands of flu vaccine contain thiomersal, a mercury-based preservative, so if you'd rather avoid this, ask your GP if it's possible to have a type that doesn't contain mercury. The flu vaccines that are thiomersal-free are as effective as those containing thiomersal, though availability will depend on your area.

from overreacting, thus reducing inflammation and oxidation (which are responsible for cold and flu symptoms). At the same time, vitamin D dramatically stimulates the production of cells that line the respiratory tract and help to prevent infection. Spending 20 minutes a day in the sun with your hands, face and arms exposed puts about 20,000 IU of vitamin D into your body within two days, compared with the 98 IU or so you get from milk.

Get control of your life Feeling out of control, whether at work or at home, stresses your immune system to the point where it overexerts and weakens itself, making you more likely to catch a cold. That's what researchers found when they studied more than 200 workers over three months. Even those who had control over their work were more likely to begin sneezing if they lacked confidence or tended to blame themselves when things went wrong.

Wash your hands again and again We're a world of dirty-handed people, which helps to spread cold and flu viruses. One study of 1,000 adults found that 43 per cent barely ever washed their hands after coughing or sneezing, 32 per cent didn't always wash before eating lunch and 54 per cent didn't wash long enough to remove germs and dislodge dirt effectively. In one study that measured the germ count on volunteers' hands, researchers found that washing just once, even with antibacterial soap, did little good in eradicating the culprits. So wash twice, and do it often. They found that after a year of regular washing, fewer microbes remained on volunteers' hands even after just one wash.

If you're already infected

Take time to heal Too many people try to tough out viral infections. But your body is designed to rest when it gets sick so it can focus all its internal healing resources on fighting the infection. Following your regular daily routine when you're sick denies your immune system the time and energy to focus on healing. Don't feel guilty about it. Just take a day or two off; set yourself up on the couch with a blanket, a book and plenty to drink; and let your body do the work of making you well.

Suck on zinc lozenges At the first sniffle, grab some zinc lozenges and suck on one every 3 or 4 hours for up to six days (don't chew them). According to the Common Cold Centre at Cardiff University, early treatment with zinc lozenges may shorten the duration of common cold symptoms by several days, although not all studies have shown benefits. But at least two well-designed clinical studies shown that the lozenges can reduce the severity and duration of the common cold, while another study of 66 women between the ages of 60 and 91 who had serious medical conditions found that the lozenges were safe.

See your GP if you're in an at-risk group If you're in one of the groups eligible for the vaccine, see your doctor at the first sign of flu symptoms – or even if you've just been exposed to someone affected, if you haven't had the vaccine or it hasn't yet had two weeks to start working. Your GP may be able to give you a prescription for an antiviral medication such as oseltamivir (Tamiflu) or zanamivir (Relenza). The drugs only shorten the duration of symptoms by between 24 and 36 hours, but they may help to you avoid complications. You need to start taking medication within 48 hours of the first symptom or the close contact with someone who's already got flu. In any case, see a doctor if your symptoms are severe or haven't cleared up within a week.

Have a little horseradish or hot sauce with dinner to clear out your sinuses. Who cares that it's not 'medicine'? It works!

Use a sports cream for your aching muscles Viral infections often make your muscles ache. While there are over-the-counter pain-relievers that work well, if you're looking for something that won't affect your liver or stomach, try a deep-heat rub or spray, made for sports injuries.

Start cooking When the cold season hits, it's time to make a pot of vegetable soup. Your grandmother knew what she was doing as she spooned the steaming broth into your mouth when you were a child. Not only does the steam help to open stuffed sinuses, but the antioxidants in the vegetables used to make the soup help to reduce the inflammatory response of your immune system to a cold.

Open up clogged sinuses with dinner In addition to the aforementioned vegetable soup, sushi with wasabi, roast beef with horseradish sauce and spicy chilli or curry are other delicious ways to thin mucus and clear your head during a cold.

To boost flu vaccine effectiveness

The flu vaccine works by introducing your immune system to the flu virus so it can develop an antibody response more quickly when the real thing appears. The older you are, however, the less effective the vaccine. The following can help to supercharge your immune system so the vaccine works better.

Meditate Researchers have found that people who meditate regularly show significant changes in areas of the brain related to the ability to adapt to negative or stressful events. These individuals, they also found, have much stronger responses to the flu vaccine than people who don't exhibit these meditation-related brain changes. Meditation training classes are available at community centres and recreation centres, or check with a complementary health-care practitioner.

Go for a brisk walk just before your vaccination A study of healthy young adults who boosted their immune systems with a brief bout of exercise or a stressful mental activity prior to getting the flu vaccine found that women, but not men, showed stronger immune responses to the vaccine than those who didn't get the boost. Brief periods of exercise or mental activity provide acute stress, 'turning on' the immune system in some way that makes it respond better to the 'challenge' the vaccine provides. Even though this study was conducted in young people, the results may also apply to older people, so it's worth giving it a try. ■

Flash a toothy smile, bite into juicy apple, kiss your partner smack on the lips – when your dental health's tip-top, there's no need to hesitate before enjoying life's little pleasures.

But healthy teeth are more than a social asset. Many of the world's healthiest, most disease-fighting foods are crunchy (think fruits, vegetables, whole grains and nuts) and require a good set of teeth to eat them. When your teeth hurt or fall out, your diet goes downhill. Numerous studies worldwide have confirmed that people who have lost teeth avoid hard and fibrous foods and as a result eat fewer fruits, vegetables and whole grains.

Healthy gums guard against major health problems, too. A growing stack of research shows that even low-level gum disease revs up your immune system around the clock, fuelling the chronic, low-level inflammation that contributes to clogged arteries, high blood sugar and perhaps even Alzheimer's disease.

Staying on top of oral health can get harder as we age. Most older people have receding gums, a sign of early gum disease, and half already have periodontitis, or advanced gum disease. Your natural supply of mouth-cleansing saliva also declines with age, and some health conditions and the medicines used to treat them cause lower saliva output. Less saliva is one reason older teeth 'grow' a bigger layer of sticky, colourless plaque (a mix of microscopic food particles and bacteria) faster than younger people's teeth do. As if that weren't enough, natural changes in dentine – the bone-like tissue beneath the translucent enamel coating on your teeth – may make your teeth look darker.

What's more, lower saliva production and more resulting plaque increases the risk of cavities in older people. And because the sensitivity of nerves in the teeth is also reduced, it may take longer to notice the little twinges that mean a tiny cavity's growing – just one reason why you may have more untreated cavities, or worse ones, as you get older. And if you've always been cavity-prone, you may find that you're developing new ones in surprising spots, such as underneath or next to existing fillings.

Experts now say that the most cavity-prone age group isn't the under 10s; it's the over 65s. But there's one positive reason for that: better oral health means more people are keeping more of their teeth. The fact is, as recently as 1960, two out of three people over the age of 75 had lost all of their natural teeth. That number has dropped significantly, but still, gum disease and tooth decay have conspired to claim the teeth of about *one in four* older people – and to raise the risk of cavities for the rest of us.

Your best move for reversing – or preventing – the tooth decay, gum disease, bad breath and dry mouth that accelerate as the years pass? Give your teeth and gums the extra TLC that they – and you – deserve. Here's how.

To maintain healthy teeth and gums

Brush up your expectations When Canadian researchers polled older people about the state of their teeth and gums, they got a jaw-dropping shock: most said their oral health was great, yet 49 per cent believed that tooth loss was inevitable with age. But this is simply not true. It's quite possible to keep healthy teeth for a lifetime. This is another area in which our attitudes to healthy ageing may have to catch up with the reality.

Faithfully follow the basics Unless you've been living on a deserted island for the past 30 years, you've heard this a million times: brush twice a day and floss once a day as a minimum. Use an electric toothbrush if you can – studies show they clean away plaque much more efficiently than brushing by hand.

Brush along to your egg timer Two minutes of brushing, with light to medium pressure, is the most effective way to remove the most plaque, say researchers from the University of Newcastle upon Tyne. Longer and harder isn't better – in fact, it may damage your gums as well as the softer, thinner enamel on the sides of your teeth.

'Although we found that you have to brush your teeth reasonably long and hard to get rid of the harmful plaque that causes dental diseases, our research shows that once you go beyond a certain point, you aren't being any more effective,' says lead researcher Peter Heasman, a professor of periodontology at the university. 'You could actually be harming your gums and possibly your teeth.'

To prevent overzealous brushing, use a soft-bristled toothbrush and hold it like a pencil, moving it in circles rather than up and down. Think 'sweeping' rather than 'scrubbing'.

Invest in a floss holder A disposable one-use holder or the type you thread with your favourite floss are both good choices if you find you don't have the dexterity to clean carefully between your teeth by grasping the floss with your hands. Floss once a day – it will take off plaque and leftover food that a toothbrush can't reach. Be sure to rinse afterwards.

Clean your tongue, too Use your toothbrush or a special tongue-scraper to remove filmy material gently from your tongue. In one study of 51 sets of twins by the New York College of Dentistry, twins who added tongue-brushing to their tooth-cleaning and flossing routine reduced gum bleeding by 38 per cent after just two weeks – and had less bad breath. In contrast, the twins' brothers or sisters who didn't brush their tongues had 4 per cent more gum bleeding. Cleaning your tongue helps to remove bacteria that take up residence just below the gumline, damaging gums and leading to bigger problems.

Bleeding gums and bad breath are often the first signs of poor oral hygiene that may eventually lead to further periodontal disease. And it's well worth investing in a proper tongue-scraper. In a small study at the University of São Paulo in Brazil, the chemicals responsible for bad breath were reduced by 75 per cent after using a tongue-scraper, but only by 45 per cent after tongue-cleaning with a toothbrush.

Rinse in the morning for your gums, at night for your teeth Studies show that rinsing with an antibacterial mouthwash in the morning can significantly cut your risk of gum disease. But if you've had cavities recently, have unfluoridated water at home or have a dry mouth, you should also consider using fluoride mouthwash at night. And if you're very cavity-prone, your dentist may suggest coating your teeth with a special long-lasting fluoride gel that can protect your teeth between dental visits.

Skip fizzy drinks That means diet colas, too. The sugar in standard colas is certainly bad for your teeth, but even carbonated drinks with artificial sweeteners contain such strong acids that they can erode the protective enamel on your teeth. Most fizzy drinks are nearly as acidic as battery acid. The best bet for healthy teeth: sip water or unsweetened iced tea (tea may help to guard against gum disease, some research suggests). If you must have fizzy drinks, the British Dental Health Foundation

Fizzy drinks are highly acidic, with some approaching the levels of battery acid. Imagine the corrosive effect they have on your teeth

recommends sipping them through a straw to avoid contact with teeth, and drinking only with meals. Finish the meal with cheese or milk to help to neutralise the acid, or chew sugar-free gum afterwards to boost saliva flow to wash it out. Then wait at least an hour before cleaning your teeth, so you're not brushing away the weakened tooth surface.

Chew xylitol-sweetened gum if you're cavity-prone Xylitol, a sugar alcohol made from substances found in birch trees and other woods, may help to lower levels of cavity-producing acids made by bacteria in your mouth, Swedish researchers report. Even if xylitol levels are low, they may help somewhat – and sugar-free gum can also help to remove bits of food stuck deep in crevices on the chewing surfaces of your teeth.

Stiff hands? Pad your brush If arthritis has made your finger joints stiff or painful, gripping your brush for long enough to do all the cleaning your teeth need may be a challenge. Try slipping a piece of foam tubing over the end of your toothbrush (you'll find these in a bike shop or hardware shop). Other options: try a longer-handled brush to reach the back of your mouth more easily or slip a wide elastic band over your hand and tuck your brush handle underneath it. The band will help to hold up the brush so you don't have to grip it as tightly.

Treat bleeding gums as seriously as you would a cut anywhere else You wouldn't live with a scrape that made your hands bleed every time you washed them, and you shouldn't live with gums that bleed every time you brush or floss. If this is happening to you, first make sure you're faithfully brushing and flossing, then add an anti-gingivitis mouthwash. If bleeding persists, book a dental appointment.

Watch for subtle (and not-so-subtle) signs of gum disease You may have it if you have any of these symptoms: red, swollen or tender gums; gums that have pulled away from the teeth; persistent bad breath; pus between the teeth and gums (causing bad breath); loose or separating teeth; a change in the way the teeth fit together, or in the fit of partial dentures. You know what to do: call the dentist.

See your dentist regularly Keep up with whatever appointments your dentist recommends, and ask each time if you need a professional cleaning, which removes calculus – hardened plaque that can make gums recede – even better than brushing and flossing. If your teeth bleed when you brush or floss, book an extra appointment for your dentist to check for signs of oral cancer and other problems.

Investigate colour changes Some teeth darken naturally with age, but sometimes darkening teeth can signal more than a cosmetic problem. Teeth can be discoloured by calculus, tartar or periodontal disease. Staining of the surface can also be caused by certain antibiotics or other types of medication, or through tiny cracks that take up stains. Whitening treatments are most effective for teeth that have become discoloured due to yellowing from age, tobacco, red wine, coffee or tea.

Turn in earlier – and stop smoking Japanese factory workers who slept seven to eight hours per night and who didn't smoke cigarettes were less likely to have gum disease than those who snoozed for six hours or less, say researchers. Those who didn't smoke and controlled their stress had better oral health, too. The connection? Lack of sleep, high stress and smoking all lower immunity, giving infection under the gumline free rein.

To battle dry mouth

Review your medication with your doctor Drugs that can cause reduced saliva production include antihistamines, decongestants, painkillers and diuretics. Ask if you can change prescriptions or cut back.

Buy a water bottle with a shoulder strap – then fill it up, slip it on and go Sipping water throughout the day can help to remedy decreased saliva. Carry your own so you've always got a no-cost supply at the ready. Slip the shoulder strap over your head and under one arm so you're carrying your bottle messenger-style. Simply hooking the strap over your shoulder, as you would a handbag, could lead to neck and back pain.

Check out sugar-free gum Stimulate saliva flow by chewing on sugar-free gum, especially after meals. Look for brands containing xylitol, a natural, sugar-free sweetener that can reduce levels of mouth bacteria, helping to fight periodontal disease and tooth decay as well.

Test-drive aids for dry mouths Artificial saliva products, available as sprays, gels or lozenges, may make your mouth more comfortable. Your GP may prescribe them, or some are available over the counter. ■

The human digestive system operates pretty much like a modern recycling factory. A mishmash of materials comes in, these are put on an assembly line, broken down by force and caustic chemicals, the useful ingredients are extracted, then the waste is efficiently released at the end.

It's a system that operates 24 hours a day, non-stop, for decades on end. It warrants our respect, care and – dare we say it? – admiration.

As with any relatively violent mechanical process, pieces and parts of your digestive system occasionally go wrong. There are four common breakdowns.

The gates malfunction Notice that you're burping a bit more or feel pain in your chest after meals? You may have heartburn or its more serious cousin, gastro-oesophageal reflux disease (GORD). The two typically occur when the valve that's supposed to keep the bottom of the oesophagus closed weakens, allowing digestive juices to flow up from the stomach and into the oesophagus, sometimes all the way to the back of the throat. Studies find more than half of people aged 65 and older have heartburn.

Waste backs up It's nothing to be embarrassed about, but we're all more likely to become constipated as we age. It's not because we're older but because we tend to become less active, follow unhealthier diets and take more medication. An estimated 41 per cent of older people have constipation.

Bad things get into the system The microbes that cause food poisoning are the obvious ones; they make you sick almost immediately after eating contaminated food. But we're more concerned with a type of bacteria called *Helicobacter pylori*, which is the primary cause of ulcers – sores in your stomach and intestines that can cause great pain and possibly blood loss.

The pipes get irritated As you get older, your intestinal lining becomes more prone to developing small out-pouchings called diverticula, probably caused by low-fibre Western diets. These affect around one in ten people over 40, half of those over 50 and around 70 per cent of those over 80. On their own, they cause no symptoms, but in about one in four cases they become inflamed and infected, a condition called diverticulitis. Other common causes of intestinal problems include inflammatory bowel disease and irritable bowel syndrome. All of these require medical assessment, and your doctor will probably advise on treatment. Simple lifestyle changes can also help with many digestive problems.

Most of the following steps will not only improve your condition but also help to avoid problems altogether or prevent them recurring.

To prevent and manage heartburn

Slow down Most of us eat the way we do everything else – too fast. When you eat too fast, you take in more air with your food, which can distend your stomach and lead to belching – which can also force the stomach contents upwards. Try this: take a bite, put your fork down, swallow, chat for a minute or read a page of your book, then pick up your fork and take another bite. A bonus: you'll eat fewer calories because your body has more time to sense its fullness, even though you've eaten less food.

Closely monitor your food choices Although the traditional advice is to cut out certain foods such as tomatoes, spicy foods, fried foods and alcohol if you have heartburn, the evidence just doesn't support it. Instead, learn what foods make *your* stomach burn. Grab a notebook and, over the course of a week, list the foods you eat at each meal. Then note any signs of heartburn and how long after eating they occur. Look for patterns, and if you see a suspicious food, cut it out. If your condition improves, you know what to avoid; if it doesn't improve after a week, add that food back in and cut out a different suspect.

Use gravity When you're upright, the contents of your stomach stay down, so walk instead of lying around after eating, raise the head of your bed with bricks to keep stomach acid flowing downwards and even consider eating while standing if it helps. This isn't just a folk remedy; when researchers evaluated more than 2,000 studies on treatments for heartburn or GORD, they found that 'gravity' solutions worked to prevent that burning feeling.

Lose weight The closer you are to a healthy weight, the fewer symptoms of heartburn and GORD you'll experience. Why? The primary reason is probably that extra weight increases pressure on your abdomen. Also, overweight people are more likely to develop a hiatus hernia, which occurs when the top part of the stomach protrudes upwards through the diaphragm into the chest cavity, increasing reflux.

Skip that before-bed fizzy drink – or sleeping pill It's been found that carbonated beverages and benzodiazepine drugs such as diazepam (Valium) and lorazepam (Ativan), prescribed for anxiety or insomnia, can lead to heartburn during the night, disrupting your sleep. And no, you don't have to swallow them together to get this result.

Try acupuncture A study by researchers in Australia found that applying very light stimulation to the wrist with electrical acupoint stimulation (a needleless version of acupuncture) reduced relaxation in the lower oesophagus – a contributor to GORD and reflux – by 40 per cent during the stimulation compared with no change using a dummy procedure.

See a sleep specialist A sleep specialist for GORD? Yes. It seems that the same treatment used for obstructive sleep apnoea – in which people stop breathing several times during the night – can help with nocturnal GORD, or severe night-time heartburn. The treatment is called continuous positive airway pressure (CPAP). You sleep with a mask over your nose; this is attached to a machine that delivers pressurised air to maintain an open airway. It appears to work by increasing pressure in the back of the throat and preventing the stomach contents from coming up the oesophagus. Since GORD and obstructive sleep apnoea often occur together, a visit to a sleep specialist could be worthwhile.

Make a doctor's appointment Persistent backflow of digestive juices can damage the oesophagus, possibly leading to a condition called Barrett's oesophagus, a potential precursor of oesophageal cancer. If your heartburn has moved beyond the usual discomfort and is causing a chronic cough, nausea, vomiting or wheezing, see your doctor.

Bake some muffins ...

To prevent and manage constipation

Fixate on fibre Eating high-fibre food is one of the seven key choices of full-life eating (see also page 131). One more reason to get more fibre is that it's a magic ingredient when it comes to relieving constipation. Fibre is the indigestible parts of plants. When eaten in whole fruits, vegetables and grains, it serves as a wick in your stomach, soaking up liquid and creating bulk to make it easier to move the stools out of your system. Your goal is 20–30g a day, which is easy enough to get if you have a breakfast of high-fibre cereal topped up with strawberries, then have a salad and 125g of beans or brown rice with lunch or dinner.

Bake some muffins Just mix in 2 teaspoons of psyllium seed or husk for each muffin. This grain is a natural laxative that's great for simple constipation, although it may take a day before you get relief. You can also sprinkle 2 teaspoons of psyllium over cereal or yoghurt.

Carry a refillable water bottle Actually, get two. Fill them halfway with water and freeze. Then pull one out, top it up with water and carry it with you everywhere. When it's empty, fill it halfway with water again, put it in the freezer, and take out the other bottle.

The paint-card test

Urine is mostly water plus waste products that have been filtered from the blood by your kidneys. It's naturally a pale yellow colour due to the excretion of urochrome, a pigment in blood. Since urine changes colour easily, it's a good marker of your body's hydration level.

Try this test: pick up colour sample cards of yellow paint at a hardware shop and use them to assess your level of hydration (or dehydration). Your urine should be as pale as the palest shade of yellow; if it's anywhere near the gold colours, it means your body isn't getting enough water.

Note that natural foods rarely affect urine colour, though food dyes can have a small effect (beetroot can occasionally turn the urine red or pink). Then there are the B-complex vitamins; they have more effect on urine colour than almost anything else, turning the shade to a bright, almost neon yellow. Cloudiness or murkiness usually means a urinary tract infection or kidney stone, so see a doctor if your urine is cloudy.

Older people are less likely to drink enough fluids, and dehydration – however subtle – is a major cause of constipation. Age blunts the 'thirst response', or your ability to feel thirsty. Plus, the amount of body fluid declines with age, from about 60 per cent of body weight in men and 52 per cent in women before the age of 60, to 52 and 46 per cent respectively after the age of 60. Another age-related change occurs in the kidneys, which become less able to concentrate urine, so you lose more liquid overall.

Learn to control the uncontrollable Check out biofeedback, a mind/body technique that helps you to become aware of and control involuntary processes. One study of 79 adults with a form of constipation in which the muscles used for bowel movements don't work well (particularly common in older people) found the technique worked better than

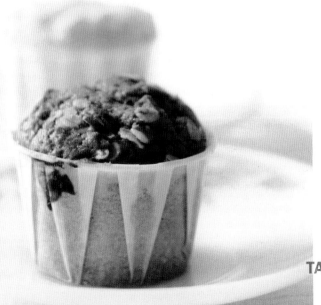

laxatives, diet and exercise for relieving constipation. In some areas the NHS runs biofeedback sessions for people with bowel and other disorders – ask your GP.

Get evaluated for depression The links between the brain and the gut are powerful. It's why you often feel nauseated when nervous or can't eat when stressed. This strong link could be why a British study of 35 women found that those who were anxious, depressed and having difficulty maintaining intimate relationships were more likely to be constipated than healthier women. The reason? Your mental state affects the function of the nerves linking the brain to the gut. The less arousal in the brain – common with many psychological conditions – the less stimulus to the gut. It could explain why low doses of antidepressants, often prescribed for gastrointestinal conditions such as irritable bowel syndrome are so effective.

Hit the gym Move, move, move. Physical movement gets other parts moving, including your bowels. But the more you sit on the couch or go from car to house to bed to car, the less likely you are to go to the bathroom.

Enjoy mornings About 30 minutes after waking up, just after that first coffee or tea, is the ideal time for a bowel movement, so find a place for it in your schedule. Instead of getting up in a rush and gulping a cup of coffee on the way out, design a routine that allows time for a natural bowel movement. Wake up, make a hot drink and a light breakfast and eat while reading the paper. Food in the stomach often prompts the urge for a bowel movement, so head to the bathroom after about half an hour. Keep doing this even if you don't initially have any luck. Remember, you're retraining your system to get it back on track. Eventually the muscle memory will kick in.

List your medication Then take the list to your GP. The following can all contribute to or be blamed for constipation: antacids containing aluminium or calcium, anticholinergics, antidepressants, antihistamines, calcium channel blockers, diuretics, iron, narcotics, nonsteroidal anti-inflammatory drugs (NSAIDs), opioids, psychotropic medications and beta-agonists such as dopamine and adrenaline.

Manage and prevent ulcers

Ditch the aspirin Taking aspirin and other non-steroidal anti-inflammatories (NSAIDs), such as ibuprofen and naproxen, is one of the main causes of ulcers not related to *H. pylori*. If you're taking daily aspirin for the health of your heart, talk to your doctor about alternatives.

Swallow some liquorice Not normal liquorice, but two tablets of deglycyrrhisinated liquorice, from healthfood shops. This herbal remedy can improve ulcers caused by NSAIDs and protect against future ulcers. It induces cells in your stomach and intestinal linings to release more mucus, which acts like armour for your stomach lining and protects it from the damaging effects of stomach acid. Studies find it may be just as good at preventing ulcer recurrence as the prescription medication cimetidine (Tagamet). It may also protect against *H. pylori*. Chew the tablets slowly 30 minutes before meals.

Protect your stomach while on NSAIDs If you need to take prescription drugs that could irritate your stomach lining, your GP may also give you a proton pump inhibitor (PPI), a drug that protects your stomach and can prevent ulcer formation. So if you're taking over-the-counter NSAIDs regularly, it makes sense to do the same – you can buy one PPI, omeprazole (Zanprol), over the counter without a prescription (it's also useful for GORD). But if you already have ulcer symptoms, talk to your GP first – there may be other drugs that would work as well without damaging your stomach.

Spoon in some yoghurt Live-culture yoghurt contains probiotics, 'good' bacteria that help to keep the proper acidic environment in your stomach. Studies find that these friendly bacteria can help your body to eradicate *H. pylori*. Eat one small pot of live-culture yoghurt (such as Yakult or Actimel) a day or take one or two probiotic capsules with each meal and at bedtime for several weeks until the ulcer heals, then take them at night for several months.

Chew on some C One effect of *H. pylori* and NSAIDs is that they increase oxidative stress in your stomach, leading to inflammation and damaging the lining, thus creating ulcers. So it

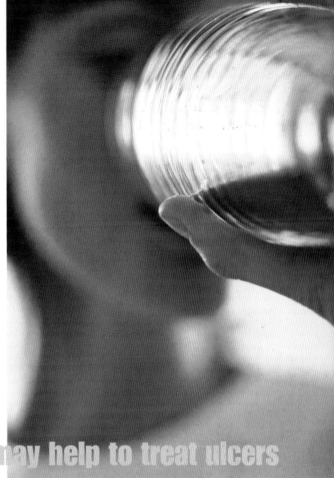

Sipping cranberry juice may help to treat ulcers

makes sense to add a powerful antioxidant such as glutathione, found in large amounts in the stomach lining. Your body makes glutathione from vitamin C, so take 500mg of either glutathione or vitamin C three times a day.

Sip some cranberry juice When 97 people infected with *H. pylori* drank ¼l of cranberry juice a day for 90 days, the bacteria were completely eradicated in 14 per cent of the participants as compared with 5 per cent of a placebo group, a significant difference.

Raid the spices Look for turmeric (*Curcuma longa*) a spice used in Indian dishes. Supplements of this spice reduce stomach acid secretion and protect against ulcers in animal studies. It works by preventing cells lining the stomach from producing histamine, a chemical that produces

stomach acid. This is the same way anti-ulcer drugs such as ranitidine (Zantac), famotidine (Pepcid), cimetidine and nizatidine (Axid) work. You can also find supplements in healthfood shops. Follow the package directions for dosage.

Get a good night's sleep British researchers monitoring 12 healthy people for 24 hours to check how their digestion worked found higher levels of the protein TFF2, which is responsible for helping to repair the stomach lining, while the volunteers slept. In fact, levels increased up to 340 times during sleep. In a second study, they found that depriving volunteers of sleep significantly reduced TFF2 levels throughout the day. Sleeping well, the researchers thought, provides more time for the protein to repair stomach lining damage, helping to prevent ulcers. For more on sleep, see page 301. ■

Fatigue

Being tired is such a fact of modern life that it's easy to forget it's not normal. Of course, if you've had a late night, have just moved into a new house, have started a new job or are ill, you're going to feel tired for a time. But if fatigue is part of your daily life, if no amount of sleep makes a dent in your tiredness, or if fatigue penetrates you to the bone, then it's a real health problem.

This deeper level of fatigue becomes more common as we age. In fact, tiredness is one of the most common complaints doctors hear from their older patients. In one study of 422 relatively healthy people, Danish researchers found that 17 per cent of men and 28 per cent of women aged 75 said they felt tired while merely doing the simple activities of daily living, such as getting dressed.

Tiredness is often a biological syndrome related to low energy reserves, less muscle mass and decreased resistance to stress-causing factors, whether environmental or physical. At other times, fatigue is a psychological reaction to social stressors. The antidote in simple cases of chronic tiredness – and this holds in the majority of cases for people young and old – is merely to push yourself to be active, with the goal of rebuilding muscle and resparking your joy and energy for life. Exercise may make you tired afterwards, but it's the best medicine of all for general fatigue and listlessness.

At other times, fatigue is a symptom of a deeper health issue, ranging from the simple, such as an infection, to the serious, such as cancer. Whether it's a symptom or the result of other issues, tiredness hints at future disability and sometimes even death. One study of 429 people found that those who felt tired doing regular daily activities at the age of 75 were three times more likely to become physically disabled over the next five years than those who didn't experience chronic tiredness.

If you feel chronically tired, take it seriously. Start by having a full physical once-over from your doctor, then add one or more of the following strategies.

To respark lost energy

Hit the gym As we mentioned, loss of muscle strength appears again and again in studies examining the causes of tiredness or chronic fatigue. You must build up your energy reserves to remedy fatigue, and the best way to do that is by building your muscle strength. It's ideal if you can start with a personal trainer, even for just a couple of sessions, to create a personalised programme designed to increase your strength gradually. If that's not possible, look for specialised classes for people who have recently been inactive, or have a gym induction to learn the best machines and weights to use. Or turn to page 202 for an introductory strengthening routine.

Get out for a walk Aerobic exercise is just as important as strength-training in alleviating tiredness. Study after study has found that something as simple as a daily walk improves fatigue in cancer patients and people with chronic fatigue syndrome, lupus and other serious medical conditions.

Turn to your faith A study of 365 older people with heart disease found that those who used religion and prayer as a way to cope, as well as those who were optimistic and felt they had strong social support, were much less likely to report physical fatigue than those who weren't religious.

Take short naps Just 10–20 minutes is all that's needed. These so-called power naps are indeed just the job for restoring energy levels. After the nap, wash your face with cold water, then go outside in the sunlight or sit, if you can, under a bright lamp while you drink a cup of tea. These post-nap activities, alone or together, will give you more energy than the nap alone.

Take a B-vitamin supplement The older you get, the harder it is to absorb vitamin B_{12}, a key energy vitamin, from food. Talk to your doctor about taking a B-complex supplement (it's best to get your Bs all in one go rather than in single supplements since they have a synergistic effect – simply meaning they 'work together').

Get screened for depression Feeling fatigued and tired regardless of how much you're sleeping is a primary symptom of depression. Ask your doctor to administer a depression screening test or just answer the following two questions, which studies find are as good as longer screenings at predicting depression.

1 Over the past two weeks, have you felt down, depressed or hopeless?
2 Over the past two weeks, have you felt little interest or pleasure in doing things?

If you answer yes to these questions, see your doctor for a more complete examination.

List your medication and take it to your doctor 'Polypharmacy', or taking multiple types of medication, is a common cause of tiredness. Ask the doctor if this could be the reason you're so low on energy.

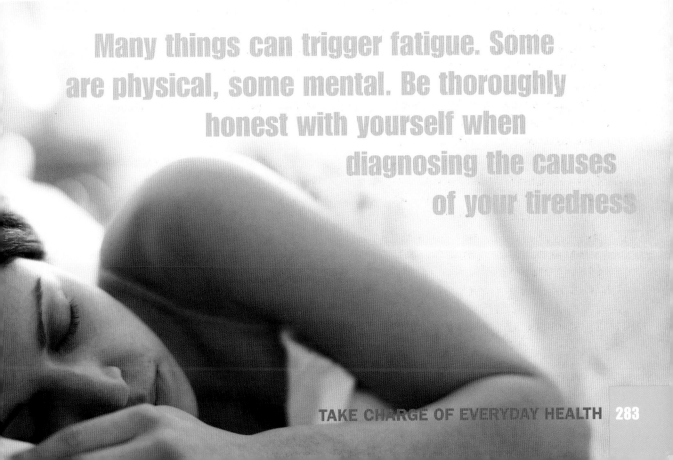

Many things can trigger fatigue. Some are physical, some mental. Be thoroughly honest with yourself when diagnosing the causes of your tiredness

when fuel runs low

Fatigue has many causes, some of which are complex. But sometimes we overlook the most obvious reason why we lack energy: we haven't provided ourselves with the proper fuels.

Often, lack of energy means nothing more than that you are hungry or thirsty. In fact, it is often a better marker that you need something to eat than any sensation emanating from your belly.

With that in mind, here are some tweaks to your food choices and eating patterns that could go a long way towards remedying low energy and daytime fatigue.

1 EAT OFTEN

Eating small meals throughout the day, or three meals and two smart snacks, helps to keep your blood sugar stable, which fends off fatigue. Try to eat something healthy every 3 hours; longer than that, and you risk a drop in blood sugar that will affect how you feel.

2 SKIP THE COFFEE ...

The caffeine in coffee is a mostly safe and natural stimulant that increases your heart and breathing rate. But its effects wear off, leaving you either craving more or feeling tired again. Many experts now say to *avoid* caffeine if fatigue is an ongoing problem.

3 ... BUT NEVER SKIP BREAKFAST

You wake up and do your morning routine, and by the time you arrive at the kitchen for breakfast, 12 hours have passed since your last meal. Even if your stomach doesn't feel hungry, your body is. Eat a small breakfast every day. Studies show that people who eat breakfast concentrate and are more productive than those who don't.

4 KEEP ON DRINKING WATER

Water is needed for the basic chemical production of energy in your body. Without enough in your diet, your body has to compensate for it in a way that can sap you of vitality. Drink a glass every 2 hours or so.

5 EAT SUFFICIENT PROTEIN

The amino acids in proteins help to increase levels of neurotransmitters in your bloodstream that play a major role in mood and alertness. A good rule of thumb is to be sure to have a serving of protein at every meal, including breakfast.

6 CONSUME FEWER SWEETS

Refined sugar is digested very rapidly and causes nearly instant blood-sugar surges – the well-known 'sugar rush' we accuse overactive children of having – followed by a crash in blood sugar that leaves people without energy. While grown-ups may not feel sugar-related surges like a child might, they often suffer from the crash. So skip fizzy drinks, cakes, biscuits; opt for proteins instead.

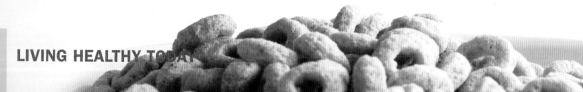

Try Siberian ginseng An adaptogenic herb, meaning it helps to strengthen your body systems to better manage stress, ginseng significantly improved symptoms among 45 people who had moderate fatigue as compared with a placebo group.

Choose the right antioxidant One that seems to help people with unexplained chronic fatigue is Coenzyme Q10. Certain medications can reduce levels of this important antioxidant in the body, particularly the widely prescribed cholesterol-lowering drugs called statins.

Tune in to yoga You're never too old to start. This ancient stretching, strengthening, mind/body regimen offers something for everyone, regardless of their physical condition. In one survey, 25 per cent of people with unexplained fatigue who added yoga to their activities found it improved their fatigue throughout the two-year study period. Try the form called pranayama. It involves breathing techniques and stretching; in one study, it significantly improved mental and physical energy in people with chronic fatigue.

Ask your GP if you could be anaemic If you're always tired, it's worth having a word with your GP to make sure you're not anaemic. This condition, in which there are low levels of oxygen-carrying red blood cells, is common in pre-menopausal women and in older people. It occurs in about 11 per cent of men and 10 per cent of women over 65. A simple blood test can indicate if you're anaemic, and a course of iron tablets or other medication can improve anaemia within a few weeks. But don't take iron supplements without consulting your doctor first, as this may not be the cause, and too much can be harmful.

Breathe deeply As we said earlier, cumulative stress could be the culprit behind your fatigue. That's why relaxation breathing may help. In one study of patients who had had stem-cell transplants, those assigned to listen to a tape that instructed them in relaxation breathing for 30 minutes a day for six weeks reported significantly lower levels of fatigue than a group who didn't listen to the tape. It may test your patience at first, but give prolonged deep breathing a try. It's the next best thing to yoga or meditation and requires no training or skill. Merely sit in a comfortable chair, close your eyes, and slowly and fully inhale through your nose, then slowly exhale through your mouth. Keep doing it for 15 minutes. For a variation, feel free to add in a gentle stretch or move your ankles in circles while performing the deep breathing. ■

Being tired is not our normal state. If you find yourself out of energy come the afternoon or early evening, you need to remedy the situation

joint and muscle pain

Twinges. Spasms. Stiffness. Aches. On any given day, the number of adults who are coping with joint and muscle pain is huge. Half of those over the age of 65 report ongoing knee, shoulder and other joint-related pain. Many more report lower-back pain and some form of significant ongoing muscular discomfort. After coughs and colds, back pain is the most common complaint that sends older people to the doctor.

As the ranks of those who suffer from aches increase, it may seem that the number of remedies available is shrinking. Several widely used prescription-strength pain pills have been pulled from the shelves due to the discovery of potential side effects. Even more worrying is that the three most common painkillers – aspirin, ibuprofen and paracetamol – have all been the subject of serious warnings in recent years.

While nearly one in eight older people still take nonsteroidal anti-inflammatory drugs (NSAIDs) – such as aspirin, ibuprofen and the prescribed drug celecoxib (Celebrex) – more and more research shows that these drugs can be dangerous. Taking aspirin or ibuprofen regularly can raise your risk of gastrointestinal bleeding and ulcers by two to nine times. These drugs can also raise blood pressure and increase your odds of a heart attack, but – perhaps most surprising of all – they may not even be all that effective against most types of joint pain.

The good news: there are many simple steps you can take to alleviate pain. Smart strategies – from ice to heat to gentle exercise – can cut the pain you're feeling now and lower the odds that it'll cause problems in future.

On page 346, we'll tell you how to protect yourself from osteoarthritis and from the inflammation of rheumatoid arthritis as well as how to cope with damage that's already been done by these chronic conditions. In this section, you'll get the lowdown on easing discomfort from the joint, muscle or back pain that can become a problem as you get older.

To relieve aching joints

Pop fish-oil capsules Omega-3 fatty acids – the 'good' fats found in fish such as salmon and in fish-oil capsules – helped people with arthritis ease pain and stiffness in more than 15 well-designed research studies. Volunteers were also able to cut back on prescription and over-the-counter painkillers. Fish oil may help with back pain, too. However, in some studies, the dosage was as high as 5,000mg of omega-3s. That's a lot of daily pills, so talk to your doctor first, and never take fish-oil capsules without a medical consultation if you're taking blood thinners, such as warfarin or aspirin.

Lose weight Dropping just 5kg (11lb) could cut your risk of developing arthritis in half and reduce pain by at least that much. For every half-kilo or pound that you lose, your knees are subjected to roughly 2kg (4lb) less pressure with every step you take, or about 2,200kg (4,800lb) less every time you walk a mile.

Strengthen your support system Strong muscles take stress off the joints and relieve pain. In a 2002 study of people with joint pain, performing strengthening exercises three times a week for 16 weeks brought pain relief as powerful as that from prescription drugs. You don't need a gym membership or fancy weight machine at home; volunteers in this study used inexpensive elastic bands.

Walk, don't run; swim, don't play volleyball
Low-impact activities with smooth movements can keep joints flexible, functional and pain-free. Sports and exercises such as stretching, swimming, water aerobics, cycling, walking on a treadmill or outside and playing golf fit the bill. Those that require quick, high-impact jumps, twists and turns – such as tennis and other racquet sports and volleyball – don't.

Try ibuprofen gel instead of tablets A recent comparative study at Queen Mary, University of London, assessed 585 patients aged over 50 with chronic knee pain and showed that anti-inflammatory gels or creams worked just as well as tablets, a finding that surprised many doctors. What's more, the gel – which is rubbed onto the area over the pain, so that it acts primarily on the part affected, with far less being absorbed into the bloodstream – had few side effects. In contrast, those taking tablets were prone to side effects such as indigestion, increased blood pressure or an exacerbation of asthma.

Wet heat helps A 'thermographic' heating pad (the type that makes 'wet' heat); a hot shower; or even hot, wet towels applied to an achy joint can loosen it up. Do easy stretching exercises as the pain subsides to restore a comfortable range of movement and ease stiffness.

Try supplementing with glucosamine and chondroitin Capsules with glucosamine (a sugar extracted from shellfish) and chondroitin sulphate (a carbohydrate taken from animal cartilage) cut joint pain by 20 per cent or more in a landmark study of 1,583 women and men with arthritis. Nearly 80 per cent of those with moderate to severe arthritis got some relief. Both substances appear naturally in human cartilage and seem to work by boosting cartilage repair and increasing joint lubrication.

Watch your paracetamol dose Easy on your gastrointestinal system, paracetamol tablets are safe and effective as long as you stick to the recommended dose. That's 500–1,000mg – usually one or two tablets – every 4 to 6 hours. But just twice this amount can be dangerous, so never take more than the recommended amount, and check labels on other remedies that could contain paracetamol to make sure you are not accidentally taking too much. Never take more than 4,000mg (usually eight tablets) in 24 hours.

Ask your GP about capsaicin cream The same compound – called capsaicin – that lends hot peppers their fiery heat can help to manage pain. Scientists think it eases pain by using up a chemical inside the nerve cells called substance P, which helps to deliver pain signals to the brain. It's available on prescription for osteoarthritis, so if you have persistent joint pain, ask your GP whether capsaicin cream (Zacin) could help.

Rub in some arnica Arnica is a herbal remedy traditionally used in creams and gels to ease the pain of bruising, swelling and sore muscles. In a recent study of patients with osteoarthritis of the hands, arnica gel was shown to be as effective as ibuprofen gel in relieving pain and stiffness.

Give acupressure a try This ancient Chinese healing art uses thumb and fingertip pressure to stimulate energy flow within the body. It works better than physical therapy at easing lower-back pain, according to a recent Taiwanese study of 129 women and men with chronic pain. For the study, 64 volunteers had six acupressure sessions, and 65 had physical therapy. When researchers checked up on them six months later, the acupressure group had 89 per cent less pain and disability than the other group. They took fewer days off from work or school, too.

To relieve muscle pain

Keep on exercising Experts have a name for the general pain you feel the day after you overexert yourself: delayed-onset muscle soreness, or DOMS. It turns out that if you were a little overzealous playing, working, exercising or even gardening, the best remedy the day after is to get moving again. Staying active works the painful chemical by-products of overexertion out of your muscle tissue and keeps muscle fibres flexible so they can't tighten up and remain sore. Light exercise helps sore muscles to heal so you'll have less pain next time.

Use ice for strains and sprains Keep a cold pack, a bag of frozen sweetcorn or peas, or paper cups filled with a few inches of water in the freezer. If it's been less than 48 hours since your injury, rub the ice in a cup over the sore muscle or 'ice it down' by wrapping the frozen veg or cold pack in a clean kitchen towel and

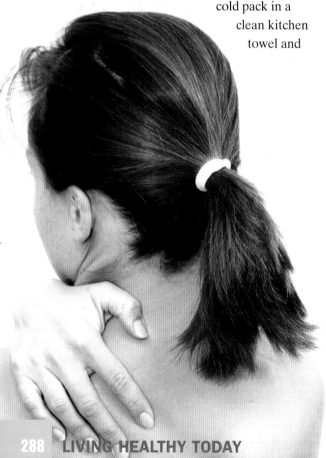

placing it over the area. Cold compresses reduce swelling and inflammation and relieve pain. Apply for 10 minutes, remove for 10 minutes, then apply for another ten; this strategy helps to protect older, thinner skin from being damaged by the ice. But skip the process if you have blood-flow issues, diabetes or Raynaud's syndrome, or if you are highly sensitive to cold.

Stretch and prop If all you have is mild soreness, movement and light exercise are the right remedies. But more severe pain is your body's signal to stop moving around or putting weight on an injured muscle. If you sense that your soreness crosses that line, stay off your feet or avoid using an injured arm for the first day or so. If you've injured a muscle in a hip or leg, keep it raised above groin level with pillows or folded blankets. This helps your body to reabsorb fluid sent into the area and reduces swelling. Make sure an injured arm is supported, not hanging down, for the same reasons.

After two to three days, add homemade heat Warmth relaxes tight, sore muscles and relieves pain. Fill an old knee sock or long tube sock three-quarters full of raw white rice, tie off the open end tightly with a rubber band and microwave it for 2 minutes. Lay it over a sore spot or use it to massage gently a healing muscle that feels tight. This do-it-yourself hot pack is reusable and works for muscle cramps as well. Add cinnamon sticks and cloves or dried lavender buds for a spicy scent.

Stash stick-on heating pads in your medicine cabinet and glove compartment Single-use heat wraps and patches that you can

Pain is inevitable. Chronic, health or situation, there

stick on right over the sore spot are great for fast relief – and they come in shapes and sizes that fit particular high-ache areas perfectly. Inside are chemicals that warm up when the package is opened and they're exposed to air. The low-level heat is safe to use for up to 8 hours, sometimes longer.

Or soak it Sink into a warm tub, Jacuzzi or whirlpool bath and add 15 drops of relaxing lavender essential oil or muscle-warming ginger essential oil to the water along with half a cup of Epsom salts or Dead Sea salts. (This is great for muscle cramps, too.)

Treat yourself to a rubdown Try this on a warm muscle a few days after an injury: rub the length of the muscle, moving from the point farthest from your heart towards the point closest to your heart. Research shows that post-exercise and post-injury massage can reduce pain and speed healing. It can reduce inflammation, too.

Listen to your body Never push through pain or fatigue. The truth is, tired, stressed muscles are injury-prone. Pay attention when your arms or legs feel fatigued or your back feels tight. These are signs that it's time to rest and relax. Pushing too hard could lead to cramps and pulled muscles.

Check your 'D' supply A vitamin D deficiency can cause muscle weakness, aches, pains and even balance problems. Skin produces D in the presence of sunlight, but older skin makes less – and virtually no one (of any age) living in the UK gets enough from sunshine during the winter months, anyway – the rays are too weak. Older people need at least 600–800 IU of vitamin D a day, and some experts say 1,000 IU would be even smarter. You can't get that much every day from food, so add up the amount in your multivitamin and take a supplement to cover any shortfall.

Muscle cramps? Fight them with this breakfast bowlful Low levels of potassium, calcium and magnesium – which act as message-carrying electrolytes in your body – can raise your odds of having sudden, painful muscle cramps. Get more of all three important minerals by spooning up some whole-grain cereal with milk and sliced banana at breakfast and by taking a multivitamin. And drink plenty of water throughout the day, since cramping can also be a sign of dehydration.

To reduce back pain

Get up and move Once, experts (as well as know-it-all relatives) said that bed rest was best for bad backs. Not any more. Study after study shows that movement helps to keep muscles supple and boosts circulation, bringing oxygen and nutrients to heal strained spots. Don't expect to play tennis tomorrow; do expect that after a brief rest, you'll rise and go about as much of your daily routine as possible, taking it as easy as you need to.

Then stretch and strengthen Add in stretching and gentle strengthening exercises, too. After a few weeks, start doing easy abdominal exercises like those in our three full-life fitness routines (see pages 200–37). These will strengthen your core – the 'inner ▷

debilitating pain is not. No matter what your age, are always ways to treat ongoing pain

hot or cold?

Confused about when to use ice or heat on a muscle injury? Here's what you need to know.

ICE

When? Within 48 hours of a sudden injury or the repeat injury of a chronic problem spot.

How? Ice cubes in a sealable bag, a bag of frozen peas or corn or a freezer pack designed for injuries. Wrap it in a small towel to avoid damaging the skin.

How long? Up to 10 minutes at a time, but stop sooner if your skin turns pink. Typically, you can reapply it about 10 minutes after the end of the previous icing session.

Key effects Curtails swelling and reduces pain.

Warning Don't use ice if you have circulation problems or easily damaged skin.

HEAT

When? More than 48 hours after a sudden injury or before starting an activity that may hurt a weak, frequently injured area. (Heat loosens up tight, injury-prone muscles.) Also good for arthritic joints.

How? Use a heating pad set on low, a flannel dipped in warm water, a single-use heat pack available from pharmacies and designed for specific areas, such as your neck or lower back, or a reusable microwaveable hot pack.

How long? 20 minutes at a time.

Key effects Draws blood to the area for nourishment, healing and muscle relaxation.

Warning If the heat causes pain, remove it immediately from your skin to prevent damage. The heat should feel comfortable and pleasant, not scalding.

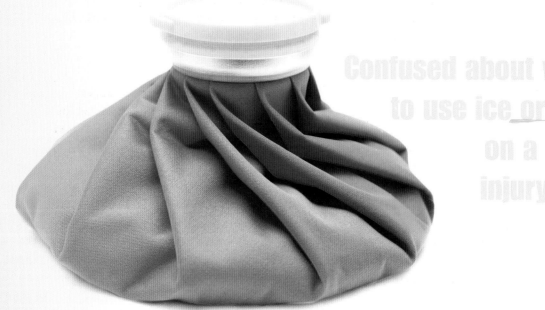

Confused about when to use ice or heat on a muscle injury?

corset' of muscles that steadies your spine. (Go easy on back exercises, though. One study found that walking provided more relief.) Aim to exercise for roughly half an hour, five days a week – it doesn't matter whether you walk, swim, do aerobics or participate in some other activity you enjoy.

Find time for relaxing stretches such as yoga Many of us unconsciously hold years of tension in our upper and lower backs. There's some evidence that mental stress can cause physical stress that could push back muscles past the tipping point, leading to pain. If chronic stress is tensing you up, you need regular doses of healing stretches. Yoga is the perfect form, but regular, slow stretching will work fine, too. Better yet, don't let anger, frustration and other strong emotions affect your physical well-being.

Walk while you talk on the phone In one study of 681 people with lower-back pain, those who walked briskly for 3 hours a week felt better physically and mentally, while those who performed regular back exercises had more pain. Movement of any kind improves the flow of oxygen and nutrients to muscles and redistributes the gel inside the shock-absorbing discs that cushion your vertebrae. In contrast, sitting allows the gel to squash to one side or the other, leaving you with uneven cushioning between the joints of your spine.

When you do sit, relax Forget everything you've been taught about the desirability of sitting up straight. In fact, that ramrod position places an unnecessary strain on your back, according to studies at Woodend Hospital in Aberdeen. Researchers used a new form of magnetic resonance imaging (MRI) scanner that allows people to move around during the test instead of having to lie flat. The 22 volunteers tested three different sitting positions: slouching hunched forward, upright with the body at 90° to the thighs and leaning back with a 135° angle. Scans revealed that spinal disc movement, a measure of the amount of strain on the spine, was worst with the bolt-upright posture. The least wear and tear on the spine occurred when people adopted the relaxed position, leaning back at 135°, with their feet flat on the floor. The researchers suggest that this is the sitting position that places the least strain on the spinal discs and associated muscles and tendons, so is the best sitting position for your back.

If you're sitting, take a break to stretch every 20 minutes Sitting still for hours deprives your back muscles of oxygen and nutrients, allowing the discs between vertebrae to bulge if you're not using perfect posture. Over time, the muscles grow tight, and a bulging disc can press on the nerves, causing pain.

Lift smarter Instead of using your back as a crane, bend your knees, pick up the object, then stand up. And get help moving heavy objects – another person or two, or something like a wheelbarrow will all work.

Reconsider the myth of the firm mattress Spanish back-pain sufferers who slept on medium-firm mattresses for 90 nights cut their morning aches more than those who snoozed on firm beds. Beds with a bit of 'give' seem to support and cushion stiffer muscles and joints better than harder, less yielding mattresses – especially for people with lower-back pain.

Women, lighten your handbags Oversized handbags, often made with heavy quilted leather and decorated with equally weighty

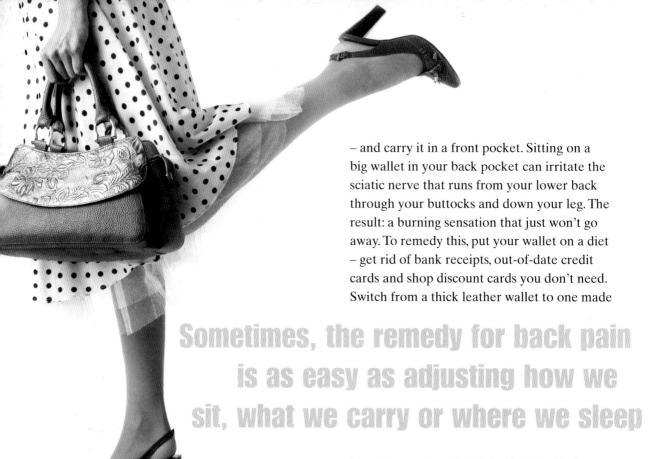

– and carry it in a front pocket. Sitting on a big wallet in your back pocket can irritate the sciatic nerve that runs from your lower back through your buttocks and down your leg. The result: a burning sensation that just won't go away. To remedy this, put your wallet on a diet – get rid of bank receipts, out-of-date credit cards and shop discount cards you don't need. Switch from a thick leather wallet to one made

Sometimes, the remedy for back pain is as easy as adjusting how we sit, what we carry or where we sleep

chain handles, are great for carrying everything under the sun – but experts find that they can weigh 3–4.5kg (7–10lb). At that weight, these over-the-shoulder suitcases throw off your back's finely balanced architecture. You force up one shoulder, putting stress on your neck, upper back and shoulders, which leads not only to upper-back pain but also to a stiff neck.

A better fashion move: invest in a small, lightweight handbag just large enough for a small wallet, mobile phone, lipstick, tissues and car keys (and while you're at it, pare down your key ring to the essentials). A backpack or over-the-body messenger-style bag distributes the weight better than a traditional shoulder bag.

Men, lighten your wallets In fact, consider swapping an overstuffed wallet for a money clip

from the new breed of thin, flexible fabric, or use a money clip. Cheapskate trick: use a thick rubber band or a bulldog clip to hold your bills, driver's licence and credit cards together.

Switch from old-fashioned high heels to stylish flats Walking in heels is like walking downhill all day – you have to lean back to avoid the feeling that you're falling forward, a move that compresses the discs in your lower back. When engineers compared muscle tightness in five women wearing flat heels, medium-height heels or stilettos, they discovered that the higher the heel, the more the women's lower-back muscles tightened up. Save your back by switching to shoes with heels that are less than an inch high. Look for a snug, firm heel counter – the part of the shoe that supports the sides and back of your heel. This gives you better foot control while walking and actually helps to support your arch. ■

Peripheral arterial disease

Millions shrug off the problem as merely part of the ageing process, but despite its name, there's nothing 'peripheral' or unimportant about this disease.

About one in five people over the age of 65 develop the aches, pains and risks of peripheral arterial disease (PAD), a circulation problem that can cause intermittent claudication, a sort of 'angina of the legs' – clogged arteries that cause sharp pain when you move and even, in later stages, when you lie down to rest. Your legs and feet may grow cold, numb or even discoloured. You may develop sores that won't heal (due to reduced blood flow and a lack of oxygen and nutrients to mend the tissue and fight infection). The long-term risks: once PAD becomes painful, your odds of having a fatal heart attack or stroke within ten years rise to nearly 50 per cent.

A slow, progressive disorder of the blood vessels throughout the body, PAD is another manifestation of atherosclerosis, a generalised 'furring up' and hardening of the arteries around the body. So the chances are that if you have PAD, you also have narrowed arteries in your heart and brain – which is why you have a higher risk of heart attack and stroke.

The same risk factors that contribute to atherosclerosis elsewhere also underlie PAD – smoking, high blood pressure, high cholesterol, lack of exercise, diabetes and a high-fat diet. The good news? Just as changing your lifestyle can help to keep the arteries in your heart clear and help to control blood pressure, so adopting healthier habits can improve the flow of blood

through the miles of blood vessels that supply every cell in your body with oxygen and nutrients.

So if you start to feel even the mildest symptoms of PAD – a cramping pain in your calves when you walk that gets better when you rest or slow down – take it as an early warning sign that should be heeded. If the arteries in your legs are clogging up, so too probably are those in the rest of your body.

Just one in four people with PAD know it – and tell their doctors. Half haven't experienced the classic aching fatigue in the muscles of the thigh, buttocks or calves that may grow worse over the months or years. Many who have felt it never tell the doctor, and often, those who do don't get the urgent head-to-toe care they need to stop PAD in its tracks before it's too late.

You need more than pain relief if you have PAD. Fortunately, all the lifestyle steps that protect your heart can slow, stop or even reverse this all-over artery clogging so you can walk where you want, when you want and cut your risk of heart attack and stroke. You may also need medication – but don't wait for your doctor to offer it. In one shocking university study of 553 people with PAD, only those who'd had heart problems in the past got all the cholesterol and blood pressure-lowering medication they needed – even though every person in the study was at high risk.

If you've had unexplained leg pain for at least a week, see your doctor. If you know you have PAD or other related circulation problems – or would like to avoid them – the steps on the pages that follow can help.

To beat peripheral arterial disease

Stop smoking The best strategy to quit? A combination of nicotine-replacement products, a prescription antidepressant and counselling. It's worth it. In one study, smokers with PAD who kicked the habit doubled or even tripled their pain-free walking distance. In another, 16 per cent of smokers who didn't quit went on to develop severe PAD in just a few years, compared with none of those who quit. Ditching the cigarettes also lowers the risk of amputation (about 4 per cent of people with PAD eventually require this grisly procedure) and cuts your odds of having a heart attack or stroke.

Walk, walk, walk We know it hurts. But this is one time when pushing yourself a little (but not too much) does yield real benefits. That's because after quitting smoking, exercise is the most powerful move you can make to cut the pain and immobility PAD can cause – and to reverse the artery clogging that makes it worse.

Exercise works its magic by lowering levels of inflammation in the bloodstream, making the artery walls more flexible, and improving the way the muscles use oxygen. It encourages smaller blood vessels in the legs to open up, and new ones to develop, helping to deliver more oxygen and nutrients to hungry muscles.

Walking has been shown to be the best exercise to help PAD, as long as you do it regularly. That means a daily walk, or at least a walk on most days of the week, of about 30–60 minutes. Start by walking until you get the pain, then have a rest, then start again. Next, try to push yourself a little further, walking through the pain for a short time. You can't damage your muscles, and this will encourage blood vessels to grow. If you have trouble sticking with a daily walking routine, try to find a walking companion in your neighbourhood.

Studies have shown that most people with PAD can stop symptoms getting worse if they quit smoking and exercise regularly, and most experience an improvement in symptoms and an increase in the distance they can walk without pain – which also means they have a lowered risk of heart attack and stroke. People who walk for less than 90 minutes a week may see their symptoms get worse, on the other hand. Be patient; it may take six months or more to see dramatic benefits. And if you can walk for longer than 30 minutes, do so. Some experts say that hour-long sessions ultimately provide more pain relief.

Make all your dairy foods fat-free Fight clogged arteries by getting rid of the building material for gunky plaque: LDL cholesterol. The body uses saturated fats to build cholesterol particles, and we get most of the saturated fats in our diets from milk, cheese, ice cream and yoghurt. Promise, right now, that you'll buy only dairy products labelled 'skimmed' or 'fat-free'. (If you love margarine, look for brands that contain low saturated fats and no artery-blocking trans fats.)

Invest in sharp kitchen scissors – and then use them It's far easier to trim away globs of fat clinging to pork chops, chicken breasts and steaks with scissors than with a knife. Kitchen scissors needn't be expensive; just make sure they're sharp so the job's fast and easy. Cutting fat off meat (and removing skin from poultry) will subtract another substantial source of saturated fat from your diet – a move your arteries will love.

Evening munchies? Snack on walnuts, not ice cream Enjoying a small handful of these nutty nuggets every evening may seem luxurious, but the good fats in these yummy

Part of the elixir of long life is frequent, pleasurable walks

morsels have a unique ability (rare among foods) to raise your HDL cholesterol. You could see a two to three point rise in HDL that will cut your risk of heart attack and stroke by up to 18 per cent.

Double up your servings of fruit and veg every day Compounds found in fruits and veg can help to prevent the artery clogging that causes PAD and worsens it. How? Antioxidants shield particles of 'bad' LDL cholesterol from oxidation by rogue oxygen molecules called free radicals. Oxidised LDL starts the chain of biochemical events that leads to the formation of gunky, blood vessel-narrowing plaque in artery walls.

Sip orange juice at breakfast and crunch a spinach salad at lunch Nothing's easier than grabbing a carton of 100 per cent orange juice and a bag of pre-washed spinach leaves at the supermarket. Both are rich sources of folate, a B vitamin that helps to lower high levels of heart-threatening homocysteine in people with PAD. And both supply vitamin C – an inflammation-fighting antioxidant that seems to be depleted swiftly in the bodies of people with more severe PAD, say researchers from University Hospital in Ghent, Belgium.

Try ginkgo The herbal remedy ginkgo biloba can improve circulation. Studies in people with PAD have shown that it may increase the distance they can walk before the pain sets in. ■

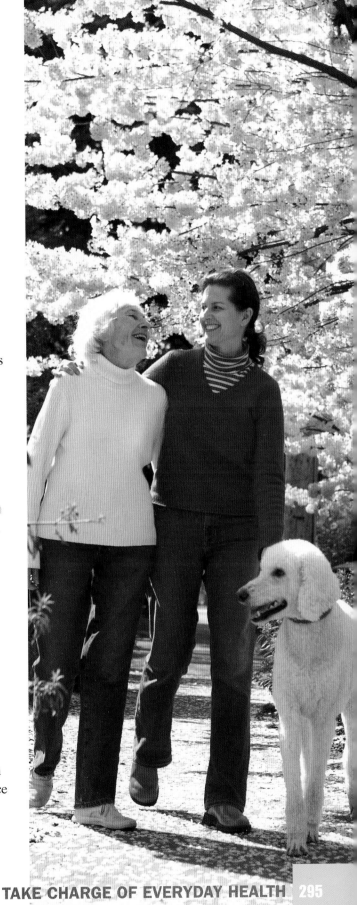

4 must-ask questions for your doctor

1 Should I take aspirin or an anti-clotting drug? Although it won't help your symptoms, aspirin could cut some of your extra risk of heart disease and even stroke. That's why most GPs will recommend that you take a low-dose (75mg) aspirin tablet each day. But aspirin raises your odds of developing a stomach ulcer or gastrointestinal bleeding. So if you've had problems with these in the past, or if you already take other pain-relievers every day (such as ibuprofen or a prescription nonsteroidal anti-inflammatory drug, NSAID), or if there's some other reason why you can't take aspirin, your doctor may prescribe an alternative medication with similar anti-clotting effects.

2 Can you help me to lower my blood pressure? If your blood pressure remains above healthy levels despite several months of improved eating, exercise and even weight loss, ask your doctor whether it's time to add blood pressure-lowering drugs to reduce your chances of a heart attack or stroke.

3 What can I do about my blood cholesterol? Changing your diet to reduce saturated fat should help you to slash your 'bad' LDL cholesterol levels. And if you stop smoking, take some exercise, lose any excess weight and have one or two alcoholic drinks (but no more) each day, you can raise your levels of 'good' HDL, the type of cholesterol that mops up the bad stuff. Your GP will probably take a blood test to check your 'bad' cholesterol levels and if they're raised you will probably be prescribed a statin drug to reduce them. In fact, some studies suggest that statins are beneficial even if your cholesterol levels are normal, so your GP may recommend them anyway. Statins can improve PAD symptoms, increasing both your overall and pain-free walking distance, as well as reducing your stroke and heart attack risks.

4 How's my blood sugar? A scary fact: people with diabetes who have PAD are six times more likely to develop dangerous skin infections and twice as likely to have PAD-related leg pain even when they're resting. If you have diabetes, keeping your blood sugar at healthy levels around the clock can lower your odds of these big problems. If you don't, getting regular blood sugar checks (as often as your doctor recommends) can help you to catch pre-diabetes early, in time to slow the development of full-blown diabetes by years – perhaps decades. (For more ways to control blood sugar, turn to part 4 of the book.)

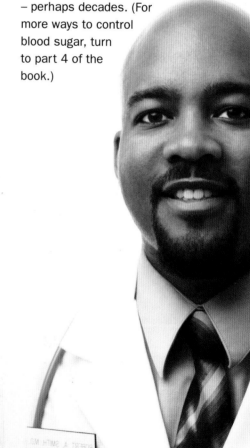

LIVING HEALTHY TODAY

Say the words *skin* and *age,* and you probably think about wrinkles. Listen up – forget about wrinkles. Normal, age-related wrinkles do you no harm. You are beautiful with them; don't let advertising, plastic surgeons or shallow, vain friends convince you otherwise. Years of sun exposure, not discovering moisturiser until your 30s and a persistent rosy flush on your face – *these* are the skin issues that adults over 40 should be most concerned with.

Consider this: when you're young, your top layer of skin typically turns over every 26–42 days. From around the age of 30, that turnover rate slows. By your 80s, your skin takes 50 per cent longer to renew itself. And that's the problem. Now the protective outer layer of your skin is just hanging around for longer, and its function is impaired.

That in turn leads to a host of skin-related problems, including dryness and a greater susceptibility to irritation. It also means that dead skin cells stay on the surface for longer, giving your skin a dull appearance and rough texture. That dryness and flaking can also make your skin itchy, sometimes resulting in red, scaly patches of eczema. Plus, your oil glands produce less oil, which also contributes to dryness.

Your skin also thins with age, with one study finding that women over 65 had lost about 20 per cent of their skin thickness. This is why skin becomes more sensitive to creams and oils with age. Just a little permeates the skin more completely and may lead to the itchiness and rashes of contact dermatitis.

This time of life is also when the sunbathing of your youth returns to haunt you. Any time the sun hits your skin, it creates an inflammatory reaction that breaks down collagen – the binding material in your skin – as well as elastin fibres. That's why people who spent a lot of time in the sun when they were younger may have that leathery look.

Ageing also delivers two other challenges to the skin.

Shingles is a painful skin condition in which the nerves just under the skin become inflamed. It's caused by the chickenpox virus, which has lain dormant in your system all these years just waiting for your immune system to weaken. About 20 per cent of people aged 60 and older who get shingles are left with a painful condition called post-herpetic neuralgia.

Rosacea starts out looking like blushing or ordinary skin redness, but, eventually, tiny pimples and very noticeable blood vessels may appear, particularly on your nose and cheeks. Rosacea affects about one in ten people in the UK, more women than men, and typically strikes between the ages of 30 and 50. Scientists don't really understand what causes it, but 'leaky' blood vessels, sun damage, a reaction to a skin micro-organism, or abnormal immune or inflammatory responses may be involved.

While these last two conditions require medical treatment, usually in the form of laser therapy and/or prescription medication, there are certain lifestyle steps you can take either alone or as an add-on to your doctor's care, to protect your skin.

To manage dry, itchy skin

Skip the soap If your skin is showing signs of ageing, then your days of using soap are probably over – most soaps are simply too drying for older skin. The British Association of Dermatologists (BAD) recommends that older people avoid soap, bubble bath and shower gels, which strip the skin of its natural oils. Instead, use moisturising soap substitutes, and apply the lotion directly to the skin with a flannel or sponge. Rinse with warm water – not hot or cold – and apply a moisturising cream afterwards.

Slap on the moisturiser Forget fancy ingredients and £100-an-ounce anti-ageing treatments. Any basic moisturiser will do a good job. Use on still-damp skin, to lock in water, and moisturise at least twice a day – when you first step out of the shower, before your skin is completely dry (the moisturiser will form a film over your skin, locking in liquid), and again before you go to bed after cleansing your face with a moisturising cleanser. Use moisturiser on your whole body – you need about 30g all over the skin for each application, says the BAD – so be sure to buy a big tub.

Hydrate the air It's common sense that dry air is bad for dry skin, and if you have a modern, centrally heated home with double glazing, the air indoors may become quite dry in the winter. If so, moisturise the air and your skin with a humidifier. You can have a humidifier installed as part of your heating system or use a portable version. Another way to put more moisture into the air in winter is to hang just-washed clothes to dry in the house. A final spin in the dryer helps to remove any stiffness and wrinkles.

Exfoliate at least weekly Exfoliation is the process of removing dead cells from the skin's surface to reveal 'younger', fresher-looking skin below. It helps to get rid of the dull look that ageing can bring, as well as shrinking the appearance of large pores and removing any flakiness from dry skin. Typically, you use a cream exfoliant to do the job. But if these are too harsh for your skin, try a cleanser with 10 per cent alpha-hydroxy acids (AHA), naturally occurring acids that act as exfoliators. If you use products with AHAs, look for over-the-counter brands with glycolic acid, which seems to penetrate the skin best.

Wear gloves Not for warmth, but for skin protection. Use rubber gloves for washing dishes, doing housework and handling household cleaners. Even better, switch to gentler, 'green' cleaners that aren't made with harsh chemicals, or use natural ingredients such as vinegar for cleaning. But still wear the gloves.

Take your vitamins Antioxidant vitamins (A, C and E) help to combat skin damage from free radicals, whether they come from our diet, sunlight or pollutants in the air. Ensuring a good intake of antioxidants from foods can help skin-repair processes, boost collagen production and help to retain moisture. But take your vitamin E in a skin cream, not as a supplement – there's some evidence that vitamin E supplements taken by mouth can be hazardous for older people.

Take a warm bath Add ten drops of chamomile oil to bathwater, then soak for 10 minutes. Other bath additions to help itchy skin include oatmeal and geranium, hyssop, peppermint and myrrh essential oils (use ten drops of one type). Don't forget to slap on the moisturiser afterwards, and make sure the water is warm, not hot. Hot water tends to dry out the skin.

Swallow some evening primrose Several studies find that taking this omega-3 fatty acid significantly reduces itching and rashes related to dry skin, most likely by increasing levels of anti-inflammatory chemicals in the blood. Take four 500mg capsules twice a day until your condition improves.

To manage rosacea

Cool off flare-ups When the redness of rosacea appears, combine several drops of soothing herbal oils such as rose, lavender and chamomile in a basin of cool water. Soak a washcloth in the liquid and lay it over your face for 10 minutes. Repeat as necessary. These herbs are often used to reduce skin irritation.

Breathe deeply Stress is a common trigger for rosacea, so practising stress-reducing deep breathing can help to avoid flare-ups. Learn to breathe from your stomach, so that each in-breath is deep enough to expand your abdomen, while each out-breath lowers it. When you start to feel the blood rising in your face, continue with this form of breathing for 3 minutes, ideally with your eyes closed.

Swallow some fish oil Fish-oil supplements are rich in anti-inflammatory omega-3 fatty acids. Since rosacea is related to inflammation, these inflammation-dampers can help to reduce flare-ups. Take 1,500mg or less

twice a day. You can also try 500mg of evening primrose oil three times a day.

Use green-tinted make-up The green helps to cover the red. This won't get rid of your rosacea, but it will stop people from asking if you've had too much sun lately.

Skip the alcohol Take this test: after a glass of wine or a gin and tonic, look at your face in the mirror. Is it as pink as a glass of rosé? Alcohol dilates the blood vessels, and since facial blood vessels are so close to the skin, you get the telltale flush of rosacea.

Watch your diet Spicy foods, hot liquids and even mature cheeses can trigger a flare-up.

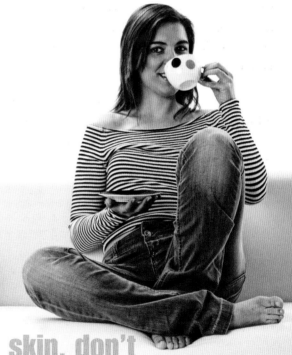

When it comes to skin, don't confuse beauty with health. Focus on caring for your skin from both the inside and outside

Try hypnosis Several studies reported in medical journals found that hypnosis can help patients to control the flushing of rosacea.

Ask your GP to test you for *Helicobacter pylori* This bacterium is the primary cause of stomach ulcers. However, a growing body of evidence suggests it may also be linked to rosacea. In one study, in Madrid, of 44 patients with rosacea and *H. pylori* infection, completely eradicating the bacteria in 29 volunteers led to a complete or significant improvement in rosacea in 19 patients – or 65 per cent.

Talk to your doctor about intense pulse light (IPL) Just two or three sessions of this therapy could make a huge difference to your rosacea. It's not generally available on the NHS, though it is offered by many private clinics.

To manage shingles

Start an antiviral At the first sign of shingles, get a prescription for an antiviral medication such as acyclovir (Zovirax), which was approved for the treatment of herpes viral infections almost two decades ago. Studies find that taking this or other antiviral medicines early can prevent the lingering pain that often occurs after a shingles outbreak.

Ice yourself down When the pain is bad, apply an ice pack wrapped in a small towel to the affected area for 10 minutes, take it off for 10 minutes, then reapply for another 10.

Take an antihistamine Some people get terrible itching with shingles. If you have itching, try an over-the-counter antihistamine such as chlorphenamine. Take it at bedtime as it will help you to sleep – but watch out for sedating effects the next day. Cool baths can also help.

Wrap yourself in plastic Putting on clothes over the blisters of shingles can be incredibly painful. Try covering the area with cling film so your clothes slide over the affected skin. ■

Yes, there are diseases of the skin. Yes, they can be managed. No, they need not affect your life or appearance

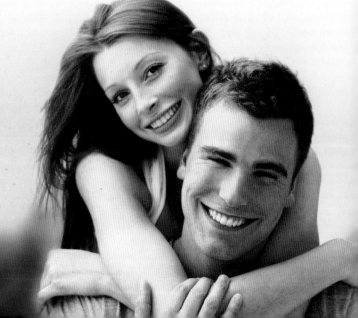

Insomnia – annoying, exhausting and mysterious – sadly becomes a common experience as we age. Sleep patterns change radically after the age of 55, when your body clock resets itself and levels of important sleep hormones drop. Diseases, medication, everyday habits and even your evening bedtime routine play important roles as well.

The good news: although you can't reverse natural and inevitable sleep changes, you don't have to settle for wide-awake nights or dog-tired days.

As people get older, these changes mean that it's more difficult to stay asleep – many people may be wide awake by the early hours of the morning, and get less sleep than their previous eight hours or so. Not surprisingly, it can then be difficult to keep going all day, so older people tend to get tired more easily in the afternoon and early evening. If you're affected, your body clock is basically running ahead of itself, with a time period of less than the normal 24 hour day.

The secret to overcoming – or sidestepping – the extra insomnia risks that come with the passing years? Everything from exercising in sunlight and saying no to an after-dinner cocktail to working with your GP to minimise the effects of health issues and medication on your sleep schedules. And the time to talk to your GP? When you're regularly feeling tired during the day and can't do the things you'd like to do or need to do. Then it's time to do something about your sleep. Getting older doesn't have to mean living with insomnia and exhaustion. There's plenty you can do about it.

Your first step? Understanding and accommodating the way your body and mind sleep now. Sleep changes don't happen suddenly. They start gradually in your 30s, but you may not notice them until you're older or retired or until other factors get in the way.

To adjust to sleep-pattern changes

Accept them It's crucial to understand that the timing and quality of your sleep does change over time. Just as you will never have the body shape and weight of 30 years earlier, you will not have the sleep patterns you once had. Be sensitive to the changes. Do you get tired earlier or are you more sensitive to morning light? Monitoring changes and adjusting to them is half the battle.

Get active during the day You'll sleep better at night if you haven't been sitting around quietly all day. In fact, although you may think that disturbed sleep is making you feel lethargic during the day, it's just as likely to be the other way round. According to a study at Loughborough University that followed a sample of elderly people at intervals for eight years, a lower level of physical activity was a significant risk factor for all types of insomnia – whereas increasing age per se generally was not. So take some exercise in the fresh air every day if you can, and generally boost physical activity levels – take the stairs rather than the lift, take up an active hobby rather than reading or watching television and if you do watch TV in the early evening, get up during the ads and do a bit of housework. You may also find that a period of bright light – preferably from sunlight or a light box – at your sleepy midafternoon period helps you to stay alert for longer.

Wind down at bedtime Just as important: once it is time for bed, let your body know. Avoid too much excitement, activity or mental exercise. Now is the time to read, chat and wind down. Give yourself at least a couple of hours of gentle relaxation before bed, and try to keep to a similar routine each evening. Start to dim the lights – your body clock was built for gradual transitions, not sudden changes in light level.

Can't drop off to sleep in an instant? Be patient – you'll get there Taking longer to fall asleep is a natural part of ageing. Older people may need 20 minutes or more to fall asleep, while younger people may need only 5 to 10 minutes. (Read on for ways to feel sleepier at bedtime and tell your brain it's time to doze.)

Don't worry if you wake three or four times during the night Once asleep, older people go through the cycles of sleep more quickly than younger people – and may wake up between cycles more frequently. Researchers suspect that lower levels of growth hormone in your system may help to explain why you spend less time in the deepest, most restorative sleep stage, called Stage Four by researchers.

Wide awake at 5am? Get up! Your body clock may have shifted to an early-to-bed, early-to-rise schedule. Turning in earlier will help to ensure that early wake-ups aren't a rude awakening.

Consider daytime naps Napping is a controversial solution for people struggling with insomnia. Some studies have shown that a short daytime nap doesn't have much impact on night-time sleep. But more than a 30 to 45 minute afternoon nap may keep you awake for too long at night. The crucial thing is not to let yourself sleep so long that you're groggy for the rest of the afternoon and then can't sleep at night. If a short siesta helps you to feel more awake and functional during the day, then take one – but set an alarm to make sure you wake up before you sink into too prolonged a sleep.

To improve your nightly sleep

Reserve your bed for sex and sleep Don't watch TV – especially not late-night thrillers – and don't work or pay bills lying in bed. It's important not to start linking your bed with activities that keep you awake or cause worry.

Create a clutter-free sanctuary Your brain deserves the balm of a soothing, organised, pleasant environment, free of worrisome reminders such as baskets of laundry that needs to be folded, stacks of magazines to be sorted or bills to be paid. Consider painting the walls a soothing colour, too.

Block the light Moonlight, street lights, late sunsets and early dawns can all interfere with the circadian-rhythm changes you need to fall asleep. Make sure you have thick, lined curtains that block out all the light, or invest in some blackout blinds to cover the windows.

Nestle on a new pillow If yours is more than six months old, or if you wake up in the morning with a sore neck and shoulders or a stuffy nose, it may be time for new head support. What's best? It depends on what works for you, but here are some pointers.
- Neck pain? Go for a thinner pillow or look for a special 'neck pillow'. In one Swedish study, a neck pillow – rectangular with a depression in the middle – enhanced sleep. The ideal neck pillow is soft and not too thick.
- Always turning your pillow over to find the cooler side? Invest in natural cool. Natural fibres – and natural-fibre pillowcases – stay

sick and tired

Without question, bad health affects how you sleep.

According to a large study by researchers at King's College London, older people with insomnia are much more likely to report worse physical health and a resulting impaired quality of life than younger adults. So if you can't sleep and you have health problems, see your GP, as treating both the insomnia and the medical problems at the same time may give the best results. Here are examples of health conditions known to affect sleep.

Pain A bad back, an arthritic knee, a pulled shoulder muscle, heartburn – any type of ongoing pain has the power to keep you awake or pull you out of a deep sleep. Talk with your doctor about pain treatments that can ensure you get a proper night's rest. Also review your prescriptions with your doctor – codeine, morphine and steroids can disturb your sleep, as can migraine drugs and other painkillers that contain caffeine.

Allergies People with allergic rhinitis – the most common form of allergies resulting from ubiquitous dust, pollen and animal dander – are much more likely to experience insomnia, wake up during the night, snore and feel fatigued when they do wake up. The French researchers who discovered this also found that those with allergic rhinitis are more likely to sleep fewer hours, take longer to fall asleep and feel sleepy during the day than those without the condition.

Gastro-oesophageal reflux disease (GORD) Studies show that people with GORD and other forms of heartburn are particularly likely to sufer from daytime sleepiness, insomnia and poor sleep quality.

cooler. In studies, 'cool pillows' – some were water-filled, and others used a mix of sodium sulphate and ceramic fibres – enhanced sleep.
● Stuffy or allergy-prone? Go hypoallergenic – and get an allergen-reducing pillowcase as well.

Move your bed Outside walls and windows in your bedroom mean more noise. Locating your sleeping spot along an inside wall could improve matters, a Spanish study suggests.

Turn your clock so you can't see the face Sleep studies show that people with insomnia often overestimate the length of time they've lain awake. It's quite possible to wake at, say, 2am, drift back to sleep, then wake again at 2.30 – and think you've been awake the whole time. And glancing at the clock every so often can make you so anxious about not falling asleep, or about how tired you'll be tomorrow if you don't, that it can actually keep you awake. So just turn the clock around. The alarm will still wake you up in the morning.

Keep bedroom reading to a minimum A few minutes of relaxing reading is a perfectly fine pre-sleep ritual. But if you get in the habit of reading in bed for a long time, or if the only time you read is at night in bed, that's a problem. You should do any prolonged reading in a chair in another room during waking hours.

Splash out on new nightware Your old pyjamas or boxers may be in good condition, ▶

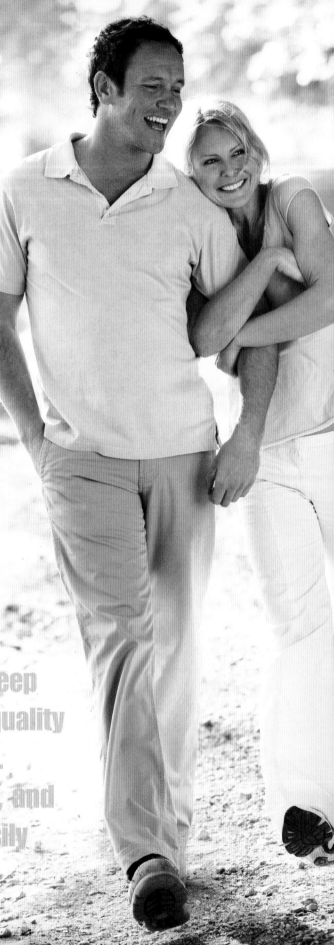

How to fix a snorer

Bedding down with a chronic snorer is bad for your sleep, your health and your hearing. Loud snorers can generate 80 decibels of noise, as loud as rush-hour traffic, researchers have shown, and snorers' bed partners actually suffered hearing loss as a result. Another study assessed noise levels in the bedrooms of 140 volunteers living near Heathrow and three other European airports and found that a snoring partner could raise a sleeper's blood pressure by as much as a low-flying aircraft. If you can't or won't sleep in separate rooms, try these remedies.

- Shop-bought rubber earplugs can screen out about 32 decibels, which is often enough to let you fall asleep.

- An audiologist can make you custom-fitted ear protectors that filter out more noise. They're expensive but worth it.

- A white noise machine, which creates a steady, soothing layer of sound, can help to mask the snoring.

- Present your partner with a box of anti-snoring strips, which work by pulling the nostrils open wider. A Swedish study found they significantly reduced snoring.

- If all else fails, pack your mate off to the GP. He or she (though it's more often a he) may be a candidate for a test called polysomnography, which is used to detect sleep apnoea.

The quality of your sleep is closely related to the quality of your waking hours. Live happily and actively, and sleep will come more easily but if they're not completely comfy, you deserve better. Invest in 100 per cent cotton pyjamas for cool comfort or cosy flannels for cold nights.

And slip on some toe-toasting socks
Got cold feet? Wear warm socks to bed. Researchers at the Psychiatric University Clinic in Basel, Switzerland, found that when blood vessels in the feet dilate late in the evening, the body can effectively cool down and get ready for sleep. Putting on socks can help to make the blood vessels widen and radiate heat.

Scent your sheets with lavender
Place a single drop of lavender essential oil on your pillow or spray your sheets with lavender water before you turn in. Studies at the University of Leicester and the Smell and Taste Research Center in Chicago found that this soothing botanical works as well as sleeping pills for quelling insomnia and tension.

Or infuse your bedroom with jasmine
Other studies suggest that a faint jasmine aroma may work better than lavender to help you to drift off, and stay more alert the following day. Try a scented oil stick or place a few drops of jasmine essential oil in a cup of hot water by your bed.

Interview your partner
Ask whether you stop breathing, jiggle your legs or wiggle your body while asleep. Millions of people have obstructive sleep apnoea, which causes brief interruptions in breathing through the night and which over time can raise the odds of getting high blood pressure and heart disease. Wiggly legs or night-time thrashing could also be signs of restless legs syndrome or another movement disorder. If your partner confirms a problem, talk to your GP. An evaluation and treatment could make all the difference to your sleep, and your health.

Kick out Fluffy and Fido
A 2002 study found that one in five pet owners sleep with their pets – or more accurately, *don't* sleep, because their pets are on the bed or in the room. It could be sneeze-provoking cat dander or the patter of little Labradoodle feet, but the study found something more incriminating: 21 per cent of the dogs and 7 per cent of the cats snored.

To live a sleep-friendly lifestyle

Take a walk after lunch, then read the paper on the patio
Exercise cuts stress, and getting exercise in the sun can help to keep your body's circadian rhythms calibrated. You need about 2 hours of daily exposure to bright sunlight to help your body to stay in tune. In the winter, or if you can't get outdoors, consider buying a light box – it radiates light that mimics the brightness and wavelengths of natural sunlight.

Or try tai chi on the lawn
In China, people rise at dawn to perform this series of ancient, gentle, dance-like movements in local parks. The sleep bonus: tai chi beat a low-impact exercise class for improving sleep in a study of 118 women and men aged 60–92. People who did tai chi three times a week for six months fell asleep 18 minutes faster and slept for 48 minutes longer each night than other exercisers.

Schedule worry time during the day, in the kitchen
We're not kidding. If your mind is accustomed to revving up sleep-robbing anxiety in bed, retrain your brain by moving your worry session to another place and time. Try midmorning at the kitchen table – pour a mug of soothing camomile tea with honey, grab a notebook and pen and write out your worries. This will clear your mind and break the link

Sleep in a pill

Sleep aids are among the most prescribed medications today, and for good reason – they are a good short-term option for insomnia, particularly if it's linked to issues such as stress. But remember – your primary remedies for chronic bad sleep are lifestyle changes and fixing the underlying causes. Vow never to rely on pills alone to solve your sleep problems.

If your doctor does recommend medication, it should be the lowest effective dose and should be taken only for a short period – tolerance to the drug's effects may develop after only a few days, which can reduce their effectiveness, and once you stop using them you may develop a 'rebound' bout of insomnia, with disturbed sleep and perhaps vivid dreams for some time before a normal pattern is re-established. Don't forget to ask your doctor whether the pill will make you drowsy the next day; several do.

If you think you need sleeping pills, it's a sign that you should see your doctor about your sleep problems. But don't be surprised if the prescription isn't for a pill but rather for cognitive behavioural therapy, a mind-over-body approach to the problem that's been proven to work better than prescription sleeping drugs in older people.

between bed, night and worry. If thoughts keep popping up to stop you sleeping at night, keep a notebook by your bed and write them down so you can think about them during the day.

Make herbal tea or water your drink of choice after lunchtime Ditch coffee as well as other caffeine sources such as chocolate, colas and other soft drinks, and black, green or white tea. Even small amounts of caffeine may keep you up late, and older people may be more sensitive to it. Caffeine blocks a brain chemical called adenosine that helps us feel drowsy and fall asleep, and the effect may last longer in older people, whose livers don't filter caffeine

as effectively. Instead, sip some chamomile tea, which contains ingredients proven to calm the nervous system and which can induce sleep.

Instead of an evening cocktail, have a glass of wine with an early supper Drinking before bed may help you to fall asleep, but as the alcohol wears off, you're likely to have light, easily broken sleep. If you enjoy a drink, have one with supper a few hours before bed.

Drink more water during the day and less in the evening If you have diabetes, an enlarged prostate, incontinence or even standard 'tiny bladder syndrome' (the bladder shrinks with age), you may get up frequently to urinate, then have trouble falling back to sleep. Try drinking more water during the day so you don't feel thirsty in the hour or so before you turn in. That way, you may have fewer slumber interruptions without risking dehydration.

To soothe yourself before bed

Soften the mood Two hours before bedtime, switch on the answering machine, turn off the television or computer, pull on your softest PJs and turn on your favourite relaxing sounds. In one recent study of 52 women over the age of 70, those who listened to quiet music fell asleep faster and had fewer middle-of-the night awakenings than before they started scheduling listening time. The best music? Whatever soothes you, whether it's Frank Sinatra, Amy Winehouse, jazz or Debussy.

Try progressive relaxation Sit in a comfortable chair with both feet on the floor or lie on your sofa or bed. Inhale and exhale naturally. After a few minutes, systematically tighten a muscle group as you inhale, then relax it completely as you exhale. Progressively loosen and tighten both feet, your lower legs, upper legs, then work your way up to your back, arms, neck, shoulders and even your face. Then continue to breathe naturally, feeling any remaining tension ebb away.

Next, combine progressive relaxation with music When 60 women and men with sleep problems listened to soft, slow music while they performed a relaxation exercise, their heartbeats and breathing rates slowed – and they slept better and for longer.

Soak in a hot bath Immersing yourself in warm water an hour or two before bed helps the blood vessels to dilate so your body can release heat – part of the natural cooling down that precedes sleep.

Take a supplement with 500mg of calcium and 300mg of magnesium Magnesium is a natural sedative – even a slight shortfall can leave you lying in bed with your eyes wide open – while calcium helps to regulate muscle movements. Getting plenty of both minerals can also cut your risk of night-time leg cramps. Take a supplement right before bed.

Enjoy a bedtime snack Have some walnuts, a banana or a glass of milk – all rich sources of the sleep-inducing amino acid tryptophan. (Bananas are also packed with melatonin, the sleep hormone.) If incontinence or frequent bathroom visits aren't a problem, have a glass of water – but not juice. In one study, people who drank juice just before bedtime became extra-alert due to the high sugar content.

Take antacids right after dinner, not before bed Some antacids contain aluminium, which appears to interfere with sleep. ■

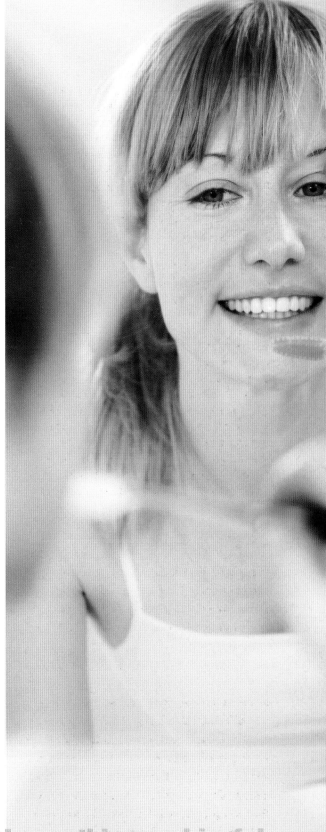

Make your pre-sleep rituals soothing and joyful

urinary problems

Sometimes you've just got to go. And it seems that the older you get, the more often this happens – with or without your conscious control. We're talking about something most people are loath to discuss, even with their doctors: urinary incontinence.

As many as 30 per cent of people over 65 have one or more of the three forms of urinary incontinence. Although women are far more likely than men to experience incontinence, by the age of 80, the gender disparity disappears. Urinary incontinence is not just embarrassing; it can affect your entire quality of life, leading you to cut out activities and friends you love and even changing the way you feel about yourself.

But here's the thing: leaking urine and sudden strong urges to urinate aren't conditions you have to live with simply because you're getting older. There are excellent medical and lifestyle treatments for incontinence. The first step, however, is admitting you have a problem and contacting your doctor or nurse.

Together, the two of you need to work out what type of incontinence you have. There are three main types – urge, stress and overflow – although you can have more than one at a time, in which case it's called mixed incontinence.

Stress incontinence With stress incontinence, you involuntarily leak urine when you laugh, run, sneeze, cough or otherwise exert yourself. This is by far the most common form and occurs especially in women, often because of childbirth. If the pelvic-floor muscles (which hold everything in your reproductive area in place) become weak, stretched or otherwise damaged during pregnancy or labour, stress incontinence often occurs. But men aren't off the hook.

Stress incontinence is often their cross to bear after prostate surgery.

Overflow incontinence This is the second most common form in men. It occurs when something blocks the urethra, the tube leading from the bladder to the outside of the body. In men, the blockage is most often caused by an enlarged prostate, medically known as benign prostatic hyperplasia (BPH). With BPH, your prostate pinches the urethra closed like a clamp would pinch a garden hose. Pressure builds up until urine finally leaks out without your voluntary assistance. Don't be embarrassed about BPH: it's the most common health problem in men aged 60 and above.

Urge incontinence In this form of incontinence, the urge to go strikes as suddenly as a summer storm – and often with similar flooding. Urge incontinence can occur if you have a central nervous system condition such as Alzheimer's or Parkinson's disease or have had a stroke. It may also be related to increased sensitivity of your bladder muscles to a brain chemical called acetylcholine, which stimulates the bladder into action.

Treatment includes medication, surgery or behavioural therapies such as exercising and bladder retraining. Lifestyle and behaviour changes are more effective overall than the medical options, but they may take longer to work, require more effort and may not provide a complete 'cure.' Here's how to get started.

To reduce incontinence

Get into training One of the best treatments for urge or stress incontinence is performing pelvic-floor muscle exercises called Kegels. The beauty of these exercises is that they can be done anywhere, at nearly any time, and you never have to break into a sweat. Start by pulling in or squeezing your pelvic muscles as if you were trying to stop the flow of urine or keep from passing gas. Count to ten as you hold the contraction, relax and repeat. That's it! Try to perform at least three sets of ten contractions a day. Start out lying down, then once you're good at them, perform your Kegels while waiting in a queue, driving, sitting in church – you get the idea. In one study comparing Kegels with medication, participants who did Kegels saw their episodes of incontinence drop by 81 per cent, compared with a 69 per cent drop in patients taking prescription medication. The combination of medication plus Kegels, however, works best for urge incontinence.

Check your medication Certain types of medication can induce incontinence, including many diuretics, asthma drugs, alpha blockers, narcotic pain relievers, anticholinergics, calcium channel blockers and ACE inhibitors for heart problems. If you aren't sure which types you take, ask your doctor for help.

Women, consider oestrogen Sometimes incontinence in middle-aged or older women is related to low levels of oestrogen. This hormone plays a role in the strength and overall health of the muscles that control the bladder as well as the bladder and urethra themselves. Talk to your doctor about using vaginal oestrogen. Because the oestrogen is inserted into the vagina via a cream or tablet, very little gets into your bloodstream, but enough gets to the urinary tract to help to reduce incontinence. One study found that 58 per cent of women receiving topical oestrogen to the vaginal area

What the doctor will say

If you want a doctor to solve your urinary incontinence problems, you may be offered either prescription drugs or surgery, depending on the type of incontinence you have.

Urge incontinence Several prescription drugs can prevent the bladder from contracting, keeping urine where it belongs until you deliberately choose to release it. Studies find that these types of medication can reduce the number of incontinence episodes by up to 70 per cent, curing the condition altogether in about 20 per cent of people.

Stress incontinence In women, surgery to tighten and strengthen the pelvic-floor muscles, followed by pelvic-floor muscle exercises, can reduce incontinence episodes by between 88 and 94 per cent. In men, however, surgical treatments may be less successful, with studies finding an improvement range of between 36 and 95 per cent. A major study comparing a minimally invasive form of surgery (in which a sling is used to hold up the urethra) to the more traditional procedure (in which the urethra and bladder are stitched to the pelvic wall) found the sling was much more effective in relieving stress incontinence.

Overflow incontinence The only real treatment for overflow incontinence is to treat whatever is blocking the urethra. In men, this usually means medication or surgery for an enlarged prostate.

three times a week had far fewer episodes of urge incontinence than a placebo group. A new treatment uses a ring impregnated with oestrogen that can be worn in the vagina for up to three months, avoiding the need for daily dosing. Be aware that some oestrogen preparations can damage the latex of condoms or diaphragms, though.

Get some training aids If you're still having trouble despite doing Kegel exercises, ask your GP about other techniques that could help you to improve the strength of your pelvic muscles. Your GP may be able to prescribe a set of

When embarrassment calls

'I have stress incontinence but I'm embarrassed to tell my doctor about it. How can I get the medical treatment I need if I can't even discuss it in a face-to-face examination?'

Join the crowd. More than half of all women with stress incontinence don't share their symptoms with their doctor, and by the time they're diagnosed, most have suffered with this condition for at least four years, studies show. Often, they don't bring it up because they don't think anything can be done, assuming it's a normal part of ageing. But incontinence is *not* a normal part of ageing and there are numerous treatments available to improve it. Instead of starting from scratch during a surgery visit, write your doctor an email or letter outlining your concerns and your symptoms. Include a schedule of all your bathroom usage and all the incontinence issues you experience over the course of a few days. Then make your appointment. When you turn up, your doctor can ask you any questions not answered in your letter, then the two of you can discuss treatment options.

vaginal cones. You insert a cone into your vagina for about 15 minutes, twice a day, and try to keep it in. You start with the lightest-weight cone then increase to the next weight up, like a sort of internal strength-training exercise. Other vaginal devices may help to support the bladder neck and stop involuntary outflow.

Get on a schedule Your GP may refer you to a specialist for bladder training. This approach takes about six weeks and aims gradually to increase the length of time between your feeling the urge to urinate and actually doing so. Initially, you urinate every hour or two whether you need to go or not, then you gradually reduce the frequency, thus training your bladder to hold urine. This approach is best for urge incontinence, with studies finding

that it is more effective than the major medication prescribed for the condition.

Ask about biofeedback This technique helps women to learn to exercise the correct pelvic-floor muscles to improve incontinence. A physiotherapist or continence adviser will show you how to use a special device that you insert into the vagina and which bleeps (or makes some other signal) when you are contracting the right muscles. Biofeedback plus pelvic-floor exercises seems to produce especially good results when combined with bladder training.

Get mildly shocked Your doctor can prescribe electrical stimulation, in which an electric current is applied directly to the pelvic floor, causing the muscles to contract and strengthening them.

Be lightly pricked Acupuncture appears to be a safe, effective treatment for urge incontinence, reducing symptoms in four to six weeks of treatment. However, the relief is likely to be short term, and you may need additional follow-up treatments.

Lose a few pounds If you're overweight or obese, there's more pressure on the neck of the bladder, increasing the risk of incontinence. Losing weight can help.

Skip the tea We're not sure why, but tea drinkers seem more likely to experience incontinence than coffee drinkers. Although it's obviously not due to the caffeine, researchers aren't sure what causes it.

Stub out the cigarettes Several studies have found a strong link between smoking and incontinence, particularly heavy smoking. ■

enlarged prostate
– that man thing

Men, are you noticing that it's taking a bit longer these days to, well, go? Do you find yourself looking for the nearest bathroom like you used to look for attractive women? Are you producing a urine stream that's weaker than your sense of humour? Don't be embarrassed. Every other man your age probably has the same problem.

Technically, you're dealing with benign prostatic hyperplasia (BPH), commonly known as an enlarged prostate. It's the most common health problem in men aged 60 and older. The prostate, in case you didn't already know, is the gland that creates and releases the fluid that makes up much of your semen. This gland surrounds the urethra, the thin tube that carries urine from your bladder to outside your body. As you age, your prostate gets larger (a bit like your ears, and no, we don't know why that happens), pressing on the urethra and, like a clamp on a garden hose, turning a stream into a trickle.

Check first with your GP to rule out a more serious problem, like prostate cancer. If your GP confirms BHP, you may be offered medication or surgery, or you may be able to handle it yourself by doing the following.

Stop drinking – at least before you go to bed Set the alarm on your watch for 2 hours before your normal bedtime. That's your signal to stop drinking so you can sleep through the night.

Choose decaffeinated One cup of coffee in the morning is fine. But after that, ask for decaf. And leave out the caffeinated tea, chocolate and aspirin, too. Caffeine is a natural diuretic.

Check your pills If you're taking diuretics for high blood pressure or heart failure, talk to your doctor. A lower dose or even a different medication could help to reduce your frequent trips to the loo. Along those same lines, ditch the decongestants and antihistamines. An unintended effect of these is to tighten the band of muscles around the urethra, making it harder to go.

Don't wait Don't try to hold it in. Visit the loo at the first urge so you don't overstretch your bladder.

Follow a heart-healthy lifestyle The same things that increase your risk of heart disease – being overweight, lack of exercise, high blood pressure, high cholesterol and diabetes – also increase your risk of BPH and make your symptoms worse. For specific recommendations on avoiding heart disease or diabetes, check out our suggestions on pages 316 and 363.

Try saw palmetto An analysis of 21 clinical trials involving more than 3,000 men concluded that the herb worked better than a placebo at improving symptoms of enlarged prostate and inadequate urinary flow and worked about as well as a widely prescribed medication. Follow the package directions for the dose.

PROTECTING

4

Preventing the diseases of ageing

Get the most from your health care

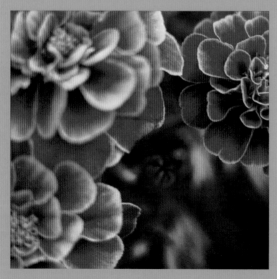
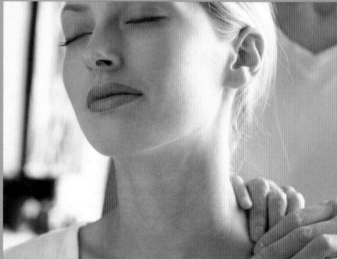

FUTURE HEALTH

Each of us has the capacity to avoid the diseases of ageing. **It just takes a little** preventive medicine – usually in the form of active, mindful living. **Here's your guide**

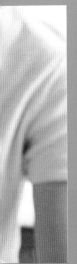
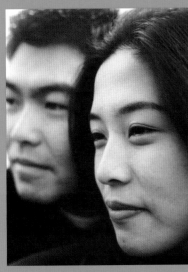
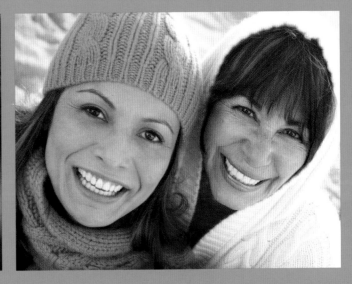

... high blood pressure   ... colds and flu

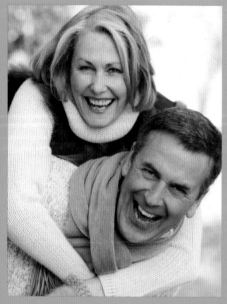
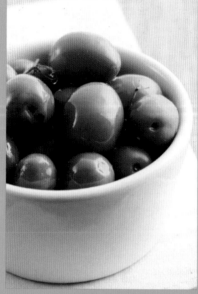
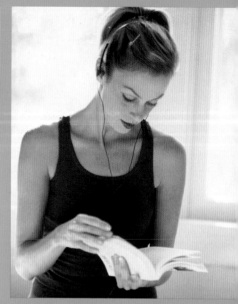

... balance   ... sleep problems

... joint and muscle pain

Preventing the
diseases of ageing

When it comes to looking at the reasons why people die, we are entering what some consider to be a 'third age'. It is a fascinating time and a wonderful development.

For most of history, viruses, bacteria or injuries were humankind's main causes of death. This was the 'first age', and it continued well into the 20th century. But with the discovery of vaccines, antibiotics and general medical knowledge regarding how to fix a broken body, we began to control many killer diseases and repair what once would have been fatal injuries. As a result, this 'first age' ended, and average life spans began to rise incredibly quickly in modern countries.

This new-found expertise in combatting disease and injury was a huge leap forward. What was still ignored or misunderstood, however, was the science of *good* health. Many of us – including doctors – smoked, overindulged in alcohol, ate fatty foods, embraced the emerging comforts of modern life (such as television) and didn't think at all about exercise. The result was the 'second age', spanning much of the past 60 years, in which heart disease and cancer rates grew to epidemic proportions and replaced viruses and bacteria as the leading causes of death in modern nations.

But something amazing has happened in just the past two decades. Researchers have started to understand what makes a heart go wrong, and to figure out some of the ways to fix it. We have even begun to understand and successfully treat some forms of cancer. Today, a diagnosis in either area carries with it a greater measure of hope and recovery than ever before. And, along the way, we discovered how nutrition, exercise, stress and compulsive habits such as smoking and drinking affect our bodies and cause disease.

Welcome then to the 'third age', in which we are living longer and more healthily than ever before. But with this new era has come a

For one component of the 'third age' of health is an unprecedented understanding of the underlying causes of good health. Fifteen years ago, issues such as chronic inflammation weren't understood. Today, we know that an immune system perpetually on the attack is a major cause of age-related disease. We also didn't know the subtleties of 'good' cholesterol or the complex changes in your body caused by stress and relaxation, or the power of micronutrients in our food to fight age-related disease and decline.

The goal: to take good enough care of your body that one part doesn't wear out ahead of the others

fresh crop of health problems that threaten to rob our later years of vitality and happiness. Generally, these are conditions caused by wear and tear. They are often the outcome of a long life led without health in mind.

For example, arthritis is frequently due to years of abuse to your joints. Diabetes, in many cases, is the result of years of poor eating and the gradual breakdown of the energy-transfer process within the cells in your body. Vision and hearing problems are often due to decades of overuse and abuse. Osteoporosis is a long, gradual decline in bone density; it, too, is a disease far more of the old than the young. And chronic pain, including back pain, is often an unwelcome side effect of a life long lived.

Living a long life

Just because you are likely to live longer doesn't mean that you are destined to suffer from these diseases and conditions of ageing.

With all this new understanding, we are on the verge of achieving not just long life, but also long health. However – and this is a major caveat – it is up to you. Doctors and the health-care system cannot deliver long health; it doesn't come in a pill. Only you can make it happen.

Forgive this car analogy, but it makes the point well: what makes one car break down at 75,000 miles for one owner, and the same model last 150,000 miles for a different owner? That's easy: regular maintenance, smart usage and constant loving care by the second owner.

It's no different for your body.

This final section of this book delves into the causes of ten of the most common diseases and conditions of ageing. More important, it provides the newest methods for preventing their onslaught. Many of these preventive measures are surprising and easily achieved. So take action! ■

Heart attacks and strokes

Once, doctors believed that the biggest risk factor for heart attacks and strokes was getting old. Conditions such as high blood pressure, out-of-balance cholesterol levels and large amounts of blood fats called triglycerides were seen as unfortunate, yet normal, parts of the ageing process.

But that was then, and this is now. The evidence today is overwhelming: making healthy lifestyle changes – as simple as an

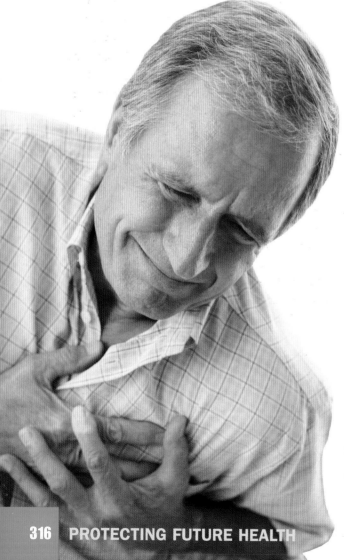

after-dinner stroll, a tropical-fruit dessert, a night out laughing with your best friends, even a glass of fine wine – can powerfully reverse those three threats and others that are the underlying causes of heart attacks and strokes.

That's the happy conclusion of hundreds, even thousands, of medical studies conducted around the world. And it holds true for people of all ages and health levels – whether you have arteries that are in tip-top shape, are taking medication to control somewhat problematic blood pressure or cholesterol levels, or have already had one heart attack or stroke and want to avoid a second.

You've no doubt heard the dire warnings already: heart attacks and strokes kill or alter the lives of more older people than any other health problem. And the cause of the damage sounds so simple: a clot comes loose in your bloodstream, stopping the flow of blood and oxygen to vulnerable heart muscle or brain cells. A clot can change your life in a matter of seconds.

But here's the information you need to know: making small, healthy changes *at any age* can dramatically lower your risk of a life-altering clot. Just four basic heart and brain-healthy lifestyle habits could make a five-fold difference to your risk of dying from cardiovascular disease, according to a major study by the Medical Research Council and the University of Cambridge. Researchers assessed the lifestyle habits of 20,000 people aged between 45 and 79 living in Norfolk and followed them for over 11 years. Each was given a lifestyle score of between 0 and 4, with one point each for not smoking, consuming moderate alcohol (1–14 units a week), eating five portions of fruit and vegetables daily and being active (either 30 minutes of exercise daily or having a non-sedentary occupation, such as a plumber or nurse). Those who had scored zero were five times more likely to have died from cardiovascular disease by the end of the follow-up than those who scored the full four.

The overall risk of dying from any cause was four-fold higher in those who scored 0 compared with those who scored 4. What's more, a 74 year old who scored on all four healthy habits had the same risk of dying as a 60 year old who scored zero, implying that just adopting these basic lifestyle habits could add an incredible extra 14 years to your life.

Previous studies have looked at the impact of single lifestyle habits, but this is the first to assess the major heart-healthy habits altogether. The researchers conclude that a large proportion of the population could gain real health benefits from moderate lifestyle changes.

When it comes to the heart, most of us do need to work to gain these benefits. At least half of all older adults have out-of-balance cholesterol levels, and 90 per cent of us will develop high blood pressure in older age, experts say. These and other threats team up to fill artery walls with heart and brain-threatening plaque, and to make blood vessels stiff and prone to damage that leads to clots.

Controlling, reversing or preventing these dangerous conditions can dramatically lower your odds of big problems: if everyone with high blood pressure got their condition under control, for example, the number of strokes would be cut nearly in half. And adopting healthier habits could cut your odds of a heart attack by up to 82 per cent.

The key? Don't rely on drugs or surgery alone. Make these healthy – and enjoyable – steps the foundation of your personal heart and brain protection plan.

Cholesterol: the new thinking

If you think automatically that cholesterol is bad for you, here's some news: at healthy levels, this natural substance isn't a demon at all. Your body uses this soft, waxy material daily to build cell membranes and to produce sex hormones, vitamin D and fat-digesting bile acids.

But modern-day cholesterol levels are out of balance – and it's not simply a matter of too much. We eat too many 'bad fats' – saturated fats and artificial trans-fatty acids that raise levels of heart-threatening LDL cholesterol. We also consume too little of the 'good fats' – the unsaturated fats and omega-3 fatty acids found in foods such as fish, nuts and some seeds – that protect levels of 'good' HDL cholesterol. And we skip exercise, the key to keeping LDLs lower and HDLs higher.

The result? Not just dangerously high total cholesterol but also dangerously out-of-balance levels of good HDLs and bad LDLs. The latest research on heart health shows that ignoring this balance, by focusing solely on lowering your cholesterol, can lead to trouble. Cutting-edge cardiologists are finding that the higher your HDLs *and* the lower your LDLs, essentially, the closer you can come to the 'natural' cholesterol balance human beings were meant to have. It's the most powerful way of lowering your risk of clogged arteries, heart attacks and strokes. At the same time, maintaining healthy levels of another important, though less well-known, blood fat called triglycerides, is important, too.

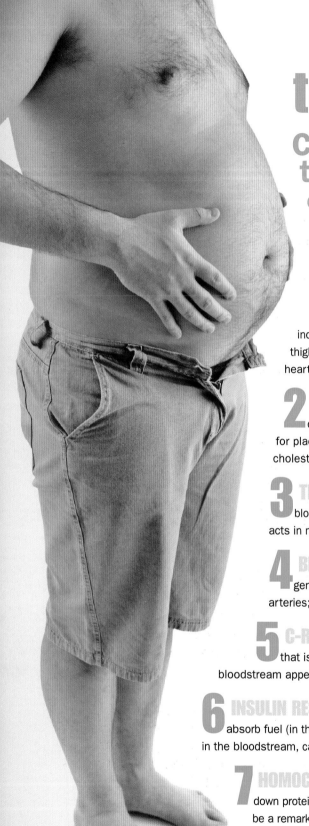

the 7 evils

Current science points to the following closely connected health factors as primary causes or indicators of future heart attacks and strokes.

1 BODY FAT New research reveals that an excess of visceral fat around your internal organs greatly increases your chances of heart disease. Interestingly, hip, thigh and bottom fat are more benign when it comes to your heart; a pot belly or wide waist is the real danger signal.

2 CHOLESTEROL Excessive amounts of 'bad' LDL cholesterol in your bloodstream provide the foundation for plaque to build up on artery walls. A shortage of 'good' HDL cholesterol is equally problematic.

3 TRIGLYCERIDES These are a type of fat found in your bloodstream. They have an important function, but an excess acts in much the same way as bad cholesterol.

4 BLOOD PRESSURE Compare a raging river to one that is gently flowing. High blood pressure creates the former in your arteries; that makes dislodging a clot far more likely.

5 C-REACTIVE PROTEIN This is an immune-system chemical that is created in response to inflammation. An excess in your bloodstream appears to contribute to the creation of plaque.

6 INSULIN RESISTANCE Insulin signals to each cell of your body to absorb fuel (in the form of blood sugar). When cells reject insulin, it builds up in the bloodstream, causing a chain reaction of unhealthy events for your arteries.

7 HOMOCYSTEINE This amino acid is created when your body breaks down proteins in your diet. High levels in your bloodstream have proven to be a remarkably good predictor of future heart disease.

9 ways to lower LDLs

Tiny, spherical LDL particles are your body's cholesterol delivery trucks, bringing liquefied cholesterol directly to the cells. But when too many LDLs crowd your blood (thanks to a diet high in saturated fat, too much weight, inactivity and, sometimes, your genes), extra particles burrow into the delicate lining of the artery walls. Free radicals – rogue oxygen molecules from cigarette smoking, digestion or ageing – damage the LDLs. A pool of fatty, gunky plaque builds up in the artery wall. If it ruptures, it causes a blood clot that could lead to a heart attack or stroke.

Put simply, high LDLs raise your risk of a heart attack or stroke. Low levels reduce your risk. For every 1 mmol/l (1 millimole per litre) fall in LDLs there is a 21 per cent fall in the risk of major cardiovascular problems. The safety zone: a desirable LDL level in a blood sample taken after an overnight fast (before you have breakfast) is 3 mmol/l or less. If you have heart risks such as diabetes, high blood pressure or a family history or personal history of heart disease, or if you smoke, your doctor may prescribe statin drugs to try to lower your LDL cholesterol to below 2.6 mmol/l – and some experts think that the target should be less than 2 mmol/l.

Research has shown that pushing LDL levels below 2.6 mmol/l can halt the progression of heart disease and cut mortality rates by 28 per cent. While doctors use statin drugs, you can take powerful lifestyle steps to cut your LDLs significantly – whether or not you also use medication. Here are nine great tips for starters.

1 Cut out trans fats Eat chopped veg instead of crisps, and fruit instead of biscuits or cakes and pastries. Choose margarines that clearly state on the label that they contain no trans fats, too. Why? Trans fats are worse for your heart than saturated fats because they boost levels of 'bad' LDL cholesterol and decrease 'good' HDL cholesterol. Avoiding these processed fats could cut your heart attack risk by 55 per cent, studies show.

2 Keep your slow-cooker on the worktop – and use it Eating leaner cuts of meat can cut your LDLs because you're getting less cholesterol-raising saturated fat in every bite. Low-fat meats can be tough, though; cooking them in a slow-cooker is an easy way to tenderise them without adding lots of fat.

3 Make your own salad dressing Use olive oil and vinegar or lemon juice, spices and crushed garlic. You'll get more cholesterol-lowering unsaturated fat and avoid the trans fats and saturated fats swimming in most bottled dressings – especially the creamy types.

4 Sit down to a bowl of porridge most mornings Porridge oats are packed with a soluble fibre called beta-glucan that whisks excess cholesterol out of your body. Having a large bowl of porridge (200g) on a regular basis could lower your LDLs by 12–24 per cent.

5 Have a pear or half a grapefruit every morning Both are rich in pectin, another soluble fibre that helps to lower LDLs. Other great pectin sources are apples and all types of berries. Grapefruit contains a substance that can interfere with the absorption of many medicines, though, so check with your doctor before making it a regular part of your morning routine.

6 Do 10 minutes of resistance-training exercises a day Women who did 45–50 minutes of muscle-building resistance-training exercises three times a week lowered their LDL levels by 14 per cent. Even just 10 minutes a day of the easy exercises on pages 202–13 will help.

7 Eat six small meals a day You'll get there if you follow the long-life eating approach. In a large British study, people who 'grazed' throughout the day had lower cholesterol levels than those who ate big meals twice a day. The difference was big enough to give the small-meal aficionados a 10–20 per cent reduction in their risk of heart disease.

8 Add a half teaspoon of cinnamon to your coffee before brewing Pakistani researchers have found that this amount (about 6g) reduced LDL levels by 30 per cent in people who had type 2 diabetes.

9 Avoid saturated-fat traps Your body uses saturated fats to produce LDLs. Overeating foods such as cheesecake, cheeseburgers and sausages provides far too much raw material for producing this heart-threatening stuff. A better plan: always stop and think before saying 'yes' to the foods heavy with animal fat. Ask yourself: what could I have instead? The answer might be a fruit salad, a lean steak, a piece of grilled chicken or fish, or a small helping of low-fat or fat-free frozen dessert such as sorbet or reduced-fat frozen yoghurt.

6 ways to raise HDLs

HDL, or 'high-density lipoprotein' cholesterol is the body's LDL cholesterol clean-up crew, actually fusing with the bad type of cholesterol and carrying it to the liver for disposal. New evidence suggests that HDLs also act as antioxidants, shielding LDLs from the type of damage that promotes plaque.

Long ignored by doctors, HDL is now taken seriously by researchers and clinicians as a heart-protection factor. Studies show that low HDL levels are an independent risk factor, and research suggests that for every 0.03 mmol/l increase in HDL, cardiovascular risk is reduced by 2–3 per cent. HDL can remove cellular cholesterol, and has anti-inflammatory, antioxidant and anti-clotting properties. Together, these inhibit atherosclerosis and improve the health of arterial linings, so reducing cardiovascular risk. This even applies to patients taking statins who have already achieved target levels of LDL, say cardiologists at University College London.

The new thinking: higher is better. Women after menopause should aim for levels of 1.3 mmol/l or higher, while men should aim for at least 1 mmol/l. Here are some ways to increase your levels.

1 Give up smoking Kicking the cigarette habit can raise your HDLs.

2 Enjoy one alcoholic drink a day A glass of wine with dinner could increase your good cholesterol. But skip this step if you also have high triglycerides – alcohol can make them soar and would cancel out the benefits.

3 Snack on walnuts or pecans You'll enhance your HDL level if you regularly snack on a small handful of walnut halves or pecans, report researchers from Shiraz University of

Medical Sciences in Iran and from Loma Linda University in California.

4 **Achieve a healthier weight** If your doctor approves of your weight-loss plans, gradually moving to a healthy weight could raise your HDLs, experts say.

5 **Walk briskly, three times a week** You can raise your HDLs with a fast-paced stroll (just vigorous enough that conversation is a little difficult) lasting half an hour, on three days of the week, studies show.

6 **Avoid a fat-free lifestyle** You read that right. Your body needs some fat to help to maintain its HDL level. Choose 'good' monounsaturated fats, found in olive oil, avocados and peanuts, and omega-3 fatty acids, found in fish, walnuts and fish-oil capsules, to help your body to keep HDLs on an even keel.

5 ways to reduce triglycerides

Triglycerides seem innocuous: they link to excess blood sugars from the food you eat and whisk them to fat cells for long-term storage. But when levels are high, triglycerides can also become the raw material for LDLs, making them another dangerous actor in the heart-disease drama. Newer studies suggest that triglycerides alone can be used to predict your risk of heart disease, because they encourage atherosclerosis – and may be twice as dangerous for women as they are for men.

Smoking, drinking, eating too much sugar and other refined carbs and being overweight can all elevate triglycerides. These additional strategies can help you to keep your triglycerides within a healthy range.

When to get help

If your cholesterol and triglyceride numbers are only slightly elevated, talk to your GP about trying lifestyle changes for about six months. After six months, ask for another blood test to check levels. If HDLs are still low or LDLs and/or triglycerides are still high, ask about medication, including cholesterol-lowering statins and drugs that can raise HDLs, such as prescription-grade niacin.

1 **Have a 'natural' whole grain at dinner every night** Try brown rice, bulgur wheat, barley, even quinoa. Simply choosing whole grains instead of the refined type could cut your risk of heart attack by 30 per cent.

2 **Have fruit for dessert** Fruit – fresh, frozen (without syrup), canned in its own juice or dried (but not sugar-coated) – has a wealth of fibre, vitamins and minerals, plus a host of antioxidants. Have some fruit most evenings.

3 **Avoid 'liquid sweets'** Skip high-sugar fizzy drinks, processed fruit juices and sweetened iced teas. Switch to fizzy water with a splash of orange juice or lemon, plain water or, if you just love fizzy drinks, try the diet version.

4 **Take your reading glasses to the supermarket** Even canned beans, tomatoes, and pasta sauce may contain sugar. Usually, a sugar-free version sits next to it on the shelf.

5 **Set a drink limit** The limit for women is no more than two to three units a day; for men no more than three to four units a day. If your triglyceride level is in the healthy range, these amounts are fine. If your triglycerides are high, cut out alcohol, as it can actually raise triglyceride levels. Even small amounts can send levels soaring in some people.

6 supplements your heart will love

These safe, well-chosen nutritional supplements repair and protect your heart in ways that go beyond a healthy lifestyle. Adding them to your personal long-life planning could add even more healthy years to your heart.

1 FISH OIL

Two heart-friendly omega-3 fatty acids – eicosapentaenoic acid (EPA) and docosahexaenoic acid (DHA) – found in fish-oil capsules can cut heart attack risk by 73 per cent. Fish oil stabilises dangerous artery plaque so that it's less likely to burst and trigger the formation of heart and brain-threatening blood clots. These oils can also cut triglycerides by 30–40 per cent. And fish oil helps to keep your heart beating in a regular rhythm, cutting the odds of out-of-rhythm beats that can trigger a stroke and sudden cardiac death.

How to take it: Experts suggest getting a total of 1,000–2,000mg of EPA plus DHA – though less conservative experts suggest twice as much may be better. How many capsules? Read the label; it varies by brand. Take it with food, and talk to your doctor first if you have a bleeding disorder or take an anticoagulant drug such as warfarin.

2 SOLUBLE FIBRE

Soluble fibre – found naturally in foods such as oatmeal, barley, beans and many fruits – forms a thick, cholesterol-trapping gel in your digestive system. Get enough and you could lower your 'bad' LDL cholesterol by 5 per cent – enough to reduce your heart disease risk by 10–15 per cent. While we need at least 8g a day – and up to 25g if you have elevated cholesterol – most of us barely take in 4g, about the amount in a bowl of porridge and a handful of strawberries. That's where a soluble fibre supplement comes in.

How to take it: Fibre supplements come as flavoured powder you mix with water, as capsules and even as wafers. Soluble fibre supplements can be made from ground psyllium seeds (the most extensively researched fibre supplement for cutting cholesterol), from beta-glucan (the same fibre that's in oatmeal) and also from fibres called inulin, methylcellulose and polycarbophil. Aim for 7–10g soluble fibre from supplements a day – and take half in the morning, half at night. Always drink a full glass of water with it. Check the product you choose; each has a different fibre content.

3 NIACIN

Megadoses of this B vitamin can raise your 'good' HDL cholesterol by a respectable 15–35 per cent, while lowering triglycerides by 20–50 per cent. But this supplement should be taken only as a prescription drug. The side effects of high-dose niacin include severe, painful facial flushing and potential liver damage.

How to take it: If you have low HDLs and high triglycerides, talk to your doctor about a modified-release niacin supplement. Some are formulated to reduce flushing and go easy on your liver.

4 ASPIRIN

Aspirin's pain-soothing, inflammation-cooling active ingredient – acetylsalicylic acid – is also a potent heart-protector that works by cutting clot risk. A daily, low-dose aspirin can cut your risk of a heart attack by a huge 33 per cent. But new evidence suggests that the benefits are far greater for men than they are for women.

How to take it: Generally, the recommended dose for prevention is 75mg/day (lower than a standard 300mg aspirin). Higher doses don't offer more protection, and more than 100mg/day may double the risk of gastrointestinal (GI) bleeding – take with a meal to cut the risk. But talk to your doctor before you start taking it as a preventive measure, especially if you also take anti-clotting agents such as warfarin or an anti-inflammatory like ibuprofen, or if you have had indigestion or an ulcer.

5 COENZYME Q10

Found in every cell in the body, coenzyme Q10 (CoQ10) boosts the effectiveness of enzymes that help cells to produce energy. Getting sufficient CoQ10 ensures that heart muscle cells will pump efficiently; it can also cut symptoms of heart failure and shield cells from free-radical damage. It may help to lower blood pressure, too. If you take a cholesterol-lowering statin, ask your doctor about adding CoQ10 daily; statins can block production of this enzyme by the liver.

How to take it: Scientists aren't yet sure how much CoQ10 is needed to gain benefits, so suggested doses range from 30–300mg daily. For best absorption, look for capsules or tablets with CoQ10 in an oil base. Take it with a meal containing a fat, such as salad dressing or peanut butter, to further enhance absorption.

6 PHYTOSTEROLS

Found naturally in soya beans, rice bran and wheat germ, plant sterols and stanols – known collectively as phytosterols – block the absorption of cholesterol from the food you eat. Now, these ingenious substances are available in capsules and in special cholesterol-lowering margarines, cream cheeses and yoghurts. A daily phytosterol supplement can lower your 'bad' LDLs, reducing your risk of heart problems.

How to take it: Experts recommend 2–3g a day – equivalent to 2–3 tablespoons of phytosterol-enriched margarine – to lower high LDL cholesterol levels. They are also available in pill form. Since phytosterols could block absorption of beta-carotene, get an extra serving of beta-carotene-rich foods every day (such as carrots, sweet potatoes and yellow squash) – and eat it at a meal when you're not using a phytosterol supplement for better absorption.

High blood pressure: the new thinking

As mentioned before, doctors once shrugged off high blood pressure in their older patients as a normal sign of ageing – a medical lapse that some believe has contributed to the high rates of heart attacks and strokes in people over the age of 55.

Today, all that has changed. While your odds of high blood pressure do rise with every passing birthday – experts estimate that 90 per cent of us will have elevated blood pressure at some point after the age of 55 – lowering it has never been easier.

Why bother? High blood pressure, also known as hypertension, is a silent killer that plays a role in 75 per cent of heart attacks and strokes. When modern living and genetics team up to stiffen artery linings, the blood pressure increases. This faster, harder flow of blood damages blood vessel walls, making it easier for heart-threatening plaque to form. At the same time, the extra pressure can cause plaque build-ups to break off; these are the clots that kill. When clots block the arteries that feed fuel and oxygen to your heart, that's a heart attack. When clots block the blood vessels to your brain, that's a stroke.

Scary stuff, yet there's more. High blood pressure can also enlarge and weaken your heart, and even damage your eyes and kidneys. It's also a risk factor for aortic aneurysm, a swelling of the major blood vessel carrying blood to the lower part of the body. If it goes undiagnosed and untreated, in extreme cases an aneurysm can rupture, which is usually fatal.

Lowering your blood pressure can cut your odds of major health problems significantly: stroke, by 30 per cent; heart attack, by 23 per cent; heart failure, by 55 per cent; dementia risk, by 50 per cent. At the same time, it can prevent or delay kidney damage and guard your eyes against vision loss brought on by severe hypertension.

So where once doctors didn't worry too much about mildly raised blood pressure, now if your blood pressure is persistently raised above 140/90 on at least three occasions, your doctor will assess your degree of cardiovascular risk – and determine a treatment plan accordingly.

Blood pressure readings are given as two numbers: the first represents systolic pressure, the force of blood against the artery walls during a heartbeat; the second number represents diastolic pressure, which measures pressure when the heart is relaxed between beats. Both numbers are expressed as mmHg, or millimetres of mercury. A desirable reading is 120/80 or below. If your reading is between 140/90 and 160/100 and you have no other risk factors and no signs of existing damage to your organs from high blood pressure, your doctor may suggest lifestyle modifications to try to bring it down. Suggestions may include losing weight, taking more exercise, eating a healthy diet, cutting down on salt and drinking alcohol in moderation.

Again and again, research confirms that high blood pressure is a major health risk, and that lower levels are almost always better

If your blood pressure is persistently above 160/100, or if you have existing cardiovascular disease or organ damage, or a high risk that these will develop, you will probably be offered medication as well. This may include drugs to lower cholesterol and treat diabetes as well as to reduce blood pressure, and a daily low-dose aspirin tablet to lower the risk of clots.

A complicated formula is used to assess your risk, taking into account factors such as your age and sex, whether you smoke, your blood pressure and blood cholesterol level. You may be told your overall risk in percentage terms. For example, a 20 per cent risk means that without treatment you have a 20 in 100 – or one in five – chance of developing cardiovascular disease (such as angina, heart attack, stroke or peripheral arterial disease) in the next ten years. Effective treatment can reduce this risk substantially, so your GP will monitor your blood pressure carefully to see that intervention is working. For example, it is estimated that lowering a raised diastolic pressure by 6 mmHg reduces your risk of heart disease by 20–25 per cent, and your risk of stroke by 35–40 per cent. So it's worth taking all the small steps you can to reduce your risk.

12 steps to better blood pressure

Even if you take drugs for blood pressure, adding these steps can lower your blood pressure even more – and allow you to get the most benefit from the lowest dose of medication.

1 Make reduced-sodium products your first choice Cutting your sodium intake by just 300mg (the amount in about two slices of processed cheese) reduces systolic pressure by 2–4 points, and diastolic pressure by 1–2

Fast clot-buster

If you or someone you're with has sudden heart attack symptoms, have them thoroughly chew and swallow one regular-strength aspirin tablet immediately. Chewing delivers aspirin's clot-stopping powers to your bloodstream in just 5 minutes; in contrast, swallowing the aspirin whole delays clot-stoppers for 12 crucial minutes.

points. Cut out more sodium, and your pressure drops even lower. Processed foods, not table salt, are the biggest source of excess sodium in our diets. You'll find more tips on reducing your sodium intake on page 162, but here are a few to jog your memory. Omit salt from recipes; fill your salt pot with a salt substitute; rinse foods canned in salted water or brine twice before cooking; select frozen meals with the least salt; and give unsalted or reduced-salt crisps and condiments a try. Read the labels on over-the-counter remedies carefully – some, such as antacids, can be surprisingly high in sodium. Your pharmacist can help you to find lower-sodium options.

2 Quit smoking Yes, you've read this advice in almost every part of this book, and have heard it for years. And for so many reasons. Here's the blood pressure reason: the nicotine in tobacco constricts blood vessels, immediately raising the pressure within them.

3 Have a banana, a slice of melon or a handful of dried apricots every day All are rich in potassium, nicknamed the *un*salt by experts because of its ability to keep blood pressure down. Other high-potassium foods include spinach, sweet potatoes and avocados.

4 Snack on soya nuts About 30g of crunchy roasted soya beans (called soya nuts) cut systolic blood pressure readings by 10 points in one study. Look for unsalted varieties in your supermarket or healthfood shop.

5 **Sprinkle 2 tablespoons of ground flaxseeds (linseeds) on your morning cereal** Then mix 2 tablespoons into your spaghetti sauce or yoghurt, or sprinkle over a salad later in the day. This could lower systolic pressure significantly, one study found. The secret ingredient? Probably the omega-3 fatty acids in flax.

6 **Have tea tomorrow morning (and afternoon) instead of coffee** For every cup of tea you drink in a day (up to four), your systolic blood pressure could fall by 2 points and your diastolic pressure could drop by 1 point, an Australian study suggests.

7 **Stroll four times a day** Exercise cut systolic pressure by 5 points and diastolic pressure by 3 points in one study of 21 women and men. But volunteers who took four brisk 10 minute walks a day kept blood pressure low for a whopping 11 hours, versus 7 hours for those who exercised for 40 continuous minutes once a day. Frequent activity keeps artery walls more fit and flexible.

8 **Avoid overuse of pain-relievers** Cut back on nonsteroidal anti-inflammatory drugs (NSAIDs), such as ibuprofen. Studies show that these popular pain-relievers can raise your blood pressure if you take them frequently.

9 **Go for garlic** A daily dose of garlic – as powder, oil or extract – produces significant reductions in systolic blood pressure, according to a review of 11 separate studies by Australian researchers. In some people, the fall was as much as that seen by taking antihypertensive drugs.

Generally, the higher the blood pressure at the start, the greater the fall when taking garlic – so garlic reduced systolic blood pressure by 4.6 mmHg on average, but in those with high blood pressure the reduction was an impressive 8.4 mmHg.

10 **Buy a home blood pressure monitor** A study presented at a recent European Society of Hypertension conference found that people who checked their blood pressure at home had lower blood pressure readings than those whose only checks were at the doctor's surgery. Relying on your doctor's tests alone misses 9 per cent of high blood pressure cases, another study has found. When you are shopping for a monitor, make sure the cuff is the right size (ask your doctor or pharmacist what size you need); be sure you can read the numbers on the monitor and hear the heartbeats if it uses a stethoscope; and take the monitor to your doctor's office to compare results with a professional model.

11 **Turn off your mobile phone – and forget about it** When 20 British students were asked to talk about their mobile phones to researchers, their systolic blood pressure jumped 8 points – a sign that a ringing phone in your pocket or bag is stressful. After the students gave up their phones for three days, the same exercise increased blood pressure by just 3 points. Silence, it seems, is healthy, says lead researcher David Sheffield, PhD, of Staffordshire University.

12 **Rediscover (low-fat) milk** Around the world, milk consumption is dropping as we sip more fizzy drinks and other sweetened soft drinks. But milk and other dairy products are important for blood pressure control because they contain calcium, which helps to regulate fluid levels in the bloodstream.

3 other risk factors

Even if you keep tabs on blood pressure and cholesterol, new evidence reveals that little-known threats could still be setting you up for trouble. The more researchers investigate, the more it seems that a number of chemical markers in the body are linked with your risk of cardiovascular disease. Yet your doctor may never mention these hidden risks, underestimate the danger or not even know about them yet. But if you're aware of them, and of what you can do to reduce multiple possible risk factors, you have a much better chance of staving off the potential consequences – and perhaps of saving your life.

The good news: taking control can be as easy as snacking on walnuts (instead of processed snacks) or taking a multivitamin every day.

risk 1
C-reactive protein

This chemical is made in the liver when part of your body is inflamed. Studies show that high levels of C-reactive protein (CRP) can raise your risk of heart disease even if your cholesterol level is healthy. High CRP is a warning signal of plaque building up in the artery walls.

So what causes high levels of CRP? Mostly, low-grade infections in your body, such as gum disease, and other ongoing irritants that mean your immune system is constantly doing battle. This is the 'chronic inflammation' problem talked about more and more in health circles.

Because blood levels of CRP can be raised by a wide variety of inflammatory conditions, measuring them has limited value in predicting risk of heart disease. However, studies have

Check your pulse

Another heart problem increasingly common with age is atrial fibrillation (AF), a condition that causes a fast, irregular heartbeat. Symptoms may include palpitations, dizziness, breathlessness or the chest pains of angina – or it may go undetected until your doctor takes your pulse.

AF affects about 1 in 200 people aged 50–60 but 1 in 20 over 65 and almost 1 in 10 of those aged over 80 in the UK. It can be caused by other heart diseases, high blood pressure, various medical conditions or something as simple as drinking too much alcohol or coffee. Its danger lies in the fact that up to 15 per cent of people with AF suffer ischaemic strokes each year – and often, they're severe.

The unsteady heartbeats of AF create turbulent blood flow within the heart that may allow blood to pool and tiny clots to form. If these get taken in the bloodstream to the brain, they can cause a stroke. The risk of stroke in someone with AF is four to six times higher than normal.

Finding, and fixing, AF could cut your risk of a stroke by 60 per cent. To check for an irregular heartbeat, find your pulse at your neck or wrist with the flat pad of your fingertip. Repeat the rhythm out loud: dum-dum-dum-dum. If what you get is more like dum-dum-da-dum or some other variation, report it to your doctor. You may need treatment with drugs or electrical stimulation (cardioversion) to regulate your heartbeat, and clot-preventing drugs such as aspirin or warfarin.

shown that lowering CRP slows the rate of progression of atherosclerosis – so it's well worth taking measures to keep your levels low. Here are three top ways to help to tame your CRP.

Brush, floss and rinse every day Even tiny pockets of gum disease increase inflammation levels throughout your body, raising the odds of a heart attack and even a stroke. Studies show that brushing carefully, flossing well, then rinsing with a gum-protecting mouthwash all help to protect your cardiovascular system.

Make all your sandwiches on wholegrain bread Research shows that getting 32g of fibre a day could slash CRP levels by half. You'll get there if you also choose high-fibre cereals, beans, lentils and wholegrain pasta.

Snack on a handful of walnuts instead of a chocolate bar Rich in fibre and 'good' omega-3 fatty acids, these nuts slash CRP levels.

risk 2
metabolic syndrome

As many as one in four people in the UK have a dangerous cluster of heart attack and stroke risk factors that doctors now dub the metabolic syndrome. It's also called insulin resistance, because a major feature is a combination of high blood sugar levels with high insulin levels.

Make all your sandwiches on wholegrain bread

Whereas normally insulin acts to increase the uptake of glucose by cells, so reducing levels in the blood, in this condition, the fat, muscle and liver cells fail to respond properly to insulin. The body pumps out more and more, in an attempt to reduce blood glucose levels, but they remain high – so a metabolic imbalance develops.

Metabolic syndrome also includes high blood pressure, out-of-balance blood fats, with increased levels of triglycerides and reduced HDL, and central obesity – the dangerous laying down of fat around the abdomen. All of these promote widespread inflammation and increase the tendency of the blood to clot – dramatically raising the risk of heart attacks and strokes. And if you don't deal with the features of metabolic syndrome, you're also at high risk of diabetes, liver and kidney disease, gallstones and other complications.

While a doctor may treat particular problems such as high blood pressure, blood fats or blood sugar, there is much *you* can do to lower your risk. Nearly every healthy eating and exercise tip in this book will help to reduce your chances of getting metabolic syndrome and prevent or delay its dire complications. And here are three steps that are guaranteed to help to make a difference.

Get 30 minutes of exercise a day It forces muscle cells to take up extra blood sugar and also makes them more sensitive to insulin.

Trim belly fat Eat whole grains, fruits and veg, and make time to exercise – these strategies can shrink dangerous abdominal fat, which wraps itself around your internal organs and raises your odds of metabolic syndrome.

Snack on fruit not sweets High-sugar, low-fibre processed sweets send blood sugar levels soaring and trigger the release of loads of insulin to bring levels down. A high-sugar diet taxes your body's ability to control blood sugar, especially if you're overweight or inactive.

Could you have metabolic syndrome?
You're likely to have metabolic syndrome if you have three of these:
- A waist circumference over 94cm (37in) in men or 89cm (35in) in women
- Triglyceride levels of 1.7 mmol/l or more
- Blood pressure above 130/85 (or if you are taking drugs for high blood pressure)
- Fasting plasma glucose (blood sugar) levels over 5.6 mmol/l (or if you are taking drugs to reduce your blood sugar levels)
- HDL cholesterol levels of less than 1.03 mmol/l in men or 1.29 mmol/l in women

risk 3 homocysteine

Evidence suggests that too much of this amino acid – created when your body digests protein, especially from meat – damages the inner lining of arteries and promotes blood clotting. People with high homocysteine levels have an increased risk of heart disease. Homocysteine levels are naturally kept low by higher blood levels of B vitamins, and people who eat plenty of fruit and veg – which contain vitamin B_6 and folate (also a B vitamin) – generally have lower rates of heart disease. But vegans tend to have high homocysteine levels because they eat no meat, fish or dairy produce, the main sources of vitamin B_{12}, which also cuts homocysteine levels.

So a healthy, balanced diet is what you need – and unless you're deficient in B vitamins, it's no good just popping a vitamin pill. In the Norwegian Vitamin Trial (NORVIT), researchers from the University of Tromsø found that people who took supplements containing folic acid and vitamins B_6 and B_{12} got no benefit from supplements, even though homocysteine levels fell by up to 30 per cent. Here are some hints on keeping vitamin B levels naturally high and homocysteine levels in check:

Cut the coffee A study at the University of Bergen in Norway, showed that those who drank more coffee had lower vitamin B and higher homocysteine levels.

Have an orange at breakfast and a spinach-and-tomato salad with lunch Citrus fruits, tomatoes and spinach are all sources of folic acid, which breaks down homocysteine.

Snack on low-fat, unsweetened yoghurt People who regularly enjoy dairy products have homocysteine levels 15 per cent lower than those who avoid them, studies show.

Stir-fry peppers and broccoli for dinner In a study of 6,000 people, those who ate the most peppers (red, yellow, green or hot) and the most cabbage, broccoli and cauliflower had homocysteine levels 16.5 per cent lower than those who didn't eat them regularly. ■

Cancer

For all the fear it invokes, cancer is not an invader of your body, like a virus or bacteria. Cancer is simply your own cells running amok. It develops when the built-in mechanisms designed to destroy damaged cells fail or are overwhelmed by the extent of the damaged cells.

And so those damaged or cancerous cells keep doing what cells do – multiplying. Unlike normal cells they don't have an 'off' switch, so they keep dividing, using up valuable blood, oxygen and nutrients that healthy cells need. Eventually, the proliferation of cancer cells makes it impossible for healthy cells to survive.

These cancer cells are pretty smart. They are able, in many instances, to disguise themselves to evade detection by the immune system. They also mutate to resist the poisons designed to root them out. And, sometimes, they lay dormant for years until something – such as biochemical stress, gene mutations, toxins or trauma – triggers them into action again.

The connection between cancer and age? Maths. The older you are, the longer your cells have been dividing. The greater the number of divisions, the greater the likelihood that some mistakes will occur. The more mistakes, the greater the likelihood that one of those 'mistake' cells will survive and become a cancer. That's why 77 per cent of all cancers are diagnosed in those aged 55 and over. And it's why until about 100 years ago – when the average lifespan in developed countries finally passed the 50 year mark – cancer was relatively rare. Today, it's among the leading causes of death in developed countries, with one in three dying from cancer.

But here's the thing: about two-thirds of all cancers could be prevented – if people stopped smoking, ate better foods and exercised.

Your job, then, is to arm yourself with all known (and suspected) weapons to reduce the probability that cellular mistakes will occur and increase the likelihood that if they do occur, the systems designed to correct or destroy them work. That means reducing the production of free radicals, increasing the availability of antioxidants to fight off free radicals, and stemming the tide of inflammation.

The best ways to prevent cancer

At a cellular level, all cancers are similar. But what makes cancer so challenging is that it can develop in many places in the body, each based on different triggers and causes.

What does this mean? For example, although excessive sun is the top cause of the cellular damage that leads to skin cancer, non-burning sun exposure may protect you from internal cancers, by boosting vitamin D production. And even though your digestive system encounters many toxins and chemicals in your food that can ultimately cause cancer to develop in your stomach, oesophagus or intestines, they might have less impact elsewhere in your body.

That means one set of preventive measures cannot effectively battle all cancers. On page 334 are the top five ▶

top 5 cancer myths

Researchers from the American Cancer Society, the US equivalent of Cancer Research UK, decided to find out just how much we know about the disease. What they found might surprise you. More than 25 per cent of the 1,000 people surveyed believed the following statements were true. If you thought they were true, too, beware: lack of knowledge about cancer is itself a risk factor for developing cancer.

1 The risk of dying from cancer is increasing Not true in modern countries. In fact, the risk of dying is decreasing as we get better at diagnosing and treating cancer. Plus, the risk of developing certain cancers is also declining as people quit smoking and take other lifestyle steps to reduce their cancer risk.

2 Pollution is a greater risk factor for lung cancer than smoking No. While high levels of pollution can increase the risk of lung cancer, the increase is tiny compared with smoking: tobacco causes around 90 per cent of lung cancers, pollution causes about 3 per cent.

3 Physical injuries later in life cause cancer Not really. Although a few studies have linked injuries such as head trauma to a later risk of certain rare cancers, the vast majority of cancers have nothing to do with trauma.

4 Electronic devices such as mobile phones cause cancer Although any risk from long-term intense use is still unclear, the vast majority of studies show no risk from short-term use of mobile phones.

5 How you live when you're young has little effect on your risk of cancer later One word here: sunburn. A single serious sunburn in your teens can set you up for melanoma, the most serious form of skin cancer, 30 years later. Smoking for even a year creates genetic damages in lung tissue cells that can trigger cancerous cells decades later. In fact, some studies are now finding that the seeds of cancer could be sown in the womb – based on what your mother did when she was pregnant with you.

steps to take; they are the closest you can come to a total cancer-prevention plan. Plus, many of the other healthy-lifestyle tips shown in this book help to battle cancer. Also, it's important to try as many of the actions that follow as possible. These are the preventive measures that, in recent studies, have shown significant benefits. In each case, the type of cancers for which the action is best suited is revealed.

SIP SOME TEA Real tea – not herbal – contains powerful antioxidants called catechins that help to protect proteins and DNA from oxidative damage, the harmful changes due to free radicals and other substances produced in cellular metabolism that can lead to cells becoming cancerous. In laboratory studies, catechins stop tumours from growing and protect healthy cells. And in population studies, researchers find that people who are regular tea drinkers have half the risk of developing some cancers as those who don't drink the liquid at all, or who drink it less frequently.
BEST FOR Stomach and oesophageal cancer

SWITCH TO OLIVE OIL Not only can olive oil reduce heart disease, it's also a great way to elude cancer. In late 2006, researchers from five European countries concluded that olive oil alone may account for the significant difference in cancer rates between southern and northern Europeans. They found that north Europeans had much higher average levels of a marker of oxidative damage. But after three weeks of supplementing with 25ml of olive oil daily, north European volunteers showed a significant fall in levels of the marker – sufficient, the researchers conclude, to support the idea that 'olive oil consumption may explain some of the north-south differences in cancer incidences in Europe'.
BEST FOR All cancers

SUPPLEMENT WITH VITAMIN D AND CATCH SOME RAYS Several studies find that the 'sunshine vitamin' reduces the risk of many cancers. Vitamin D is best produced by sunlight acting on the skin, but also comes from food sources, and in winter in northern climates you can get the benefits by taking supplements.

In one study, researchers followed 1,179 postmenopausal women for four years. Half took 1,400–1,500mg of calcium alone, and half took the calcium along with 1,100 international units (IU) of vitamin D. Those getting the calcium/D supplement had a 30 per cent lower risk of developing any type of cancer during the four years than those receiving just calcium.

Other studies found that women with vitamin D intakes of more than 800 IU a day from diet or supplements had a 19 per cent lower breast cancer risk than those getting less than 400 IU. Studies also find that people in sunny climates are far less likely to develop solid tumours such as stomach, colorectal, liver, gall bladder, pancreatic, lung and prostate cancers than those from northern climates.

The bottom line: the more steady, continuous exposure you get to the sun (*not* sunburn), the less likely you are to develop many internal cancers. One reason for vitamin D's benefits may be its ability to limit cell division and to help to ensure that when cells do divide, they don't differ significantly from other cells of their type.
BEST FOR Most solid tumours (such as breast, prostate, pancreatic, colorectal, lung, stomach, liver and gall bladder)

FOLLOW A CANCER-PREVENTING DIET
The link between cancer and nutrition is so powerful that there's even a medical journal devoted just to that topic: *Nutrition and Cancer.* So as well as substituting olive oil for other fats,

as mentioned above, and loading up on tomatoes (see page 334), get plenty of these other foods.

● **Apples** Apples are packed with quercetin, an antioxidant shown to reduce the risk of numerous cancers, particularly lung cancer. One study of more than 77,000 women found that just one apple a day reduced the risk of lung cancer by 21 per cent, regardless of smoking status. Meanwhile, experiments in the laboratory showed that quercetin prevents lung cancer cells from multiplying.

● **Raspberries** Raspberries, seeds and all, contain even more antioxidants than blueberries and strawberries. Rats injected with a compound to cause colon cancer, then fed a diet rich in raspberries, developed 80 per cent fewer tumours than rats who didn't get the fruit (but who did get the cancer-causing chemical).

● **Cruciferous vegetables** These include broccoli, cauliflower, brussels sprouts and even cabbage-based dishes such as sauerkraut and coleslaw. In one major study, men who ate three or more 40g servings of these veggies a week reduced their risk of prostate cancer by 41 per cent, compared with men who ate less.

Steam the vegetables slightly and drizzle on a little olive oil.

● **Garlic and onions** These two flavoursome vegetables are jammed with cancer-destroying chemicals. Get 16 servings a week of onions (80g raw, chopped onion equals one serving) and 22 servings a week of garlic (one clove equals one serving), and your risk of oral, oesophageal, colorectal, laryngeal, ovarian, breast and prostate cancers drops precipitously.

The protective effect from both vegetables stem from the same compounds that give each their distinctive odours: organosulphur compounds. These compounds do many things: they influence enzymes that detoxify carcinogens; they prevent DNA from bonding to cancer-causing substances; and they scavenge free radicals in the bloodstream, inhibit proliferation of tumour cells and support the immune system, among other benefits. People who consume a diet rich in these compounds have been shown to be less susceptible to a variety of cancers. One hint: either use garlic raw or let it sit for 10 minutes after chopping; otherwise, heat destroys the cancer-protecting enzymes.

BEST FOR Nearly all cancers

Garlic and onions are jammed with cancer-destroying chemicals

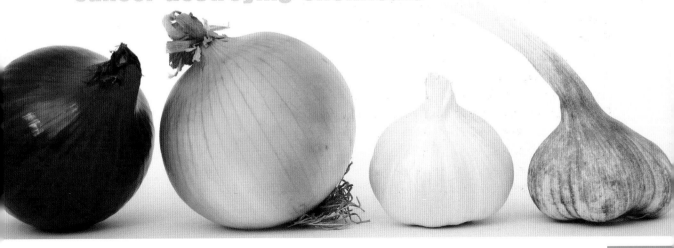

Top 5 ways to prevent cancer

1 **Stop smoking** You've heard it before. But consider this: if you smoke, you are 23 times more likely to develop lung cancer than someone who doesn't. Compare that with a woman who had a mother, sister or daughter diagnosed with breast cancer; her overall risk is only twice that of a woman with no mother, sister or daughter diagnosed with breast cancer. Yet what do women worry about most? Breast cancer.

2 **Cut back on the alcohol** Drinking excessive amounts of alcohol is a major cause of breast, bladder, stomach, oesophageal, liver and colon cancers, among others. Scientists suspect the link may be due to the effects of acetaldehyde, a suspected carcinogen that forms as the body metabolises alcohol. This compound reacts with natural compounds that are required for cell growth. This reaction can cause DNA damage to cells, which can, in turn, lead to malfunctioning cell division. Healthy limits are no more than two units a day for women, or three for men.

3 **Lose weight** About one in three cancers results from poor diet and being overweight, particularly breast, colon, rectal, stomach, prostate and pancreatic cancers. When you're overweight, your body produces more oestrogen – linked to breast, ovarian and uterine cancers; and more insulin, which can increase inflammation and free-radical damage.

4 **Eat right** Studies find that diets low in red meat and high in whole grains result in lower levels of various cancers, as do those that get seven to nine servings a day of fruits and vegetables.

5 **Get moving** Physical activity not only helps you to maintain a healthy weight, it also reduces the percentage of body fat and helps your muscles to make better use of insulin, reducing insulin blood levels and free-radical production. Specific studies find that regular physical activity can slash the risk of bowel cancer by half and the risk of uterine cancer by a third, as well as significantly reducing the risk of ovarian, breast and colon cancers.

HAVE SEX No, we're not kidding. An eight year study of 29,342 men aged 46–81 found that the more orgasms the men had, the lower their risk of prostate cancer. Specifically, those who had at least 21 orgasms a month slashed their risk of the disease by a third, compared with those who only had four to seven a month. The mechanism at work here? The prostate makes semen; the more you ejaculate, the more potentially cancerous cells you're getting rid of (and no, they won't hurt your partner). If you don't have a partner, don't worry. The benefit comes from ejaculating, which, as you no doubt know, doesn't require a partner.
BEST FOR **Prostate cancer**

SPOON ON SOME TOMATO SAUCE

Lycopene, an important antioxidant in tomatoes, packs a heck of an anti-cancer wallop. Just ten tomatoes a week reduces the risk of prostate cancer by a third and the risk of breast cancer up to 50 per cent. The thing is, you get way more lycopene if the tomatoes are cooked, which releases more of the chemical. Even just gently heating a chopped tomato will up the content.
BEST FOR **Prostate, breast and oesophageal cancer**

DRINK WATER LIKE A THIRSTY CAMEL

The more water you drink, the more you dilute toxins in food and other liquids, reducing their damaging effects on your colon and bladder. One major study found that just six 250ml glasses of water every day slashed the risk of bladder cancer by half in men; while another found a 45 per cent reduced risk of colon cancer in women who drank a lot of water throughout the day. To avoid a huge pile of plastic bottles, keep a jug of filtered water in your fridge at home and at work, and make sure you empty it at least once, preferably twice, a day.
BEST FOR **Colon and bladder cancer**

Chronic pain

Slam your finger in the car door and it hurts. No, it *really* hurts. But after a few minutes and an application of ice, the pain recedes to a dull throb. By tomorrow, only the bruise remains to remind you of the incident. You've just experienced acute pain – pain related to a short-term cause, such as a burn, bump or broken bone.

But around four in ten adults aged 65 and older have ongoing, chronic pain that doesn't go away. This becomes more common with age, and may be linked

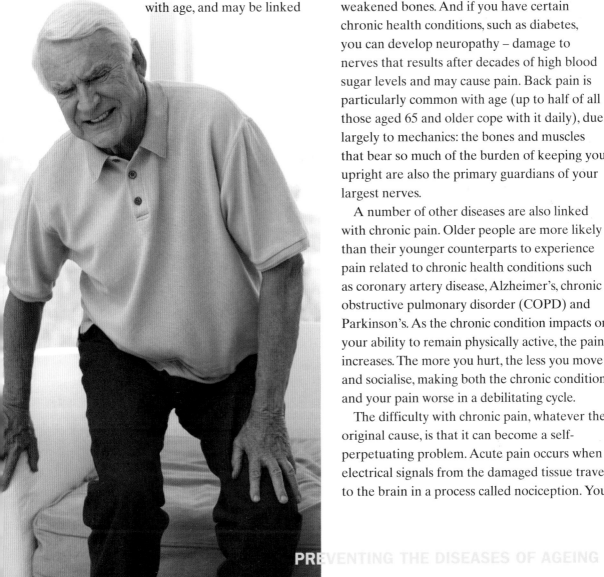

with a variety of causes, or sometimes no specific cause can be found.

Chronic pain may follow an injury (even a trivial one), surgery, amputation or a shingles outbreak. It may be part of a condition such as fibromyalgia or multiple sclerosis, related to long-term medication or it may simply come from years of wear and tear on your body. After five or six decades of active living, you naturally become more likely to experience ongoing pain from arthritis, worn joints or weakened bones. And if you have certain chronic health conditions, such as diabetes, you can develop neuropathy – damage to nerves that results after decades of high blood sugar levels and may cause pain. Back pain is particularly common with age (up to half of all those aged 65 and older cope with it daily), due largely to mechanics: the bones and muscles that bear so much of the burden of keeping you upright are also the primary guardians of your largest nerves.

A number of other diseases are also linked with chronic pain. Older people are more likely than their younger counterparts to experience pain related to chronic health conditions such as coronary artery disease, Alzheimer's, chronic obstructive pulmonary disorder (COPD) and Parkinson's. As the chronic condition impacts on your ability to remain physically active, the pain increases. The more you hurt, the less you move and socialise, making both the chronic condition and your pain worse in a debilitating cycle.

The difficulty with chronic pain, whatever the original cause, is that it can become a self-perpetuating problem. Acute pain occurs when electrical signals from the damaged tissue travel to the brain in a process called nociception. You don't actually feel the pain until the signal hits the brain. But if the pain goes on for a long time, it seems to lead to persistent changes in the nervous system – perhaps some damage to the nerve cell 'wiring', degeneration or faulty repair within the nervous system, spontaneous electrical or chemical nerve signals, faulty pain 'memory' in the brain or even an autoimmune attack on the nerves. While the exact mechanism is uncertain, scientists think that somehow the nervous system begins generating its own electrical signals – irrespective of any injury. Those messages travel to the brain and activate pain centres in a kind of feedback loop from the brain to the nerves and back again that's become stuck in the 'on' position.

This is no small thing. Chronic pain significantly affects your quality of life: it increases your risk of depression, keeps you away from the health-enhancing benefits of socialising and disrupts your sleep. It can even affect your memory and ability to learn.

That is the harsh side of the pain discussion. There is a positive side as well. Over the past decade, the medical world has made huge strides not only in understanding pain and its remedies but also in how to help to communicate with patients regarding pain. The latter point is important; it wasn't long ago that pain was seen as a side issue to other health problems, either to be coped with or dealt with via strong painkillers – many of which have been proven to have serious side effects.

Today, doctors understand much better how to manage chronic pain, and specialist, multi-faceted pain management can often make an enormous difference, especially if the pain is part of a larger health issue. So don't suffer in silence – talk to your GP about whether referral to a pain clinic or pain specialist is appropriate.

The message: no one, NO ONE, needs to suffer in silence from chronic pain.

Managing pain the smart way

It would be great to give you the perfect mix of tips to guarantee that you won't ever face chronic pain, but it's not possible. There is just too wide a range of causes, from disease to injury to old-fashioned wear and tear.

While we have to acknowledge that chronic pain becomes more prevalent with age, there are effective ways to minimise it and, in some cases, erase it. And so, here are 12 proven, smart ways to control ongoing pain. If you're already taking pain-relievers, these tips may allow you to use less medication, or to forgo it altogether.

Jump on the exercise bike Studies show that exercise can be a powerful antidote to pain. There are many reasons: strong muscles take pressure off the joints; exercise washes your body with nourishing oxygen and nutrients, and it also releases feel-good brain chemicals that provide relaxation and relief. The key is to go for more than 10 minutes – shorter bouts don't seem to help. But, in fact, nearly any type of physical exercise will significantly improve your pain – as long as you stick with it (even after you start feeling better).

Say 'ohhmmm' Okay, you don't really have to chant, but meditation can do more for low back pain in older adults than any over-the-counter drug. In a study published in the journal *Pain*, 37 adults aged 65 and older either joined a mindfulness-based meditation programme or were put on a waiting list for the programme (the control group). Those meditating significantly improved their scores on an objective pain scale and upped their activity levels compared with the control group. Another study found that people who listened to a 7 minute tape that helped them to relax, focus on the images their pain elicited, then change those images with their mind, described their pain as 'more tolerable' or 'easier to control' than a control group. These tapes are available online and from most healthfood shops.

Sign on for biofeedback Biofeedback teaches you to control involuntary reactions, voluntarily. For instance, instead of tensing when you feel pain, which can make the pain worse, you learn to relax, which stems the release of pain-inducing stress hormones. In one study, 17 participants between the ages of 55 and 78 learned to use biofeedback to relax their muscles and breathe more slowly and deeply. Not only did their pain improve, but they were able to elicit certain physiological changes that contributed to the decrease in pain. For instance, their skin temperature increased, an indication that there was more blood flow to the painful area, which helps to clear away toxins and inflammatory chemicals that may add to the hurt.

Join a group It doesn't matter what the group does, as long as you're interacting with other people. Studies find that older people who keep busy and engaged, including maintaining a strong social network, have significantly less chronic pain than those without.

Become a student of pain management Use the internet or your local library to find information about chronic pain. Simply learning the whys and wherefores of your pain can significantly improve it. Enlist the help of friends and family members so they can better understand your experiences as well as help you to find the most effective approaches.

See a therapist Cognitive Behaviour Therapy teaches you to avoid negative thinking and self-defeating behaviour (for instance, 'I hurt too

Assessing pain

Pain is so subjective that it's often difficult to describe to other people, including doctors. It's also impossible to measure – there is no 'pain' chemical or virus you can test for. So doctors often rely on simple rating systems as a way of determining the intensity of your pain. These are often as easy as rating your pain on a scale from 1 to 10, or picking a drawing of a face that best portrays the pain level (ranging from smiling happily to grimacing).

Another way doctors monitor pain is through non-verbal indicators, such as these.

Vocal complaints moans, gasps, sighs or exclamations

Facial expressions such as grimaces, winces, clenched teeth, furrowed brows or narrowed eyes

Bracing movements clutching a railing or grabbing a body part

Rubbing movements massaging the affected area

much to take a walk'), and provides positive reinforcement for achieving your goals (take that walk!). It also teaches you coping skills for better pain management. You should see results in just 6–15 sessions, but check that the therapist is experienced in working with pain patients. In some areas, your GP may be able to refer you to a therapist on the NHS.

Follow an anti-inflammatory diet Chronic inflammation is often the culprit behind chronic pain, particularly with conditions such as rheumatoid arthritis. And the cause of much of the inflammation in your arteries and the rest of your body is from free radicals, those destructive molecules that damage cells. An anti-inflammatory diet has two main components: lots of antioxidants to neutralise free radicals in your bloodstream, and plenty of healthy fats such as olive oil to reduce inflammation. So what should you eat?

- One to two vegetable and/or fruit servings with each meal (even breakfast)
- Some form of oily fish (salmon, fresh tuna, anchovies) at least twice a week
- A daily helping of soya – edamame (soya beans), 250ml soya milk, tofu cubes, even soya-based frozen desserts
- Flaxseeds (linseeds) sprinkled over salads and yoghurt and mixed into sauces
- Olive oil for cooking and salad dressings
- Foods such as asparagus, avocado and walnuts

And here's what to limit or remove entirely from your diet:

- Fats such as butter, corn and vegetable oil
- Red meats high in saturated fats
- 'Simple' carbs, particularly those high in sugar and low in fibre, such as sweets, doughnuts, cakes and fizzy drinks.

Munch some cherries Cherries are high in anti-inflammatory anthocyanins, plant-based chemicals that give the fruit its dark red colour. Some studies find that these chemicals can reduce the pain of arthritis and gout, as well as swelling and inflammation.

Have a piece of chocolate When pain is an issue, a small piece of dark chocolate may help. Like other sweet foods, chocolate can stimulate the release of pain-relieving endorphins in the brain. That's why newborns are often given sugar water to suck on during painful procedures, such as collecting blood from their heels (and perhaps why most women in one recent survey said they preferred chocolate to sex). But unlike sugar, a small amount of dark chocolate can actually be good for you – it's full of antioxidants that can help conditions such as diabetes.

Try chiropractic The evidence for the use of chiropractic for certain painful conditions, including back and neck pain, is irrefutable. Numerous studies show that it is effective – so much so that it is often now available on the NHS. Talk to your GP if you think chiropractic could help you.

Consider acupuncture This ancient healing practice, in which very thin needles, pressure or electricity are used to stimulate certain body parts, has become mainstream in terms of pain management. Acupuncture stimulates the release of feel-good endorphins into your spinal fluid, where they serve as a kind of buffer to prevent pain signals from reaching your brain. Acupuncture has been used successfully with few, if any, side effects to treat back pain, neck pain, osteoarthritis, fibromyalgia and generalised pain. One caveat: you may need repeat treatments if your pain is chronic.

Keep up your vitamin D intake According to a study of 7,000 British people aged over 45, chronic pain was more common among smokers, non-drinkers, people who were either overweight or underweight and, in women, those with low vitamin D levels. Researchers aren't sure whether supplements – rather than food or extra sunshine – could help chronic pain, but it's another good reason to make sure you maintain good levels of this vital vitamin.

3 pain-enhancers to avoid

Yes, some things you do may inadvertently make your pain worse. Here are the biggest culprits:

1 Sedentary living When you hurt, the last thing you want to do is move. But that's exactly what you must do. As stated before, studies find that regular, moderate exercise not only helps with the pain of osteoarthritis and other conditions, but may help to prevent it. For instance, strengthening your core muscles with sit-ups and other similar activities can prevent or improve back pain. Exercise can even help with the pain of neuropathy, common in people with diabetes, by making your cells more receptive to insulin and reducing the damaging effects of high blood sugar on nerve cells and blood vessels.

2 Fear of dependency If your doctor has prescribed medication to help you to manage your pain, use it as suggested. Don't wait until the pain is so severe that you can't stand it. By then, the medication probably won't help. Taking your medication before the pain breaks through makes it far more effective, as well as making your life more pleasant. It also reduces the risk of drug dependence, which is the main fear of many people, because you don't learn to associate the drug with relief from severe pain. So make sure you ask your doctor exactly how often your medication should be taken, and report back promptly if the recommended dose is not controlling your pain. Often doctors suggest taking a double dose at bedtime, specifically so that the pain does not break through overnight.

3 Depression Slightly more than half of chronic pain patients seen in pain clinics also have major depression, and low doses of antidepressants are often prescribed to treat chronic pain. The linkage may come from brain chemicals such as serotonin, dopamine and noradrenaline, which play a role in both conditions. That doesn't mean that the two conditions are one and the same; thus, it's important that your doctor treats your depression *and* your chronic pain so you can find relief from both. ■

A habit worth breaking

Next time you have a headache or your arthritis flares up, stop before you swallow those mainstay pain-relief medicines: **ibuprofen** or **aspirin**. Older people have been systematically excluded from most clinical studies on aspirin and nonsteroidal anti-inflammatory drugs (NSAIDs) – which include ibuprofen. But as it turns out, older people are most likely to experience one of NSAIDs' most troublesome side effects – stomach bleeding. The risk of **gastrointestinal (GI) bleeding** in the general population is about 1 per cent; for those aged 60 and older, it's 3–4 per cent; and for those with a history of GI bleeding, it's about 9 per cent. Older people are also more at risk from heart-related side effects of NSAIDs.

If you need medication to control your pain, you may wish to start with paracetamol, which is milder on most people's digestive systems. If prescription-grade relief is necessary, you may be better off with opioids such as codeine and morphine, low-dose corticosteroid therapy or antidepressants or anticonvulsants, depending on the type of pain you're experiencing. One note of caution: if your doctor prescribes narcotic pain-relievers, make sure you take the smallest possible dose. Older people tend to be more sensitive to the effects of these drugs, getting stronger and longer pain relief on much smaller doses than younger individuals.

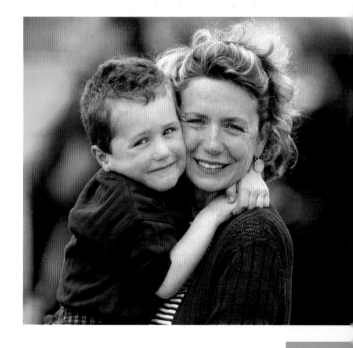

Memory problems

You've misplaced your car keys, lost your mobile phone and can't recall the name of that new book someone recommended. You listened to the weather report this morning but ... will you need a sun hat or an umbrella this afternoon? And did your doctor want you to take that new medicine twice a day – or once every other day?

The stereotype is that memory loss is a part of growing old. In one survey of older people, it was ranked as the most-feared health problem – ahead even of cancer, heart disease and diabetes. It's no wonder: until recently, the conventional wisdom was that memory glitches and fuzzy thinking couldn't be prevented – let alone fixed. Scientists thought that brain cells simply died out, never to be replaced. And what's more frightening to imagine than old versions of ourselves, physically healthy but with greatly diminished memories and mental skills?

But today the story is far more positive – and fascinating. Scientists have long known that learning new facts and skills generates new connections between brain cells – and that the number of connections is far more important in keeping us mentally alert than the absolute number of brain cells. But recent research shows that adult brains can even create new neurons in some areas, especially in sites related to memory and learning. And scientists now know that this process is highly sensitive: too much stress, or stress hormones, and fewer new neurons survive; but new brain cells are enhanced by exercise and, interestingly, by antidepressants.

So a healthy lifestyle and continued mental activity actually create stronger, more prolific connections between the brain cells at any age, and may even increase our brain cell count – and all it takes is a little physical and mental effort to make it happen.

New thinking about memory

In study after study, researchers are discovering that a wide variety of brain 'fertilisers' – from exercise to good fats in your diet, from brain-training programmes to simply socialising more often with your neighbours – can promote the development of healthy, new connections between brain cells and even spur the growth of *new* brain cells. In turn, these stronger connections and fresh new neurons may prevent or even reverse age-related memory lapses and sharpen thinking skills. Keeping your brain well-'fertilised' may even lower your risk of major problems like dementia and Alzheimer's disease.

While it's true that we all need this kind of 'fertiliser' more and more with every passing decade, Australian research seems to confirm the idea that keeping mentally active staves off the brain shrinkage traditionally associated with old age. Among people over 60, those who scored lowest on a 'lifetime experiences' questionnaire had lost more than twice the average volume of brain cells in their hippocampus – the area associated with memory. So, the researchers concluded, using your brain more stops age-related deterioration. And it doesn't seem to matter how you do it – anything from travel to learning a language to playing chess can help to preserve mental function into old age.

But if you're concerned about sudden changes in memory or thinking skills – or are worried that memory problems are interfering with your ability to live your everyday life – see your doctor (see 'When to get help', opposite). Other factors that can affect the memory include the side effects of medication (especially from sleeping pills), medical problems such as thyroid disorders or depression, dehydration, a nutritional deficiency or a head injury.

So don't just assume that gradual mental decline is inevitable – even if you already have some problems with your memory or thinking skills. In many cases these can be halted or even reversed. And if you'd like to sharpen your mind, these 16 strategies are proven winners. Be prepared for a surprise: the first few tips are all about controlling other health issues that were once considered independent of brain function, but which in recent years have been proven to have a big effect on your thinking skills.

Balance your cholesterol A growing stack of evidence links high levels of 'bad' LDL cholesterol and low levels of 'good' HDL cholesterol with memory problems. The same steps that protect against heart attacks and strokes guard your little grey cells, too. In a

When to get help

If you (or a loved one) have these warning signs of more serious memory loss, be sure to see your doctor fast.

- A sudden or significant decline in your ability to remember facts or assigned tasks
- Repeating phrases or stories in the same conversation
- Trouble making choices or handling money
- Not being able to keep track of what happens each day
- Asking the same questions over and over again
- Getting lost in places you know well
- Not being able to follow directions
- Getting very confused about time, people and places
- Not taking care of yourself – eating poorly, not bathing or being unsafe

large study of more than 3,600 British civil servants, those with the lowest levels of 'good' HDL cholesterol were 60 per cent more likely to have poor memory skills compared with people with the highest levels. And five years later, those whose HDL levels had reduced compared with the earlier test were two-thirds more likely to have had a decline in memory than those whose HDL levels remained higher.

Pampering your cardiovascular system – with all the steps outlined earlier – keeps large and small blood vessels in your brain more flexible and free of artery-clogging plaque. This helps to guard against vascular dementia – the loss of memory and thinking skills that develops when brain cells simply don't receive the oxygen and blood sugar that they need to function properly.

Tame high blood pressure Doctors have long suspected a link between high blood pressure and reduced performance on tests of mental ability. Research released by the Alzheimer's Society now reveals that people with high blood pressure are twice as likely to develop Alzheimer's disease, the most common form of dementia, and six times as likely to develop vascular dementia, the next most common form.

Untamed blood pressure restricts oxygen supply and damages blood vessels in the brain, leading to the formation of tiny blood clots that can cause mini-strokes and starve the brain cells of the nutrition and oxygen they need. The Alzheimer's Society estimates that tackling high blood pressure in midlife could reduce the number of deaths from dementia by up to 15,000 people annually in the UK.

Control your blood sugar Diabetes doubles your odds of memory problems later in life. Experts aren't sure why, but there is some evidence that the chronic inflammation that can help to trigger type 2 diabetes can also contribute to the build-up of brain tangles and plaques linked to Alzheimer's disease. The same lifestyle steps that lower your blood sugar – a healthy high-fibre, low-sugar diet plus exercise and stress relief – are good for your brain, too.

Maintain a healthy weight Extra weight was found to dim brain power in a study by the Toulouse University Hospital and the National Institute of Health and Medical Research in France. Researchers checked the body mass index (BMI) and thinking skills of 2,223 women and men, aged 32–62, twice over five years. People with high BMIs scored lower on memory tests and had bigger mental declines from the beginning until the end of the study. The cause could be reduced blood flow to the brain.

Sweat a little People who exercise for 20–30 minutes at least twice a week in their late 40s and early 50s more than halve their risk of developing dementia or Alzheimer's disease 20 years later, according to a Swedish study of nearly 1,500 people. In order to be protective,

help your brain to remember

Creating a strong memory is like taking a good holiday snap: you have to focus, capture the image, then store it so that you can easily retrieve it again later. Here's how to work with your brain's natural information-processing and storage machinery to improve your memory.

Focus on one thing (or person) at a time No multi-tasking. Your brain needs at least 8 seconds of focused attention to 'process' information and successfully send it into long-term storage.

Find – and use – your natural 'learning style' You're a visual learner if you tend to say 'see what I mean' in conversation or if you look at the pictures or diagrams most when assembling something (such as a toy or piece of furniture). You're an auditory learner if you prefer verbal or written instructions. Use your natural style when learning new info to send your brain the strongest signals.

Rehearse Hoping to remember the names of the five new people you met at the party yesterday? Practise them tonight, and again tomorrow morning, as you recall their faces. Brain scientists call this spaced rehearsal and say that it refreshes memory more effectively than trying to recall the names hastily 5 minutes before your next meeting.

exercise must be sufficiently demanding to cause breathlessness and sweating.

What's happening? Scientific studies show that exercise boosts production of a wonder chemical called brain-derived neurotrophic factor (BDNF) – a sort of cell fertiliser that encourages growth, development, maintenance and function of brain cells, making them stronger and more resistant to damage and disease. Some studies even suggest that exercise can make already damaged brain cells healthier.

Take depression seriously Low mood, lack of interest in everyday activities and lack of pleasure are warning signs of depression. But in older people, depression is often misdiagnosed as dementia and may be virtually ignored. If you or a loved one has any signs of depression, regardless of age, alert your GP and ask for help. You deserve to feel well and think clearly.

Schedule a daily 'relaxation appointment' with yourself The best time to do it: mid afternoon, when natural body rhythms are likely to make you feel like taking a break. Try 10 minutes of yoga, a cup of herbal tea and a good book, a leisurely stroll with a friend or some hands-on time at your favourite hobby. Relaxation can lower levels of the stress hormone cortisol; unchecked, cortisol can damage a brain area called the hippocampus, which is involved with processing information and, as we've said before, storing memories.

Get the sleep you need Your brain needs sleep in order to organise and store information in the memory so that you can retrieve and use it again, studies show. If you're tired during the day, it will be even more difficult to concentrate and remember important things. Sleep patterns do change with age – read all about how to get a refreshing night's sleep on page 301.

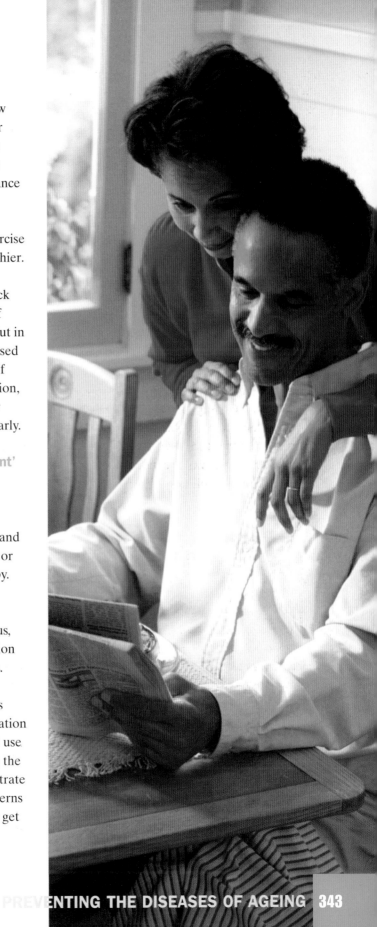

Sip cocoa Cocoa and chocolate are rich in antioxidant flavanols, which have beneficial effects on the blood vessels. When researchers at the University of Nottingham scanned the brains of 16 women after they drank flavanol-rich cocoa for five days, they found increased oxygen levels in their brains' blood flow. What's more, just one high dose of flavanol-enriched cocoa increased the blood flow to their grey matter. The researchers suggest that cocoa flavanols could be used to maintain cardiovascular health and perhaps even to treat vascular impairment in dementia and strokes.

Eat fish three times a week Higher blood levels of an omega-3 fatty acid called docosahexaenoic acid (DHA) – found in fatty fish such as salmon, sardines and mackerel – improve cognitive function and reduce the risk of dementia in older people, according to a review by researchers at the London School of Hygiene & Tropical Medicine.

Similarly, population studies have shown that increased fish consumption reduces the risk of impaired cognitive function. Two to three portions of oily fish a week should do it, but if you dislike fish, try fish-oil capsules. A 2006 Swedish study found they cut the rate of mental decline in people with mild Alzheimer's disease.

Sip 100 per cent juice There is 'hefty evidence' that regularly eating fruit and vegetables can help to prevent dementia, according to the Alzheimer's Society. And in one study of nearly 2,000 people, those who drank fruit or vegetable juice more than three times a week had a 76 per cent lower risk of developing Alzheimer's disease than those who drank pure juice less than once a week. The effect is due to the high levels of antioxidants in juices, especially polyphenols and vitamins C and E.

Have berries at breakfast Compounds in blackcurrants and boysenberries seem to block cell damage that leads to Alzheimer's disease, say researchers at the Horticulture and Food Research Institute of New Zealand. But other berries are equally rich in cell-protecting antioxidants. While a healthy diet may not ever cure Alzheimer's, scientists say it could delay its onset or even prevent it in the first place.

Dine on beans 'n' greens ... and broccoli and whole grains All are rich in folic acid, a B vitamin that improved memory and information-processing speed in a 2007 study of 819 women and men conducted at the Wageningen University, in the Netherlands.

Enjoy a glass of red wine Moderate consumption of red wine – up to two glasses daily for women, three for men – may cut your risk of Alzheimer's disease and dementia. The reason? The polyphenol resveratrol, a powerful antioxidant found in red wine, seems to protect brain cells against the build-up of harmful substances characteristic of Alzheimer's disease, according to laboratory studies at the University of Basel, Switzerland. Red wine can also improve blood flow and cut your odds of blood clots. But take it easy – overdoing it damages brain cells.

Visit, call, write to or email friends and family every day Spending time with family and friends, or volunteering or joining a group, helps to stimulate your memory, concentration and mental processing. One study showed that regular socialising cut dementia risk by 42 per cent. When researchers from Chicago's Rush University Medical Center conducted post mortems on 89 elderly residents whose cognitive function had been measured during their lives, they found something surprising: although on the whole those with more brain plaques and tangles associated with Alzheimer's disease had lower cognitive scores than others, this was not true for all of them. Some people with the same brain changes had displayed no signs of dementia while they were still alive. The difference was that these people had more extensive social networks, which seem to protect against thinking problems and, especially, memory loss.

Play brain games every day In a study in Sydney of 70 healthy volunteers aged over 60, those with higher levels of complex mental activities – in education, work, the creative arts, reading, writing, socialising and day-to-day habits – had half the level of brain shrinkage over the next three years as those with the lowest mental activity scores.

3 memory-robbers to avoid

These three factors contribute greatly to declining mental function.

1 Tobacco Smoking cigarettes or cigars constricts the important arteries that deliver oxygen to your brain. It raises your odds of a stroke and vascular dementia – due to inadequate blood flow to brain cells.

2 Endless hours of TV In one study comparing 331 healthy people with 135 people with Alzheimer's disease, TV-watchers had a higher risk of dementia. The more TV, the higher the odds. Each additional daily hour of viewing increased the risk 1.3 times. In contrast, participation in intellectually stimulating activities and social activities reduced the risk. Even a high-minded documentary doesn't stimulate thought and brain connections the

Try something new

Have you ever got dressed with your eyes closed? Turned all the photos on your desk upside down for the day? Brushed your teeth with your other hand?

Surprising your brain with these unfamiliar experiences could help to stimulate underused nerve cells in parts of the brain linked to memory and abstract thought, says Duke University Medical Center neurobiology professor Lawrence Katz, PhD. Nerve cells in these key areas tend to shrink with age, reducing the brain's ability to process new information and to retrieve old data.

Dr Katz suggests trying daily 'neurobics' – aerobics for the brain. These fun exercises use your senses and force you to think in new ways. Research shows that this kind of brain stimulation prompts the release of neurotrophins, fertiliser-like chemicals that encourage the growth of bigger, more complex dendrites – the branches that nerve cells use to transmit, receive and process information.

More neurobics to try: search for your keys in your bag using only your fingers (don't look!). Take a new route to a familiar place. Type an email or letter with one hand. Dance to music with an unusual beat. Work out how to say words or sentences backwards or play other creative word games. See how long a sentence you can make using words that all start with the same letter or two letters (try 'cr' and 'st' for starters).

way that talking to friends, pursuing hobbies, learning new things, even playing games can.

3 Head injuries Forget the roller coaster: there's evidence that high-speed rides that whip your head from side to side or up and down may cause minor bleeding inside the brain. Experts also suggest that you wear a helmet if you cycle or ski. Any injury to your brain changes blood-flow patterns, affects cellular connections and can contribute to a decline in memory. ■

Arthritis

A man walks into his doctor's surgery. The doctor asks, 'What's wrong?'

'It's my left knee,' the patient says. 'It hurts when I walk.'

'Well, you're 70,' says the doctor. 'That's what happens as you get older.'

'But doctor,' the patient says, 'my right knee is the same age, and it feels fine!'

The message? Arthritis is not an inevitable consequence of getting older, nor should it be treated that way. These days, even teenagers, particularly athletes or those who spend more time on the football pitch than in the classroom, are turning up with arthritis – and they're not old.

Yet one in four patients seen by doctors is there because of musculoskeletal problems; and among those over the age of 65, the most common complaint is osteoarthritis. The condition affects 50 per cent of people aged 65 and over, and up to 85 per cent of those aged 75 and above.

Osteoarthritis results from microscopic damage in the structure and make-up of cartilage – the soft, slippery tissue that covers the ends of the bones in a joint. When cartilage is healthy, your bones glide smoothly over one another, with the cartilage acting as a kind of shock absorber for the movement. But when you have osteoarthritis, that surface layer of cartilage has worn down, allowing the bones to rub together. The result? Pain, swelling and loss of motion. Over time, bone spurs called osteophytes might grow on the edges of the joint, and bits of bone or cartilage can even break off and float inside the joint space, increasing the pain.

Over the past 20 years, researchers have discovered far more about the underlying causes of many diseases, and that's true of osteoarthritis too. In this case, scientists now suspect that the damage lies with cells that help to maintain normal cartilage, called chondrocytes. Genetics and wear and tear contribute to chondrocyte damage, impacting their ability to maintain healthy cartilage. In particular, injury and biomechanical stress (that is, how you walk and move) are tough on chondrocytes. With each injury, additional blood and oxygen rush into the area to help to repair the damage. The metabolic processes involved accelerate the dying off of chondrocytes and promote osteoarthritis.

As little as 20 years ago, doctors primarily treated arthritis with medication and rest. Now, your doctor will probably tell you to lose weight and get some exercise, as well as offering pain relief. A comprehensive treatment plan also includes nutritional advice, relaxation and non-medical methods of pain relief.

The following provides you with some of the latest thinking on how to prevent osteoarthritis or, if you already have it, how to reduce the pain and disability without reaching for drugs.

The best ways to prevent arthritis

Focus on your weight There's no mincing our words here: if you're overweight, you're much more likely to develop arthritis, particularly of the knees, probably because excess weight puts extra stress on the weight-bearing joints, eventually damaging the cartilage. But scientists have shown that if you lose just ½kg (1lb), you put 2kg (4lb) less pressure on your knees.

The researchers also found that even 10 per cent weight loss can significantly improve overall function. While losing weight is important, studies also suggest that reducing your percentage of body fat and increasing your muscle strength are most effective when it comes to improving the pain and disability of arthritis, as well as reducing the initial risk. One of the best ways to do that is with strength-training.

Concentrate on your quadriceps These are the muscles in your upper thighs. The stronger they are, the more strain they take off your knees. Reducing the strain reduces the risk of injury to the chondrocytes. Good exercises are squats, knee extensions and step-ups (in which you use your stairs as exercise equipment).

Tilt your face towards the sun At least in the summer, about 15–20 minutes a day should do it. Sunlight is your best source of vitamin D, which is required for healthy bones. Bone strength is important for arthritis because as cartilage tries to repair itself after injury, it triggers bone remodelling – breakdown and replacement of bone cells. In winter, as we've said before, you may be advised to take a supplement if you can't head off to sunnier climes. Studies have shown that people with low vitamin D levels in their diet and blood are three times more likely to have arthritis than those with high levels. This finding is particularly important for older people, who are less able to absorb vitamin D from the sun as they age. Aim for 400–800 international units (IU) of vitamin D a day. In addition to sunlight, other good sources are fatty fish such as salmon, mackerel and sardines (about 345 IU in a 100g serving), cod-liver oil (1,360 IU per tablespoon), fortified cereals (40 IU in a 100g serving), egg yolks (20 IU in a whole egg) and beef liver (15 IU in a 100g serving).

Boil some kale Kale is high in vitamin K, which plays a key role in the development of cartilage and bone. When researchers evaluated

Habits worth breaking

Give up the high-heeled shoes. Harvard University researchers wondered if the fact that women are twice as likely to develop osteoarthritis might have something to do with the high-heeled shoes they wear. They studied 20 healthy women as they walked barefoot and in their own high-heeled shoes. Researchers found that walking in high heels increases pressure across a major joint in the knee called the patellofemoral joint and puts 23 per cent more force on the inner part of the knee, both of which could lead to joint damage and osteoarthritis. You don't have to be wearing 4in spikes; even shoes with 1.5in heels lead to greater twisting of the knee.

the diets of 672 people with an average age of 65, they found that the higher the levels of dietary vitamin K, the lower the likelihood of arthritis of the hand or knee. About half the study participants had low blood levels of the vitamin. That's not surprising given that studies in the US and UK found that people in both countries have low vitamin K levels. The best sources of this vitamin, apart from kale, are leafy greens such as spinach, turnip greens, Swiss chard and raw parsley.

How to reduce arthritis pain

Use the pool Swimming has long been recommended as a good exercise for people with arthritis; the weightlessness from the water reduces impact on your joints. But there's been very little research into the benefits of this therapy. Finally, a Taiwanese study confirms what anyone with arthritis has long suspected: working out in water significantly improves knee and hip flexibility, strength and aerobic fitness. Meanwhile, an Australian study found that such programmes also resulted in less pain and better overall function. Contact your local health club, leisure centre or swimming pool and ask about water aerobic classes or other classes specifically designed for people with arthritis.

Walk barefoot Going au naturel reduces the load on the knee joints, minimising pain and disability from osteoarthritis by 12 per cent compared with walking with shoes. That's the finding from a study of 75 people with osteoarthritis conducted by researchers at Rush University Medical Center in Chicago. If barefoot isn't an option, find shoes that mimic your natural arch and heel contour, but don't lift up the heel, which puts more pressure on the joints. Orthotic insoles may also help.

Rub on some ibuprofen If your stomach has rebelled against over-the-counter and prescription pain-relievers, attack the pain at its source with ibuprofen cream or gel. Recent studies have shown that it is just as effective as pills in relieving pain – but as only around 5 per cent of the drug is absorbed into the bloodstream, it's a lot less likely to cause side effects than tablets.

The best arthritis supplements

Whatever you think of herbs and supplements, the research results are clear: several natural supplements make a difference to arthritis relief. Here are four to consider seriously.

Glucosamine sulphate You've undoubtedly heard about the benefits of glucosamine/chondroitin supplements for joint repair. The best evidence is for glucosamine, an amino sugar required to build the substances needed to maintain and grow healthy cartilage.

Numerous studies find that it can reduce the symptoms of osteoarthritis and, although it isn't a cure, it may prevent further damage. Take 1,500mg at one time or in three divided doses, and be patient. It may take four to six weeks before you notice any improvement. A caveat: glucosamine supplements come from seashells, so avoid if you're allergic to shellfish.

SAMe (S-Adenosyl methionine) You may be more familiar with this supplement for mild depression. But it also works well in osteoarthritis, probably because of its anti-inflammatory properties. An analysis of 11 studies involving 1,442 people found that it worked as well as nonsteroidal anti-inflammatory drugs (NSAIDs) such as aspirin or ibuprofen in terms of reducing pain and improving function, with fewer adverse effects such as stomach problems. Take 600–800mg, and use it along with a B-50-complex vitamin.

Devil's claw Another anti-inflammatory herb, Devil's Claw significantly improves pain and other symptoms related to arthritis, with some studies showing that it works just as well as prescription drugs but with fewer side effects. Recommended doses vary according to the potency of the extract. Follow the dosage instructions on the label.

Boswellia This anti-inflammatory herb, *Boswellia serrata,* comes from the Boswellia tree, commonly found in India. In one study, 30 patients with osteoarthritis of the knee took the extract for eight weeks, then took a placebo for eight weeks (although neither they nor the researchers knew what they were receiving). When taking the herb, the participants had less knee pain, a greater range of motion and could walk farther than when taking the placebo. ■

the exercise cure for arthritis

Researchers from Tufts University in Boston, USA, randomly split 46 people with knee osteoarthritis into two groups. The first group was assigned a 16 week, home-based strength-training programme; the second (the control group), a nutritional education programme.

The results are hardly surprising: those doing the strength-training reduced their pain by 43 per cent and increased their physical function by 38 per cent. The comparable improvements for the control group were 11 per cent and 21 per cent.

Without question, exercise – not sitting – is the right response to arthritis. But a simple walk, while an excellent start, isn't enough. In addition to regular aerobic exercise such as walking or swimming (experts suggest doing 20–30 minutes a day, three to four days a week), you need both range-of-motion exercises and strength-training. Flexibility exercises increase the length and elasticity of your muscles, helping to reduce stiffness, increase joint mobility and prevent contractures. Strength-training reinforces the muscles that support the affected joints.

The fitness programmes in this book incorporate both types of exercises: try the 'Easy does it' routine (page 202) as a start. To get the most out of your efforts, follow this advice.

FLEXIBILITY EXERCISES

- Perform stretching exercises before bed, when your pain and stiffness are likely to be at their lowest.

- Take a warm shower or apply moist heat to the painful joint before beginning your stretching exercises to warm and relax the muscle.

- Relax before you begin, perhaps with some deep breathing exercises or focused mental imagery (imagine your muscles warming, lengthening and becoming more flexible before you even start).

- If your joint is inflamed, go easier on the stretching but don't give it up altogether.

STRENGTH-TRAINING

- Do not work your muscles to the point of fatigue. The exercises you perform should be challenging, but doable without you feeling you've reached your limits.

- Start out with one set of 4–6 repetitions of each movement twice weekly, increasing about 1 repetition a week until you reach 12.

- Breathe through each muscle contraction. For instance, if you're doing squats, keep inhaling as you squat down and hold the position; this keeps oxygenated blood flowing through your body and prevents a rise in blood pressure.

- If your joints hurt an hour after a strength-training bout, you've done too much.

Osteoporosis

We've all seen her, and it's heartbreaking: the stooped old woman whose gaze is fixed on a spot just in front of her feet. The one who has to sit down and lean back to look you in the eye. They used to call the dome shape on the backs of such women a dowager's hump. But it's certainly not limited only to rich ladies – or even women – and it's not a hump, but the result of years of compression fractures that leave the spine inches shorter and the body twisted.

The woman described above has an extreme case of osteoporosis, the most common bone disease in most countries, and one that affects an estimated 50 per cent of women and 20 per cent of men over the age of 50. Once thought to be an inevitable consequence of ageing, today we know that osteoporosis is a preventable disease, one that, even if it does occur, can be arrested in its development and even reversed.

The best way to understand what happens to your bones as you age is to think in terms of your retirement fund. If you're lucky, you've been saving money over the years, watching it grow, counting the interest, anticipating the day when you'll finally start making withdrawals. The goal, of course, is to ensure that you don't outlive your money. The same is true of bone.

Throughout your life, cells called osteoblasts busily build bone, using hormones, vitamins and minerals in a complex metabolic process to create the densest bone possible. At the same time, however, other cells called osteoclasts break down bone (a process called resorption) as it is continually remodelled to maintain living tissue. Normally these processes are in balance – but if for any reason there isn't enough calcium to supply other parts of the body, particularly your brain, muscles and nervous system, calcium will be leached from the skeleton to provide for other needs. That's why calcium intake is so important throughout your life; not so much to build strong bone, but to provide this valuable mineral for the *rest* of your body so the osteoclasts don't have to dissolve bone to get it.

During childhood and adolescence, the osteoblasts have it over the osteoclasts and you normally build more bone than you lose. But as you age, it's harder for the osteoblasts to hold their own, and the osteoclasts begin gaining until you start losing more bone than you build. This isn't so much of a problem if you have dense bone to begin with, just as retirement-fund withdrawals are fine as long as the principal remains relatively intact.

But if you never laid down enough bone to begin with, or if you're following a lifestyle that makes it easier to break down bone and harder to build up bone, at some point you may find yourself with a deficit. When this happens, your bones become lace-like, with holes and paper-thin spots, and you can fracture your wrist simply by pushing open a heavy door. That is osteoporosis.

The best ways to prevent osteoporosis

Fifteen years ago, you'd have been lucky to be evaluated for osteoporosis, let alone diagnosed. That's because there was nothing doctors could do if you had it. Today, though, a plethora of drugs and a greater understanding of the impact of our lifestyles and diet on bone health have made osteoporosis not only treatable but eminently preventable. There follows advice to help you to make a great start at preventing or slowing the onset of this disease.

Stop smoking Researchers helped 152 postmenopausal women who smoked at least ten cigarettes a day to quit. After one smoke-free year, their total hip-bone mineral density increased by 1.52 per cent, an amount more significant than it sounds. Also, the bone mineral density in the upper thigh bone increased by 2.9 per cent among the quitters.

Hit the weights Strengthening exercises build up more than just muscle; they increase bone density, too. While walking and other aerobic exercises are important for maintaining bone throughout your life, regular strength work-outs, like those beginning on page 202, provide the most significant benefits.

Load up on calcium Get it in your diet and, for good measure, take a daily calcium citrate supplement. In one seminal study, 301 healthy postmenopausal women took 500mg a day of calcium citrate, calcium carbonate or a placebo for two years. Those taking calcium citrate had small improvements in bone mineral density in their hip bones and less bone mineral density loss in their spines. Those taking calcium carbonate only maintained the bone mineral density in their hips and showed no change in the density of their spinal bone. As it turned out, calcium citrate is the form of the mineral best absorbed; take half in the morning, half at night.

Pop some D Calcium is great, but it's just one part of the nutritional needs of bone. Without vitamin D, calcium can't get into your bones, and the results can be devastating. A recent study at

the Southern General Hospital in Glasgow found that more than 97 per cent of 548 elderly patients admitted with a hip fracture had inadequate blood levels of vitamin D. Meanwhile, the Women's Health Initiative study, a 15-year-long investigation into the health of postmenopausal women, found that the more consistent they were in taking calcium and vitamin D supplements, the lower their risk of osteoporosis. It doesn't take long for the supplements to produce benefits, investigators found; just two to three years of consistent use reduced the risk of hip fracture by 29 per cent. Although study participants took 1,000mg of calcium carbonate and 400 international units (IUs) of vitamin D, the researchers suspected that they would have seen an even greater improvement if the vitamin D supplement had been upped to 600 IU. In addition to supplements, exposing your arms and legs, or hands, arms and face to the sun two or three times a week for 5–10 minutes can also guarantee sufficient vitamin D intake.

Switch to decaf A study of 96 women with an average age of 71 found that those getting more than 300mg of caffeine a day (the amount in three mugs of coffee) had much higher rates of bone loss than women getting less. The really interesting thing is that the bone loss occurred only in women with a certain gene that affects how the body uses vitamin D. If you have a

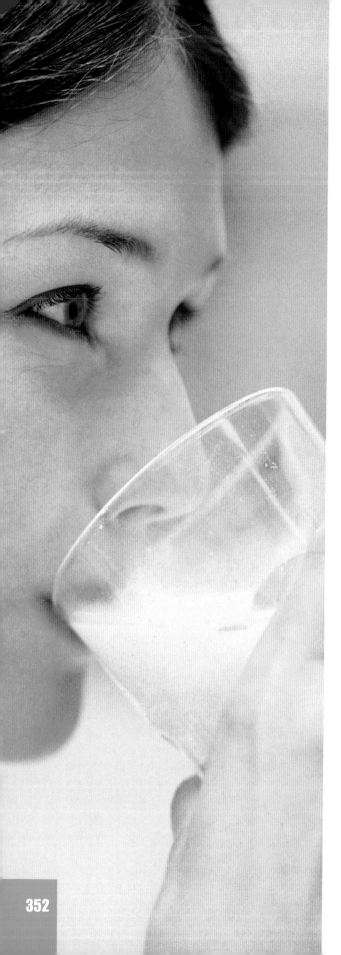

family history of osteoporosis, you may have this genotype and could significantly benefit from cutting out caffeine.

Switch from fizzy drinks to skimmed milk or water When researchers measured the bone mineral density at the spines and hips of 1,413 women, they found that those who drank fizzy drinks every day – whether standard, diet or decaffeinated – had average hip-bone mineral densities 3.7 per cent lower and spine densities 5.4 per cent lower than those drinking less than one fizzy drink a month.

Take an exercise class A planned exercise programme to increase strength, flexibility and balance can reduce the risk of falls by up to 50 per cent, even among frail older people who have already fallen once, according to research funded by the charity Help The Aged. Women aged 75–93 who took regular exercise for just 12 weeks improved the strength of their thigh muscles by 25 per cent on average – equivalent to making their thighs 16–20 years younger.

Shape up your cholesterol levels High levels of 'bad' LDL and low levels of 'good' HDL increase the risk of fractures of the vertebrae in postmenopausal women. Plus, a study from researchers at Alberta University in Canada found that women with osteopenia (a forerunner of osteoporosis) or osteoporosis of the lower spine and hip were more likely to have high cholesterol levels. Meanwhile, other studies suggest that people taking statins, the most commonly prescribed drugs for high cholesterol, have a 60 per cent reduced risk of fracture.

Cholesterol levels are also important when it comes to prevention. When researchers compared mice that had been fed a high-fat diet, designed to raise cholesterol levels, with those fed a normal diet, they found a 43 per cent decrease in mineral content and a 15 per cent decrease in bone density in the leg bones of the high-fat-diet mice. One link between cholesterol and osteoporosis may be that free radicals resulting from oxidised cholesterol molecules prevent osteoblasts from functioning normally to build up bone.

Add a fruit or vegetable to every meal

While calcium and vitamin D get all the glory, when it comes to osteoporosis prevention, a Scottish study of 62 healthy women aged 45–55 found that those who consumed the greatest amounts of foods containing zinc, magnesium, potassium, fibre and vitamin C had the highest bone mineral density. The best sources? Fresh fruit and veg.

Munch on some prunes Dried plums, known as prunes, are high in calcium and other nutrients and may hold the key to restoring bone loss in postmenopausal women. Several studies have found that supplementing your diet with around ten prunes a day improves markers of bone formation in postmenopausal women.

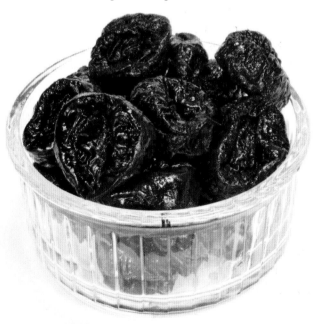

Eat more calcium

If the only time you buy milk is when you bake a cake or have young children to visit, don't despair! A glass of milk isn't the only way to get your calcium. In fact, it may actually be the *worst* form of calcium because it's so high in protein, which contributes to bone breakdown. Calcium goals are 700mg a day, and here are some of the best non-dairy dietary sources:

100g tofu	510mg
85g sardines with bones	325mg
80g steamed spinach	144mg
80g steamed kale	120mg
200g baked beans	96mg
2 slices white bread	88mg

Meanwhile, researchers at the University of Bern in Switzerland report that adding prunes to the standard diet of laboratory rats inhibited bone resorption (as did fennel, celeriac, oranges, french beans, mushrooms and red wine). Other studies have shown that when rats induced into an artificial menopause were fed prunes, it significantly restored bone mass. Researchers don't know exactly why the dried fruit has such an effect, but suspect that it's related to an increased rate of bone formation through some action of plant-based chemicals on osteoblasts.

Check your dental health The only way to diagnose osteoporosis conclusively is with a bone mineral density test. One early clue that you're at risk, however, may be tooth loss and gum disease. Conversely, if you *have* osteoporosis, you're at a much higher risk of developing gum disease and tooth loss. So if you're having dental problems, ask your doctor to test your bone mineral density. ∎

Vision problems

What if you couldn't watch your grandchildren growing up, enjoy the latest films at the cinema or even see well enough to drive your car? Once, poor vision and even blindness were accepted as inevitable parts of growing older – with truly life-altering consequences.

The thieves of sight are still with us. These are the four main ones:

- The first is the least troublesome: the loss of ability to focus on close objects. Called presbyopia, it affects virtually all adults from their 40s; by the mid 50s, the decrease usually ends, leaving many adults with reading glasses in their pockets, but no other significant damage done. The cause of this problem is merely the loss of elasticity in the lens in your eye, along with the loss of power of the muscles that bend and straighten that lens.

- The second is cataracts, in which the normally clear lens in one or both of your eyes may grow so cloudy that your vision blurs. Half of all people over the age of 80 develop cataracts.

- Third, you may develop age-related macular degeneration (AMD). A leading cause of blindness in developed countries, AMD slowly damages your retina, the thin lining at the back of the eye that collects visual images.

- Fourth, your optic nerve, which transmits images to your brain, may become damaged by too much fluid pressure inside your eyes – a condition called glaucoma. Once this damage begins, you have a 50 per cent risk of going blind in at least one eye within 20 years, unless you take action.

These are the same four concerns we've long known about – but the thinking regarding them has changed significantly in recent years. Excuse the pun, but the future is brighter than ever when it comes to the health of your eyes.

New thinking about vision

Exciting new research proves that catching these problems early – sometimes before they've done even a tiny bit of damage – and

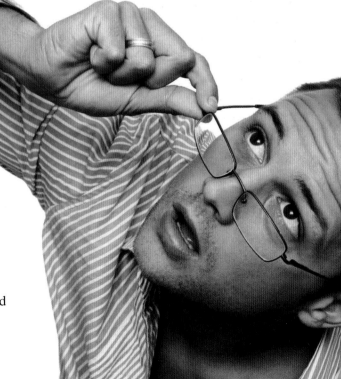

treating them with newer, more effective drugs and procedures, could save the sight of millions of older women and men. Even more exciting: pampering and protecting your eyes with smart eating and exercise, and even by choosing the right kind of sunglasses, could slash your risk of ever having these conditions in the first place.

The first rule is to see an optometrist (optician) at least once every two years, or however often your specialist advises – especially if you are at risk of conditions such as glaucoma or diabetic eye disease. And get checked out promptly if you develop any visual problems. Many people are entitled to free eye tests on the NHS.

And if your optometrist does spot a problem, take action – quickly. The earlier you get treatment for potentially blinding conditions such as glaucoma and AMD, the more likely you are to preserve your precious vision. Prescription-only eyedrops can lower inner-eye pressure (doctors call it intraocular pressure), which destroys the optic nerve in glaucoma. In studies, these eyedrops have significantly slowed or even halted the advance of this condition.

And treatment for the more advanced 'wet' form of AMD, with new drugs such as ranibizumab (Lucentis), which is injected directly into the back of the eye, can prevent wet AMD from getting worse. Treatment slows visual loss in around 90 per cent of people, and significantly improves vision in about a third of patients.

Got cataracts? Consider surgery. Replacing the eye's clouded lens with a plastic, acrylic or silicone version is one of the safest and most effective surgeries you can have. And while doctors once waited until cataracts were advanced, they now suggest having the surgery as soon as you have cataract-related vision problems, such as too much glare from oncoming traffic while driving at night. In fact, driving may be one of the best reasons to go ahead with this procedure. It could save your

life or someone else's. In one study of older drivers, those who had cataract surgery were less likely to be involved in car crashes than those who didn't have the procedure.

Ways to keep your vision clear

You can lower your odds of ever having many common vision problems by following these smart lifestyle steps.

Order bouillabaisse or pasta with clams when you eat out Shellfish, such as clams, oysters and mussels, are rich sources of zinc – a mineral known to protect against AMD. Other good zinc sources include lean meat, wheat germ, whole grains and yoghurt.

Start the day with porridge Packed with fibre, this breakfast cereal is especially adept at keeping your blood sugar on an even keel. Your eyes will thank you: in one study of 500 women aged 53–73, those who chose high-fibre foods such as oatmeal – and steered clear of white bread, sugary drinks and high-sugar desserts – cut their risk of developing early signs of AMD in half, compared with women who ate high-sugar, refined-carbohydrate foods.

Make an omelette Fast and fresh, a two-egg omelette is a delicious evening meal. The bonus for your eyes: egg yolks are the food world's richest, most easily absorbable and usable source of the eye-protecting antioxidants lutein and zeaxanthin. Even better, throw in some sweetcorn or leafy green vegetables, also excellent sources of these two nutrients. As well as their powerful antioxidant action, lutein and zeaxanthin strengthen the light-sensing cells and blood vessels in the retina ▶

moisturise dry eyes

Your eyes naturally produce tears – a mix of water, oil and mucus – to lubricate, clean and nourish the outer surface of the eye. But wind and sun, ageing and stress, and even various types of medication can reduce your eyes' natural production of tears.

The result is a dry, scratchy, gritty feeling – and even pain, redness and blurred vision.

The fix? Start with these items to protect and moisturise your eyes.

SUNGLASSES They shield your eyes from wind, pollen and airborne grit as well as sun – all factors that can dry out your eyes.

FISH OIL AND/OR LINSEED OIL CAPSULES Many large studies have shown that people who get the most good omega-3 fatty acids in their diets have the lowest risk of dry eyes. Many eye doctors recommend 1,000mg of flaxseed oil a day, but fish-oil capsules are a more potent source of these good fats. Experts suggest getting 2–3g of omega-3s from fish-oil capsules daily. (Check the label to see how many capsules you'll have to take; it varies by brand.)

BLINKING If you spend hours watching TV, surfing the Web or working at a computer, you may not be blinking enough. Studies show that while people normally blink 12 times a minute, your 'blink rate' may drop to two or three times in 3 minutes while you're watching a screen. Simply positioning your screen just below eye level could help to minimise moisture loss, because you'll close your eyes a little bit to look down. But also make a conscious effort to blink more.

A HUMIDIFIER Air-conditioning and heating systems can both dry out indoor air. If your eyes dry out at home, consider a humidifier to boost the air's moisture content. Keep the filter and water tank clean to avoid mould and bacteria.

ARTIFICIAL TEARS Look out for demulcent (anti-irritant) drops that moisturise your eyes – not types that remove redness (these can dry out eyes even more).

A WARM FLANNEL If having dry eyes is just an occasional concern, soak a flannel in water, wring it out, then warm it in a microwave for 20 seconds, or until it's soothingly warm. Then place it over your eyelids for 5–10 minutes. This will provide instant relief and will also help to get the tears flowing again. You can repeat a few times a day if you wish.

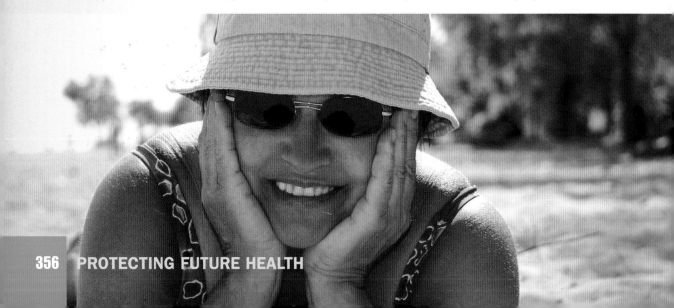

and help to protect the eyes from the sun's ultraviolet rays. People who get plenty of these healthy antioxidants have a 20 per cent lower risk of cataracts and a 40 per cent lower risk of AMD.

Add a side salad of dark, leafy greens

Adding spinach, kale, Swiss chard or other greens to salads, soups and sandwiches is a smart, eye-defending move. They're also rich in the eye-protecting antioxidants lutein and zeaxanthin, as well as beta-carotene.

Wear sunglasses whenever the sun shines

All-round protection from the sun's damaging UV rays can help to lower your odds of cataract development, as well as photokeratitis (a sort of sunburn of the cornea), pterygium (an abnormal growth of tissue on the white of the eye), corneal degeneration, cancer of the skin around the eye and on the eyelids and possibly AMD. Sunglasses act like sunscreen for the eyes.

Look for close-fitting shades (wraparound styles are best) that block at least 99 per cent of UVA and UVB rays. Good news: the price and the colour of the lenses won't affect how well they deflect the sun's damage. You can get sunglasses fitted with prescription lenses if you need these for short sight or other vision problems, as well as sunglasses that work even when you're wearing contact lenses.

Add a broad-brimmed hat You may be
especially vulnerable to sun damage if your eyes are blue, if you spend lots of time outdoors – especially at the beach, on the water or near snow, which all reflect and magnify sun exposure – or if you take sun-sensitising drugs (ask your doctor about your prescriptions; many classes of drugs have this effect). If any of these apply to you, wear a broad-brimmed hat plus sunglasses for double protection.

Snack on an orange or red fruit or veg at least once a day A tangerine, clementine,
handful of ripe strawberries, strips of red pepper … these high-vitamin C foods add a delicious sweetness and crunch to snack time and pack an eye-guarding bonus. Spanish researchers in Valencia who investigated the vitamin C levels of a group of 668 people aged 55–74, half (roughly) with cataracts and half without, have found that the people with the highest levels of the vitamin in their blood cut their risk of cataract by 64 per cent. They concluded that vitamin C may protect the lens from age-related cataracts, even in a population with already high vitamin C intakes.

Have salmon for dinner tonight The omega-3
fatty acids present in foods such as oily fish and flaxseeds may reduce the risk of AMD. In a University of Melbourne review of nine studies including a total of 88,974 people, those with the highest dietary intake of omega-3s had a 38 per cent lower risk of late AMD compared with participants with the lowest intakes. Just eating fish at least twice a week reduces the risk of early AMD by 24 per cent and of late AMD by 33 per cent. Other studies have shown that people with a high intake of omega-6 (vegetable oils) were more likely to develop macular degeneration, while those with a combination of lower omega-6 and higher omega-3 intake were less likely to have the disease.

Think about vision-protecting supplements

People at risk of AMD should consider taking eye-protecting supplements. That's the conclusion of researchers after a huge study by the US National Eye Institute of 3,640 people aged over 55 in the early stages of AMD. Those who took antioxidant supplements had a 32 per cent reduction in their risk of progressing to advanced AMD or vision loss after eight years. The results are so impressive that researchers recommend that anyone at risk should consider taking the same supplements in the same doses: 500mg vitamin C; 400 IU of vitamin E; 15mg of beta-carotene; 80mg of zinc as zinc oxide and 2mg of copper as cupric oxide (Copper is added to avoid copper deficiencies, which can result from getting high levels of zinc.) Some combined supplements contain all of these plus others, such as lutein, for maximum eye protection.

Don't take high-dose antioxidant supplements of C, E and/or beta-carotene alone – studies show that without zinc, they don't seem to help. And if you smoke, skip this supplement completely. Studies show that smokers who take beta-carotene supplements may raise their risk of lung cancer.

Keep taking the eyedrops If you have initial signs of glaucoma, your doctor may prescribe drops to stop the condition progressing and causing damage to the optic nerve at the back of the eye. It's really important to keep up with the treatment, even if you don't have any vision symptoms as yet – the eyedrops dramatically cut the risk of potentially vision-robbing complications. And if you have a family history of glaucoma, make sure you visit your optometrist as often as recommended, so the problem can be detected before it does any damage. If you have a family history, you're entitled to a free eye check every year.

Pamper your eyes If you have diabetes, high blood sugar raises your risk of cataracts, glaucoma and diabetic retinopathy – damage to the blood vessels within the eye that can lead to blindness. Controlling your blood sugar and getting a yearly eye examination in which your pupils are dilated so that the optician can look carefully at the insides of your eyes can greatly reduce your chances of future vision troubles.

Vision-robbers to avoid

Here are a few things that you can control and which can hurt your vision as you age:

Sitting disease When researchers tracked nearly 4,000 residents of a town in Wisconsin, USA, for 15 years, they found that those who climbed more than six flights of steps a day or walked round the block more than 12 times were 70 per cent less likely to develop advanced AMD than their more sedentary neighbours. So it turns out that a sedentary lifestyle – aptly called sitting disease – can even harm your eyes.

Smoking Cigarette smokers are up to four times more likely than non-smokers to be blinded by AMD later in life.

Tight neckties Seriously. In one study of 40 men, half of whom had glaucoma, wearing a tight tie raised the pressure of fluid within the eye – a risk factor for glaucoma – significantly in both groups. That's on just one measurement – no one knows the long-term effects of wearing constricting neckwear daily for years, but it could raise your risk of glaucoma or make an existing condition worse. So if you do wear a tie, make sure you can easily slip two fingers inside your collar. If you can't, loosen your tie. ■

Hearing problems

Deep within your inner ear, tiny 'hair cells' are dancing to the soundtrack of your life. Whether you're listening to the quiet strains of a violin solo or the roar of a chainsaw, these microscopic bristles quiver, quake and shimmy – and convert sound waves into electrical signals for your brain. But when they die off – the result of too many loud concerts in your younger days, too many lawns mowed without ear protection, even too many nights with a snoring bed partner – they're gone. And so is some of your hearing.

Most of us will have a little hearing loss as we get older. By the time you're in your 20s, you may already have lost the ability to detect extremely high-pitched sounds. In later years, as hair cells die a natural or unnatural death, you may have difficulty hearing lower tones as well. So if you find you're asking people to repeat themselves, or if you frequently turn up the volume on the TV or don't always notice that the phone is ringing, you're in good company. Between 24 and 40 per cent of adults over the age of 65 have difficulty hearing, as do up to half of people over 75. By the age of 85, 30 per cent are even deaf in one ear.

The problem is that modern Western lifestyles make it almost impossible to stop all hearing loss. And once it's gone, you'll need a hearing aid to get it back. The good news is that much hearing loss can be avoided – and it's never too late to preserve what you have.

If you're planning to use all the strategies at your disposal to live a long, happy, healthy life – from eating well to exercising frequently, from socialising often to keeping your mind active with cultural and educational activities – you'll need your ears. But when researchers at the London School of Hygiene and Tropical Medicine asked more than 32,000 people aged 75 and over about their hearing, they were shocked to find that 42 per cent said they had difficulty hearing. And when they conducted a whispered voice test on almost 15,000 of them, 23 per cent failed – and more than half of those did not have a hearing aid. Yet hearing loss has a major impact on quality of life, they say – and it can lead to social isolation and depression.

In contrast, a survey of 2,069 people with hearing problems and their families underscores how vitally important sharp hearing is for good health and a long life. Among those who made the decision to wear a hearing aid, 71 per cent said life was better, 35 per cent felt more self-confident, 40 per cent were involved in more social activities including sports and clubs, 53 per cent had better relationships with family, 28 per cent said their physical health improved, 35 per cent were less dependent on others … and 13 per cent said their sex lives improved.

14 ways to preserve your hearing

Most medical issues are complicated; hearing problems, by contrast, are pretty simple. In the majority of cases, they are caused by – you guessed it – prolonged exposure to loud sounds.

Sadly, modern living is decidedly noisy. Whereas most of human history lacked engines, machines and amplified music, today's life exposes us to a never-ending parade of loud sound. Some of that is to do with lifestyle choices – living in an urban environment, a love of rock music, frequent flying. For many others,

When to get help

Your GP may be able to find an easily rectified cause for any hearing loss – for example, by removing ear wax, or changing any medication that could be causing it. Or you could be referred to your local audiology clinic for a hearing test. So don't delay if you have sudden or bothersome hearing loss.

- **Get emergency help if you suddenly lose most or all of your hearing in a short time –** such as three days or less. Doctors suspect that the cause of sudden hearing loss is a viral infection of the inner ear or of important nerves related to hearing.

- **See the doctor if you seem to be having more difficulty hearing than in the past.** Make an appointment if you're having problems hearing people on the telephone, following conversations involving several people, understanding what's happening in a noisy room, hearing the speech of children or women, or if other people seem to be mumbling or if family or friends tell you that you're turning the TV up too loud.

it's job-related: just a week as a firefighter, police officer, factory worker, farmer, construction worker, musician or working in the military or heavy industry can damage your hearing.

Your first move? Do all you can to protect the hearing you have right now. The first few tips are common sense – protect yourself from loud noises. But these may be the hardest to take action on: many people worry that earplugs and hearing aids will make them look old or silly. Wrong. With the rise of mobile-phone usage and MP3 players, there's hardly any adult – or teenager – who doesn't have ear gadgets of some type. No one notices, and no one cares, if you have a hearing aid or sound-blocking tool in your ear! With that in mind …

1 Buy earplugs and keep them in your home, garage, car and bag Wear them when you'll be exposed to any sound over 85 decibels – such as lawn equipment, loud concert, wedding or social event with loud music, an afternoon target-shooting, even time in a loud health club. Don't rely on cotton-wool balls or bits of tissue stuffed in your ears; they'll screen out only about 7 decibels of sound, while foam earplugs can block up to 32 decibels. Need more protection? Look into custom-made earplugs from an audiologist, or special sound-deadening earmuffs.

2 Love your headphones? Ask a friend if he or she can hear the music, too Your tunes are turned up TOO LOUD if others can hear the sounds from your ears or headphones from a metre (3ft) away, warns the Royal National Institute for Deaf People (RNID). And listen to music piped directly into your ears for only about 1½ hours a day at normal volume – just 5 minutes at top volume. Beyond that can cause hearing loss.

3 Change seats at a noisy event If it's too loud where you are – at a concert, meeting or social event – move. Do the same if you can't hear someone who's just a couple of feet away, if you have to raise your own voice to be heard or if the sounds around you begin to seem muffled. Again, there's nothing old-fashioned about removing yourself from overly loud situations.

4 Wear earplugs at holidays celebrated with a bang, too Fireworks and loud, booming rockets are a staple of festivities around the world. Enjoy them to the fullest – with your eyes. Meanwhile, keep earplugs firmly in place in your ears.

5 Keep earplugs on your bedside table A small Canadian study found that bedmates

Have orange juice

of snorers suffered hearing loss in the ear closest to the person making all that night noise. Snoring can reach 80 decibels – as loud as someone yelling for help – or even 90 decibels – equivalent to heavy traffic noise.

6 Get your medication checked Many prescription and non-prescription drugs can damage the ear and cause hearing loss. These include high doses of aspirin, anti-malarials and antibiotics, including erythromycin, vancomycin, tetracycline, gentamicin and streptomycin.

7 Ask about earwax Embarrassing but true: sometimes, hearing loss is simply the result of a gradual accumulation of earwax. It can block the ear canal and prevent the transmission of sound waves. Ask your doctor to check your ears and remove any build-up.

8 Control your blood sugar When specialists from Whipps Cross Hospital in London tested the hearing of 102 diabetic patients compared with people from the general population, they found that the diabetics were significantly more likely to have hearing loss, especially at low and mid-frequencies. Hearing thresholds got worse the longer the duration of the diabetes. High blood sugar levels damage the tiny nerves and blood vessels in the ears – and throughout the body – giving people with diabetes one more reason to keep their sugar levels healthy.

9 Snack on pumpkin seeds In scientific studies, magnesium deficiencies seem to stress cells in the ear. A two-month study of army recruits found that a little magnesium seemed to protect them from some permanent noise-related hearing loss. Pumpkin seeds are a rich source of magnesium, as are Swiss chard, halibut, flaxseeds and brown rice.

10 Have a glass of orange juice at breakfast In a Dutch study of 728 older women and men, those who got 800mcg of folic acid a day had less hearing loss after three years

How loud is too loud?

Unprotected, your ears will be damaged by just 1 minute of exposure to a chainsaw – or any other sound at 110 decibels or higher. Your damage threshold is 15 minutes for sounds at 100 decibels and just a few hours at 90 decibels. A smarter plan: always wear ear protection around these potential deafeners.

Gunshot (peak level)	140–170	decibels
Jet taking off	140	decibels
Crying baby, rock concert, chainsaw, diesel train	110–120	decibels
Motorbike, lawnmower, workshop tools, heavy traffic	90	decibels
Snoring spouse	30–90	decibels

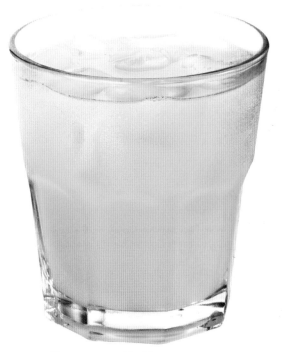

at breakfast

than those who didn't. Split-pea soup, wholegrain bread, spinach and fortified breakfast cereals are also great sources of this important B vitamin.

11 Enjoy a glass of wine, in silence
Soothe and protect your ears at the same time. Some research suggests that a little alcohol somehow slows age-related hearing loss.

12 Get moving! Exercise improves blood flow to all body cells – including the ever-so-delicate hair cells inside your ears. But don't listen to loud music on headphones while you walk or work out. A Swedish study found that even at a moderate volume, exercisers with headphones had hearing loss after just 10 minutes.

13 Stop the buzz of tinnitus Ringing in the ears is a problem for 10–14 per cent of older adults – often, the noise sounds like a squeal, a roar or a whistle or hiss. Controlling your blood pressure and lowering your cholesterol can help. So can avoiding alcohol, which increases blood flow to the inner ear. Quiet 'white noise' such as a fan or soft radio static can help to mask the buzz.

14 Have a bowl of vegetable soup and a fruit salad topped with nuts Laboratory studies suggest that extra vitamins A, C and E may protect against ear damage caused by exposure to loud noises. Skip the supplements, though. Get extra vitamin A from sweet potatoes, carrots and turnip greens as well as mango, papaya and apricots. Soak up extra E in almonds, pistachios and wheat germ. For vitamin C, how about citrus, strawberries and red peppers?

3 hearing thieves to avoid

These three habits have been shown to have a particularly bad effect on your hearing.

1 Caffeine Make your morning blend decaffeinated. Caffeine can worsen tinnitus, another problem associated with hearing loss.

2 Excess sodium Choose low-sodium foods and take the salt cellar off the table, too. There's evidence that controlling your sodium levels can help to reduce your odds of a vertigo problem called Ménière's disease, which is also linked with hearing loss. Too much salt can alter the pressure of fluids in your inner ear.

3 Smoking Exposure to tobacco smoke – from your cigarette or someone else's – raises your odds of more severe age-related hearing loss. ■

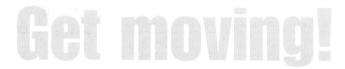

Get moving!

Diabetes

If you haven't heard the word 'epidemic' linked to the word 'diabetes', then you've clearly chosen to avoid the TV news, the newspapers and even the internet. For few health stories have had as much coverage in recent years – and rightly so – than the growing menace of type 2, or 'adult-onset' diabetes.

As the World Health Organization – an international agency not known for its bold pronouncements – puts it: 'Diabetes is a common condition and its frequency is dramatically rising all over the world.' Today, at least 171 million people worldwide have the disease, a figure likely to more than double by 2030 as populations age. And just who are these people? Primarily, those 'above the age of retirement', according to the World Health Organization. In other words, older people. In fact, one in five people aged 75 and over has diabetes.

But let's be clear: diabetes is not merely a side effect of ageing. Yes, it's true that as we age, our bodies become less efficient at producing and using glucose and insulin – the two key factors in type 2 diabetes. But this natural decline isn't enough to cause the disease. Instead, look at the other major lifestyle issues of our time.

Not too long ago, many people – and doctors – blamed a diet high in sugar as the cause of type 2 diabetes. Today, we know that's not the real issue (though, yes, eating lots of refined sugar and refined carbohydrates does cause troublesome peaks and troughs in your blood sugar levels that make diabetes problems worse). More recently, doctors have shown that being overweight is a major risk factor for the disease.

But here's the breakthrough news, based on an increasing body of evidence: the amount you exercise – not just how much you eat – in large part determines your risk of developing diabetes or its precursor, insulin resistance. Put simply, sedentary living, coupled with excess body weight, are the real culprits. And you control both.

To prevent diabetes, then, you need to take action. And the first step is to become educated about the disease.

Understanding insulin resistance

To start, there are two types of diabetes. Type 1 starts in childhood and is usually related to a malfunctioning pancreas. It requires a lifetime of careful management and, often, daily insulin injections. Type 2 is far more common, and is the form of diabetes that is rising in epidemic proportions, due in large part to the growing unhealthiness of our daily lives.

Type 2 diabetes usually progresses along a predictable pattern. Before there is diabetes, there is insulin resistance. It works like this. Every time you eat, your body signals to the 'beta' cells in your pancreas that it's time to pump out the hormone insulin. Insulin's job is to shepherd the energy extracted from your food – in the form of glucose, commonly called blood sugar – into each living cell of your body.

Insulin does this in a kind of lock-and-key process by fitting into molecules on the surface of cells called insulin receptors. Once 'unlocked', the cell performs its energy exchange, either pulling in glucose from the bloodstream to use or store, or sending out stored energy – as either fat or glycogen (the stored form of glucose) – to be used by other parts of your body when they have depleted their own energy stores.

Once a cell is filled with fat or glycogen, or if the cell has been inactive for a long time, it moves the insulin receptors deep within, effectively making it impossible for insulin to reach them. But as the cell uses up its energy stores, it becomes thinner, and those insulin receptors move to the cell's surface again. And the cycle resumes, with the receptors ready to bond with insulin and usher in more glucose to the cell.

But if you're overweight and/or sedentary, more of those insulin receptors stay hidden within the cell. The result? Glucose and insulin build up in your bloodstream. Those high levels of glucose signal to the beta cells in your pancreas to pump out more and more insulin, vainly trying to move that glucose into the cells. Eventually, thanks to sheer numbers, some insulin links up with the insulin receptors and some glucose gets in. But this process gets more difficult every year until, finally, your beta cells wear out like an overworked engine. The next thing you know, your body lacks the capacity to make enough insulin to carry energy to all your cells. And that is why many people develop diabetes and require treatment with drugs or even insulin shots.

The relatively simple relationship between glucose and insulin becomes more complex as you age because of the presence of a second hormone called glucagon. While pancreatic beta cells react to high glucose levels by issuing insulin, their neighbours, the alpha cells, react to low glucose levels by issuing glucagon. This hormone attaches onto receptors in the liver, telling it to release glucose into the bloodstream to provide energy for the rest of the body.

The thing is, alpha cells learn about the state of blood glucose levels only from signals they receive from the beta cells. In older people

with insulin resistance or type 2 diabetes, communication breaks down between alpha and beta cells in the pancreas. So even while beta cells are releasing insulin in response to high blood glucose levels, alpha cells are releasing glucagon, stimulating even more glucose to be released into the bloodstream. You can see how this can become a real mess. And the mess is called diabetes.

Once you have diabetes, you become subject to a range of complications as you age, including blindness, chronic nerve pain, nerve damage, incontinence, impotence, memory loss and, of course, the biggie: heart disease. If you have diabetes, you're more likely to have a heart attack than a lifelong smoker – even if you've never taken a puff yourself. Diabetes is also the strongest predictor of functional decline in older people, that is, how they handle the day-to-day tasks of life such as walking, dressing or house-cleaning. Plus you're more likely to be depressed or to develop dementia and Alzheimer's. And it means you're twice as likely to be in hospital and require other medical services as people the same age who don't have diabetes.

6 ways to prevent diabetes

The good news is that insulin resistance and, in some cases, type 2 diabetes can be reversed through generally healthy living, as prescribed throughout this book. Not only that, but a healthy lifestyle can prevent the disease – even if you already have insulin resistance. The following tips have been proven in studies to have particularly strong preventive powers.

1 **Strengthen your muscles** Work out with hand weights six days a week. It's the best ▶

the best diet

Advice on what and how to eat when you have diabetes is constantly changing. At one time, people with the disease were forbidden to eat any foods with sugar. At another, they were told to cut nearly all the fat from their diets.

Today, the advice focuses more on an overall diet than on any specific food or food ingredient. The British Diabetic Association recommends the following:

1 Eat three regular meals a day. Avoid skipping any, and evenly space your breakfast, lunch and evening meal over the course of the day. This not only helps to control your appetite, but also helps to regulate your blood glucose levels.

2 At each meal include starchy carbohydrate foods such as bread, pasta, chapattis, potatoes, yam, noodles, rice or cereals. The amount of carbs you eat is important to control your blood glucose levels. Try especially to include those with a lower glycaemic index as they won't affect your blood glucose levels as much.

3 Cut down on the fat you eat, particularly saturated fats as this is the type linked to heart disease. Choose unsaturated fats or oils, especially monounsaturated fat (eg olive oil and rapeseed oil) as these are better for your heart.

4 Eat more fruit and vegetables. Aim for at least five servings in total a day to provide you with vitamins and fibre as well as to help you to balance your overall diet.

5 Include more beans and lentils such as kidney beans, butter beans, chickpeas and red and green lentils, as these can help to control your blood glucose levels and blood fats. Try adding them to stews, casseroles, soups and salads.

6 Aim for at least two portions of oily fish a week. It contains omega-3 polyunsaturated fat, which helps to protect against heart disease. Oily fish include mackerel, sardines, salmon and pilchards.

7 Limit sugar and sugary foods. This doesn't mean you need to stick to a sugar-free regime, though. Sugar can be used in foods and in baking as part of a healthy diet. However, opt for sugar-free or diet squashes and fizzy drinks, as sugary beverages cause blood glucose levels to rise quickly.

8 Reduce salt in your diet to 6g or less a day – more can raise your blood pressure, which can lead to stroke and heart disease.

9 Drink alcohol in moderation only – a maximum of two units a day for women and three units a day for men. Remember: alcohol contains empty calories, so think about cutting back further if you are trying to lose weight. Never drink on an empty stomach, as alcohol can make hypoglycaemia (low blood glucose levels) more likely to occur when taking certain diabetes medications.

10 Don't be tempted by diabetic foods or drinks. They offer no benefit to people with diabetes. They are expensive, contain just as much fat and calories as the ordinary versions, can have a laxative effect and will still affect your blood glucose levels.

thing you can do to prevent diabetes. See the fitness routines on page 201 to get you started. Every time you stress the muscle cells with strength-training, you increase their need for glucose, thus reducing insulin resistance. The more muscle you build, the more glucose they need. That means more insulin receptors on cells, and less glucose in your bloodstream.

2 Maintain your level of activity If you're using aerobic activities such as walking, playing tennis and cycling to maintain healthy glucose levels, don't give up. When you're young, the boost in insulin sensitivity you get from one bout of aerobic exercise can last up to four days. But once you pass the age of 40, that boost has a shorter and shorter time span. This makes it crucial that you get some type of activity almost every day.

3 Drink tea A compound in black, green and oolong tea called epigallocatechin gallate substantially increases the ability of cells to take in insulin. Just skip the milk; adding just a teaspoon of semi-skimmed milk reduced the benefit by a third. Also stay away from non-dairy substitutes and soya milk, which also significantly reduced the benefits.

4 Get your grains Whole grains – whether wheat, quinoa, rice, rye or oats – should be considered as diabetes prevention in a plant. Because these grains haven't been stripped of nutrient-containing components and fibre, they pack a powerful nutritional punch. How powerful? A study of nearly 43,000 male health professionals found that those who had the greatest amount of whole grains in their diets were 42 per cent less likely to develop type 2 diabetes than those who got the least amount of grains. Whole grains' benefits probably come from their ability to slow the release of glucose into the bloodstream, thus tempering that post-meal insulin rise. Thus, studies find, diets high in fibre naturally improve insulin sensitivity and reduce insulin secretion.

5 Load up on magnesium Found in high amounts in whole grains (yet another reason for that morning bowl of oatmeal), magnesium influences the release and activity of insulin, and plays a role in your body's ability to use carbohydrates. When blood sugar levels are high, your body loses magnesium. Numerous studies, including two that followed more than 170,000 health professionals for up to 18 years, found that the risk of developing type 2 diabetes was much higher in men and women with low dietary levels of magnesium than in those with high levels. Other

Drinking tea increases

good sources include halibut, almonds, cashews, soya beans and spinach. Just 30g of almonds or cashews provides 20 per cent of your recommended daily intake of magnesium.

6 Choose chicken When researchers evaluated 37,309 healthy and non-diabetic women aged 45 or over, they found that the risk of developing type 2 diabetes over the average 8.8 years follow-up was increased by higher consumptions of animal protein, red meat and cholesterol. The most dangerous habit was frequent consumption of processed meats, which raised diabetes risk by 43 per cent. Bacon and hot dogs emerged as particular culprits.

4 ways to stabilise blood sugar

Already struggling with insulin resistance or diabetes? These four tips have been shown to have a wonderfully stabilising effect on blood sugar levels.

1 Switch to soba Instead of pasta, ladle your tomato and other pasta sauces over soba noodles, made with buckwheat. Canadian researchers found extracts of the grain reduced blood glucose levels by 12–19 per cent in diabetic rats, and a similar effect appears to occur with people. You can find soba noodles in the oriental food section of some supermarkets.

2 Pop some cherries These sweet-and-sour fruits are filled with powerful antioxidants called anthocyanins that can increase insulin production by up to 50 per cent, according to animal studies.

Time to supplement

Studies find that older people with diabetes tend to have low levels of magnesium and zinc. Taking supplements of these minerals has been proven to improve blood glucose control. Additionally, taking supplements of antioxidant vitamins such as vitamins C and E can help to improve blood sugar control, probably by reducing inflammation and oxidation within your bloodstream. Talk to your doctor about the right amounts for you.

3 Get a good night's sleep If you don't get enough sleep, or you toss and turn all night, your blood sugar levels may be higher than normal the next day. One study of 161 people with type 2 diabetes found 67 per cent had poor sleep quality. Lack of sleep and poor sleep wreaks havoc with a multitude of hormones responsible for metabolising glucose and regulating appetite, studies find, so much so that some researchers suggest our 24 hour society may, in part, be contributing to the current diabetes epidemic.

4 Try tai chi Researchers from Taiwan had 32 people with type 2 diabetes participate in a 12 week tai chi programme. This ancient Chinese martial art uses a combination of movement and breathing exercises to strengthen the body and mind. After 12 weeks, participants showed a significant decrease in their haemoglobin A1c levels, a marker of glucose levels, over time, and fewer pro-inflammatory chemicals.

Another study, from the University of Queensland in Australia, involved 12 people with type 2 diabetes who practised qigong and tai chi three times a week for 12 weeks. At the end, participants' blood sugar levels had significantly improved, and they'd lost weight, were sleeping better and had more energy.

the ability of cells to take in insulin

Lung disease

Chronic Obstructive Pulmonary Disease (COPD) is called the forgotten killer, even though it is currently the fifth leading cause of death in the UK and globally. In 2005, it killed more women than breast cancer. And it's the only common cause of death still increasing in prevalence – by 2020 it's expected to be the third leading cause of death worldwide, exceeded only by heart disease and stroke.

COPD is a collection of chronic lung diseases, including emphysema and chronic bronchitis, that blocks the airways and restricts oxygen flow throughout your body. The condition has long been linked with cigarette smoking, and smoking remains its top cause. But researchers now know that some cases of COPD are also the result of exposure to dust, fumes and secondhand smoke; decades of living with asthma; poor diet; and even a wily bacteria that shifts just enough to outwit continually the antibiotics used to vanquish it.

Researchers also think COPD is more than just a disease of the lungs. In an editorial in the medical journal *The Lancet*, doctors from the Netherlands and Italy suggested that, in many people, COPD is part of a cluster of conditions, all related to chronic inflammation in the body. This systemic inflammation is probably responsible for the high blood pressure, diabetes, coronary artery disease, heart failure and even cancer that tend to exist along with COPD. They recommend that people who tick at least three of the following be diagnosed with what they call Chronic Systemic Inflammation Syndrome, not just a single disease:

- Smoking for more than ten pack-years (the equivalent of smoking one pack a day for ten years; or two packs a day for five years)
- Symptoms and abnormal lung function of COPD
- Chronic heart failure
- Metabolic syndrome
- Increased levels of C-reactive protein, an inflammatory marker, in the bloodstream.

Other evidence that COPD is often part of a broader syndrome comes from several British studies showing that people with the disease develop arterial stiffness, or atherosclerosis, far earlier than those without COPD. Researchers also found high levels of inflammatory chemicals in the arteries of people with COPD. All of these add up to one thing: COPD, whether on its own or as part of a cluster of conditions, is scary stuff.

The best ways to prevent COPD

Who wants to lose their ability to breathe? As with so many other serious health conditions, the answer to that question is determined by how you choose to live each day. Lead a healthy, energised life, and the chances of COPD ever becoming an issue for you will be remote.

Stop smoking Cigarettes are by far the number one cause of COPD. There are so many arguments for quitting, and this is yet another big one. If you continue to smoke, and want to stop, turn to page 62 for guidance.

Follow a Mediterranean diet This healthy approach to eating, with its emphasis on fruits, vegetables, healthy oils, fish and whole grains, can reduce your risk of COPD by 25 per cent. In contrast, following a typical Western diet high in refined grains, cured and red meats, desserts and chips increases the risk by 31 per cent. Meanwhile, other studies find that diets high in starches and sodium also significantly increase the risk of a person developing COPD. The Mediterranean diet's anti-inflammatory effects may be one reason for its impact on COPD risk.

Live a fit life Exercise, particularly aerobic exercises such as walking, cycling or swimming, helps your lungs to become more efficient at providing your body with the oxygen it needs. Not only do your heart and lungs benefit from the more robust breathing, but so do all the muscles and connective tissues in and around your lungs. If you get winded easily, it's time to take daily walks and build up your aerobic fitness.

Become a healthy breather Too many people take lots of small breaths as they go about their business. Rapid breathing also becomes the norm in stressful times. But for better lung health – and overall health, for that matter – learn to breath more deeply and less frequently, mainly using your diaphragm. Inhale through your nose slowly and fully; most movement should come from your abdomen. If only your chest moves, your breathing is too shallow. Exhaling should take twice as long as inhaling, and the more you clear your lungs out with strong exhalations, the healthier and fuller your inhalations will be. While there's no agreed standard, try to reduce the number of breaths you take in a minute to just six. Deep breathing not only improves lung function but can also lower blood pressure and provide relaxation, even in stressful times.

The wrinkle factor

If you smoke and are still on the fence about quitting, look at yourself in the mirror. Is your face heavily lined with wrinkles? If yes, then you really need to quit. A study by researchers at the Royal Devon and Exeter National Health Service Foundation Trust found that middle-aged smokers with heavily lined faces were five times more likely to have COPD than smokers with fewer wrinkles. They were also three times as likely to have more severe emphysema than those with less-lined faces.

If you still insist on smoking, make sure that you're getting as much exercise as possible. A study by researchers in Barcelona, Spain, evaluated the chances that 928 smokers would develop COPD over 11 years; those who got moderate to high levels of physical activity were 21 per cent less likely to develop the lung disease than the couch-potato smokers.

Natural remedies for COPD

If you have COPD, the chances are that your doctor has prescribed various medications and programmes to help you to cope. But there are simple lifestyle improvements you can also make to battle back against the disease.

Ventilate your indoor spaces High levels of indoor air pollution caused by smoking, indoor fires and indoor toxins can significantly exacerbate COPD symptoms, say researchers from Aberdeen. The scientists measured concentrations of indoor air pollutants in the homes of 148 people with COPD, and found that levels were up to four times higher than experts say is acceptable. The higher the levels of indoor air pollution, the worse the individual's COPD. As expected, the highest ▶

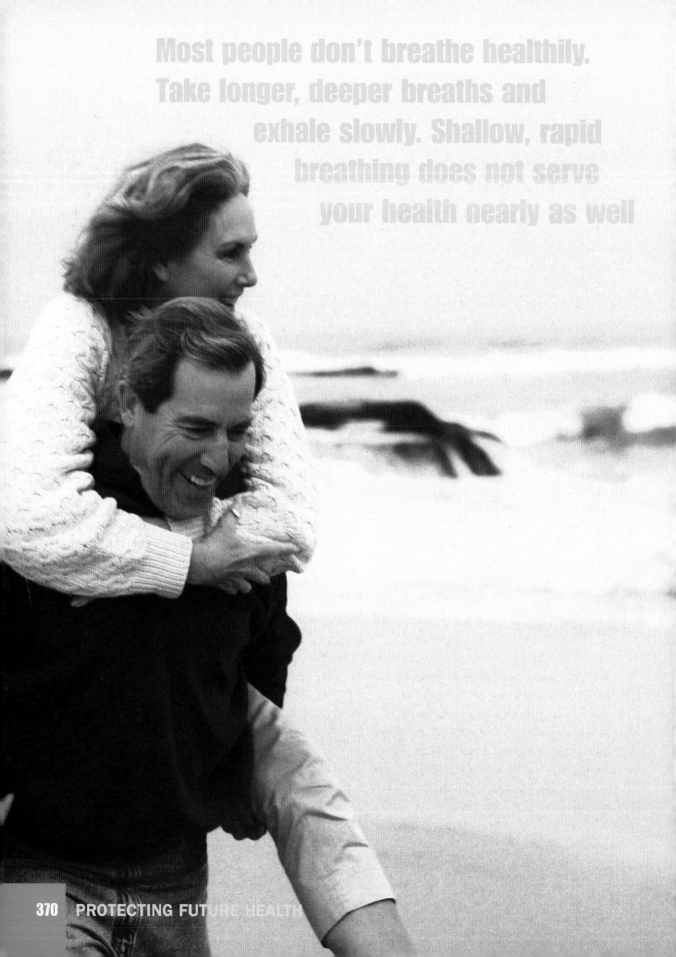

Most people don't breathe healthily. Take longer, deeper breaths and exhale slowly. Shallow, rapid breathing does not serve your health nearly as well pollution levels were found in homes in which someone smoked.

Get at least 20 minutes a day of moderately intense exercise It could be riding a stationary bicycle, briskly walking or swimming. Not only will this improve your breathing capabilities but, chances are, you'll feel mentally sharper afterwards. That's what researchers found when they evaluated the effects of just one session of exercise on 58 adults, half with COPD and half healthy. The COPD group was able to process and retain information better than before they exercised, while the healthy subjects didn't show any improvement. The improvement in the COPD group was probably due to the fact that the exercise increased their lung capacity – sending more oxygen to their brains. The healthy group already had good lung capacity; a 20 minute exercise session wasn't going to affect them that much. A follow-up study in which participants were tracked for a year found that those who continued exercising maintained their cognitive gains, while those who didn't lost physical, cognitive and psychological functioning.

Pop some fish oil Two grams a day should do it. Take half in the morning and half in the evening. When Japanese researchers had 64 people with COPD supplement their diets with about 400 calories a day of an omega-3-rich supplement or one without omega-3 fatty acids for two years, they found numerous indicators of improved lung function in the omega-3 group, but no change in the placebo group. They also found much lower levels of inflammatory chemicals called cytokines in the omega-3 group. Omega-3 fatty acids are potent anti-inflammatories; their ability to quell the inflammation of COPD probably prevented further lung damage during the study.

Mind over breath

Shortness of breath, or **dyspnoea**, is one of the most debilitating and frightening symptoms of **COPD**. People describe it as a sensation of chest tightness, suffocation, not getting enough air and smothering. The fear of dyspnoea leads many with COPD to cut their activities and do as little as possible, one of the worst things they can do. If you feel that horrible sensation of not being able to breathe, don't panic. That only makes the feeling worse. Instead, slowly close your eyes and focus on your breathing. Then envision a calming, peaceful place that makes you happy. Don't just see it in your mind, however; try to engage all your senses. For instance, if you picture the ocean, let yourself hear the waves, taste the salt, feel the grittiness of the sand. This is guided imagery relaxation, and numerous studies find it can help people with COPD to reduce the number and severity of episodes of breathlessness. One way in which it does this is by stimulating your body to release natural brain chemicals called endorphins. These activate part of your nervous system to relax your body and reduce your blood pressure, respiration and heart rate.

Maintain a healthy weight Being overweight puts more pressure on your heart and lungs, increasing breathlessness. It also makes it harder to exercise. But being underweight – a common problem as COPD progresses and eating a full meal becomes more difficult – is linked to an increased risk of death. Aim for a body mass index (BMI) of between 20 and 25. If you're having trouble maintaining your weight:
- Talk things through with your GP and ask for nutritional advice
- Ask about calorie supplements that can help you to maintain weight
- Eat several small meals throughout the day rather than three large ones
- Increase your calories in each meal. For instance, if you eat yoghurt, make sure it's the full-fat variety. ■

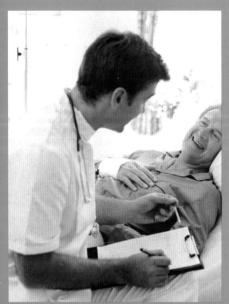
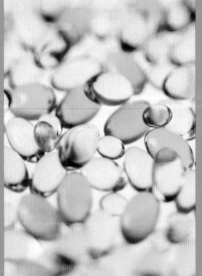
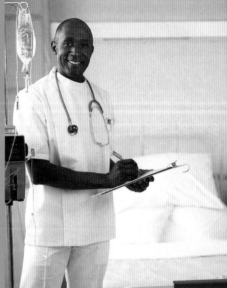

... seeing the doctor   ... hospital stays

... right dosages

Get the most from
your health care

A compassionate doctor. An early, accurate diagnosis. Effective drugs and treatments that work, with minimal side effects. You deserve all this – and more – from your health-care system.

But the reality can be far different: your doctor's appointment may be shorter than a TV ad break; your doctor may interrupt you and have no interest in listening to you; at the hospital, the staff who care for you may forget to wash their hands – raising your risk of a hospital-acquired infection; and you may receive prescriptions that cause unwanted side effects or that interact with other medication and remedies you're taking. Like any other service industry, there are many terrific doctors and hospitals,

but plenty of mediocre ones, too, and, on any given day, someone is going to a make a mistake.

But there's the other side of the health-care equation. As patients, we don't always hold up our end of the bargain. Studies show that half of us don't take prescription drugs as directed, and many of us skip them entirely. One in three of us is reluctant to ask questions. And many of us withhold important information from the doctor, either intentionally or without giving it a second thought. But ultimately you're responsible for your own health, and it's up to you to get the best from any medical consultation. Sometimes patients need to speak up – about their problems, needs and concerns – to secure the best outcomes.

Your first step in making sure you receive top-quality health care? Believe that you deserve it. Don't dismiss your health problems simply as signs of ageing. If you take care of problems that come up as readily as you would have at a younger age, or even sooner, you're most likely to stay healthy and active as you age.

Your second step? Follow these strategies to get the care you need – and deserve.

Visits to the doctor that work

Experts have found that doctors tend to interrupt patients just 20–30 seconds after they begin speaking during a consultation. But the truth is, bossy doctors are just one reason you may feel short-changed when you leave your doctor's surgery. Your visit itself may feel way too short: in a study published in the *British Medical Journal*, Belgian researchers found that the typical visit in Germany and Spain lasted less than 8 minutes; in the United Kingdom and the Netherlands, around 10 minutes; in Belgium and Switzerland, about 15 minutes.

On top of that, we don't always use our time with the doctor to our best advantage. A Dutch study found that half of all visitors to the family doctor hadn't decided in advance what they wanted to talk about; 77 per cent did absolutely nothing to prepare for their visit; and 80 per cent didn't bring a list of questions with them.

Given the brevity of most appointments, being ready to give – and get – information should be your top priority. Information is a powerful weapon. And having a good relationship with your doctor is important. You should be comfortable discussing your lifestyle and health history so that your doctor can best address your health concerns and keep you healthy. ▶

Beyond the doctor

Your doctor is the main person in your health-care team: he or she makes the diagnosis, decides on medication and treatments and oversees your progress. But the doctor is not the whole team. You'll get better sooner when you're ill, live more happily with chronic conditions and avoid medical problems if your team includes at least some of these health-care all-stars.

The practice nurse For straightforward problems, health-monitoring or routine screenings – such as having your blood pressure taken, keeping an eye on your weight or having a cervical smear test – you may be offered an appointment with the practice nurse instead of the GP. Often the nurse can devote more time to your appointment and may seem more approachable.

A nutritionist If you have diabetes or heart disease, meeting with a registered dietitian is an important way of finding out what you should be eating on a daily basis – and how to come up with strategies to make it happen. A nutritionist should also be on your team if you're overweight or underweight, have trouble eating due to an illness or if you're having trouble sticking with a healthy-eating plan.

Physiotherapist If you have back pain, joint pain or chronic muscle pain, a physiotherapist can help you to work your muscles in ways that ease the ache and build strength so that you'll stay pain-free.

Pharmacist This unsung member of the team can check for potential drug interactions when you get a new prescription dispensed – but only if you have all your prescriptions supplied at the same pharmacy (a highly recommended move). Pharmacists are willing to discuss side effects to watch out for and can help to suggest alternatives if an over-the-counter medication is causing you some problems.

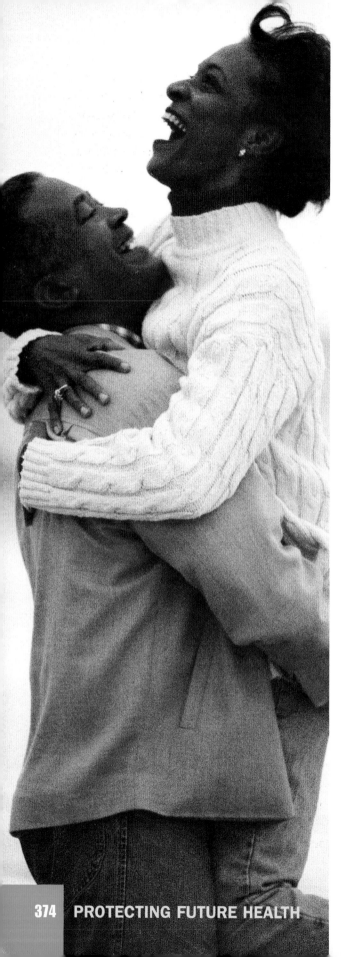

Here's how you can prepare for your visit, and feel more confident about asking questions.

Swot up before your visit Research your medical conditions and concerns by reading reputable websites. Generally, government health websites and those maintained by medical associations, large non-profit-making groups dedicated to a single medical condition, and university medical centres have the most trustworthy, up-to-date medical information. Make notes and create questions, but don't hand your doctor a huge sheaf of printouts and expect a response to them during your visit. Nor should you try to diagnose your symptoms or self-prescribe your remedies. It's still up to your doctor to do that.

Make a list of questions, then prioritise them You'll feel more confident when talking to your doctor – and you'll get the answers and information you need. The bonus: in one review of 33 studies of surgery visits, researchers found that people who brought checklists even got more time with their doctors.

Once you're in the examination room, don't be afraid to give your doctor the list. That way he or she can make sure that important questions aren't left for the last minute of your visit, and can check that the most serious issues are covered. It's okay to ask your doctor to give you the list back so that you can refer to it.

Rehearse In one study, older people who practised their questions were nearly twice as likely to speak up during the visit than people who didn't rehearse. Ask your spouse, another relative or a close friend to play doctor while you voice your health concerns, and ask every question on your list, out loud. The best time to do this is in the hours before your appointment.

Bring a family member or friend along
Another person who knows about your health and your concerns can help you to listen carefully, take notes, ask the right questions and even help you to make important decisions during a doctor's appointment.

Carry a tape recorder Replaying an audiotape of your visit could assist you in better understanding instructions and information that you may have missed or not fully understood at the time. Just let the doctor know you are recording for that purpose.

Be sure that your doctor knows these three important things about you If you haven't done so already, give your doctor your past health history, your family's health history and your own lifestyle history at your next consultation. When discussing your own past, include major illnesses, allergies and drug reactions. Family history? Summarise major illnesses your close relatives (parents, aunts and uncles, grandparents) have had, and pay special attention to medical conditions such as diabetes that seem to run in the family. Tell your doctor about your own lifestyle – explain how much you exercise, how you eat, whether you have a pet, how stressed you are, whether you smoke tobacco or drink alcohol, and any over-the-counter or prescription drugs (from another doctor) that you take regularly. Do you bungee-jump, skydive or ski? Include details of any risky sports that you enjoy, too.

Evaluate your doctor Is she too bossy? Is he too deferential? Does your doctor interrupt or not take your views as seriously as you'd like? Try discussing your concerns first, and make a good-faith effort to build a relationship of trust and respect with your doctor. But if it's not working out, don't feel obliged to stay.

Patients who don't trust their doctors simply don't get well as quickly, studies show, probably because they're less motivated to follow their advice and treatments. Request to see another doctor in the same practice, or ask friends and family for recommendations for a new doctor.

Get the right dose

It was an eye-opening study: when researchers listened in on recorded conversations between 44 doctors and 185 patients, they uncovered a dangerous silence in relation to prescription drugs. When doctors prescribed new medication, they neglected to mention side effects 65 per cent of the time, didn't tell patients how long to take a new drug in 66 per cent of cases, skipped instructions on how often to take it 42 per cent of the time, and didn't explain the drug's purpose in 23 per cent of instances They even left out the name of the drug 26 per cent of of the time.

Doctors often fail to communicate critical information about medication use – and this could contribute to patient misunderstandings, researchers say.

This communication gap helps to explain why half the time, people don't follow directions when taking medication. And that, in turn, could contribute to dangerous side effects. A recent review from the University of Manchester found that 6.5 per cent of all UK hospital admissions are due to adverse reactions to medication, with higher rates in elderly patients – those who are most likely to be taking multiple medications for long-term illnesses. And such adverse reactions are often due to prescribing errors, most of which are avoidable – so be sure you know just what you're supposed to be taking, and in what dose, and check that your prescription and the medication dispensed accords with the name and dose of each drug. ▶

full-life health project
keep your own health records

Maintaining your own health-care records will make it easy for you to provide your doctor with important information – and could even save your life. You can store your medical info in this simple, colour-coded folder system, or opt for software to keep records on your computer or even online. The best system: the one that's easiest for you to complete and maintain. Here's what to include.

Red folder Must-have information
Keep this folder of basic and emergency information at the front of your medical records.

- **Emergency health information:** keep a list of life-threatening allergies or other health conditions that medical personnel should know about immediately in case of an emergency. Put this info into the folder, label it 'EMERGENCY INFO', and make sure it's the first file in your folder of medical records.

- **Contact information for your health-care team:** make a note of your GP's name, and the surgery name, address and telephone number. Also note the name and contact details of any other health-care professionals that you see, such as physiotherapists or hospital consultants.

- **Emergency contact info:** list the names, phone numbers and addresses of relatives and friends who should be contacted if you or your spouse has a medical emergency.

- **Copies of any advance directive:** if you have made an advance directive specifying treatments that you would refuse in certain circumstances – a so-called 'living will' – or have appointed a health-care proxy (someone to take decisions should you be incapable of doing so), keep a copy of the paperwork here. Remember to give a copy to your GP as well, and to tell your next of kin that you have made such a statement.

Blue folder Doctor's records
This is where to keep information about doctor's visits, hospital stays, procedures and test results. From now on, ask for copies of reports on tests, procedures and important visits to the doctor as they happen, so that your file will be up to date.

- **Current records:** ask each of your current doctors for copies of your health records. If you've seen one doctor for many years, ask if the office can create a summary for you. Include your dentist, optometrist and any specialists you see regularly.

- **Reports from specialists:** your GP's records will probably contain details of any hospital or specialist treatment you have had. You can also ask each hospital you've attended for a full copy of your records relating to your treatment there. There will be a charge.

- **Immunisation records:** include current immunisations and, if possible, past immunisations.

- **Spectacles prescription:** this is the place for a copy of your vision prescription.

- **Test results:** keep copies of X-rays, blood tests and other results in a separate file.

- **Doctor's reports on medical procedures:** if you've had outpatient or inpatient hospital treatments, surgery or other procedures, ask the institution for copies of your records.

Green folder Medications, remedies and supplements

- **Copies of prescriptions:** for each drug you take, file a copy of the prescription and contact details for the pharmacy where it was dispensed.

- **Over-the-counter remedies:** keep a list of any that you use on a regular basis, such as low-dose aspirin. If you see your doctor for a specific health complaint, be sure to bring along a list of any non-prescription remedies you've been taking along with your prescription drugs.

- **Vitamins and other supplements:** keep a list of supplements – such as multivitamins, calcium, vitamin D, fish oil or herbal supplements – that you take on a regular basis. Note the type, brand name and the amount you take each day.

- **Side effects list:** on a separate sheet of paper, note anything you've taken that's caused side effects. Include the name of the drug, remedy or supplement; when and how much you took; details about the side effects; other drugs and remedies you were using at the same time.

- **A list of drugs you've been told not to take.** If you've ever been told you have an allergy or have had a serious reaction to a drug, make a note of it. Include any relevant test results or other info here, too.

Yellow folder Your own health notes

Here's the place to track vital statistics, such as your weight, as well as the results of ongoing home testing – such as blood sugar tests for diabetes, home cholesterol checks, home blood pressure checks and so on. Your yellow folder should include:

- **Your height and weight, tracked over time:** log both four times a year. Watch for diminishing height – a warning sign of osteoporosis of the spine. Take weight changes seriously, too. Unintended weight gain or weight loss could be a sign of an underlying health problem and warrants a call to your doctor.

- **Your waist measurement:** experts now know that your waist circumference can help to determine whether you're at risk of metabolic syndrome – a collection of symptoms and conditions that raises your risk of heart attack, stroke, diabetes and more. You're in the danger zone if your waist measures more than 89cm/35in (for women) and more than 94cm/37in for men. A waist of more than 102cm/40in is a serious threat.

- **Your BMI:** short for 'body mass index', this number reveals whether your weight is healthy for your height. A BMI of 18.5–24.9 is healthy; 25–29.9 is overweight; 30-plus is obese. The best way to figure out your BMI is with an online calculator (the maths is fairly complex). Most health websites have one.

- **Results of ongoing home testing:** keep track of your blood sugar levels, blood pressure, cholesterol levels and other common health measurements, whether taken at home, at work, at the doctor's office or elsewhere. This will help you to notice trends and provide info you can show to your doctor in case the numbers move in an unexpected direction.

To get the full story when you're prescribed a new drug, ask these crucial questions.

1 What is the name of the drug? Is it a brand-name drug or a generic?
2 Why is it being prescribed?
3 How, when and for how long should I take it?
4 Will I need a repeat prescription? How can I get one?
5 What are the side effects, and what should I do if I have any adverse effects?
6 How soon should it start working? How will I know?
7 Will I need a smaller dose because of my age or because I'm a woman?
8 Do I need to take it all, or can I stop when I feel better?
9 Should I avoid any foods, beverages (including alcohol), medication or supplements while taking it?
10 What if I miss a dose?
11 How should I store it?

The next step in smart medicine management: have all your prescriptions dispensed by one pharmacy. Your pharmacist can maintain a list of all your medicines and screen for drug interactions to avoid problems.

Survive your hospital stay

Each year, a surprisingly large number of people die in hospitals – not as a result of a medical condition but due to medical mistakes such as a wrong diagnosis, inappropriate treatments or hospital-acquired infections. In the UK it has been estimated that medical errors contribute to 72,000 deaths a year. According to the National Patient Safety Agency, about one in ten patients admitted to NHS hospitals is harmed, to some degree, by their medical care – and this despite admitted under-reporting of medical errors. Adverse events are more likely in men, elderly people and emergency patients. These steps can help you to prevent something from going awry the next time you require overnight medical care.

Choose the best hospital in your area When you need a scheduled procedure – or before, if you want to be armed with information just in case – check out and compare your local hospitals on the NHS choices website (www.nhs.uk/pages/homepage.aspx). New rules mean that if your doctor says you need to see a specialist you can choose from any provider of NHS treatment. This may not apply, though, to accidents and other emergencies where you are taken to hospital by ambulance, or to conditions where your GP deems that you need to see a specialist quickly. Nor does it apply to mental health and maternity services.

Look for a 'high-volume' surgeon New studies show that doctors who have had more experience performing specific procedures really do get the best results. In research published in the *Journal of the National Cancer Institute*, prostate cancer patients treated by highly experienced surgeons were much more likely to be cancer-free five years after surgery than patients treated by surgeons with less experience. Ask your doctor how many times he or she performs the procedure in a year, and how many overall.

And a study of more than 11,000 older women treated for breast cancer found that those who went to high-volume hospitals were less likely to die than those whose surgery was performed at lower-volume hospitals.

Before a procedure, confer with your GP Find out what tests, drugs and processes to

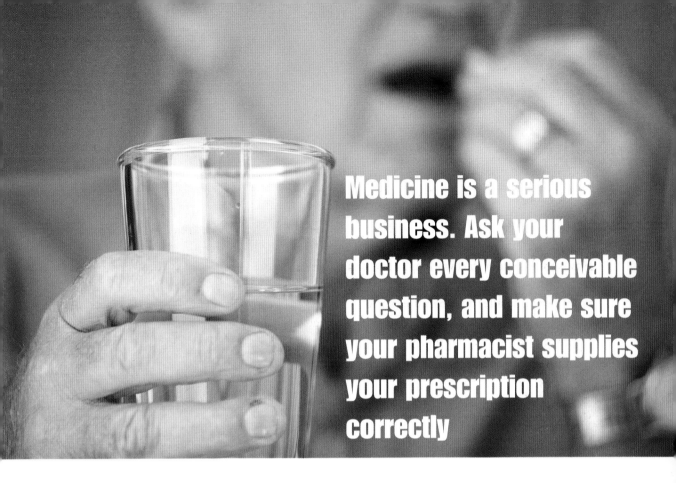

Medicine is a serious business. Ask your doctor every conceivable question, and make sure your pharmacist supplies your prescription correctly

expect – and whether there are any drugs you should avoid. Write down what you find. During your stay, you or a family member or friend should consult the list each time you are given a drug, a doctor's review or a treatment. If it's not on the list, find out more about the drug and why you need it. Not satisfied? Ask for a delay while hospital staff consult your doctor.

Find out who will be taking care of you
Once you're on the ward, find out from a nurse which doctors and other nurses will be taking care of you. Later, if a nurse or junior doctor is doing something that you're not sure is right for you, you can find out who ordered it. If the doctor's name isn't on your list, the procedure may be meant for someone else.

Ask questions Always ask about any procedure or treatment that seems unusual.

Make them scrub up Less than half of all hospital nurses and doctors clean their hands between patients – one reason millions of people contract hospital-based infections each year. Studies show that its more likely that health-care professionals will wash up, and even use more soap, if someone asks them to. The government has campaigned to get hospitals to improve their hygiene procedures, and many now supply a bottle of hand-sanitiser gel for each patient's bed. If yours doesn't, take your own – and don't be afraid to ask staff to use it every time.

Don't leave without instructions Before you're discharged, ask the doctor caring for you for written instructions on how you should care for yourself. Look over the instructions and ask questions, or have a friend or family member do it for you. ■

smart screening

Most diseases don't just happen, like the switching on of a light. They develop gradually and imperceptibly. By the time you finally feel or observe a symptom, it's likely to have been progressing for a long time. It's a scary thought.

But modern screening tests can often inform doctors about what's going on internally even before symptoms occur. Even better, you can check many aspects of your health yourself, in the privacy of your own home.

checks you can do yourself

check your ... Weight

Check your weight every two to four weeks and report to your doctor if you gain or lose more than 2–2½kg (4–5lb) without obvious cause.

check your ... Urine

It should be clear and light yellow, nearly straw-coloured. If it's dark, you're either not getting enough fluids or you may have some blood in your urine.

check your ... Stools

These should be a medium brown. If they're black and tarry, or there are signs of blood, let your doctor know.

check your ... Breasts

Many breast lumps are found by women themselves, or by their partners. As breast tissue can feel different at different times in your monthly cycle, you are the best person to detect any changes from normal. So make sure you stay 'breast aware'. The best way to feel for any changes is in the shower. See your GP at once if you find an unusual lump, or if you develop any nipple changes, bleeding or discharge.

check your ... Testicles

Even young men should check their testicles regularly for any unusual lumps or bumps that could signal cancer or other problems. Any sudden onset of pain should be reported to your GP promptly.

check your ... Moles

Examine any moles for changes to their size, shape or colour, which could signify cancer.

check your ... Hearing

You can take a hearing test by telephone with the RNID (see the Resources section for details).

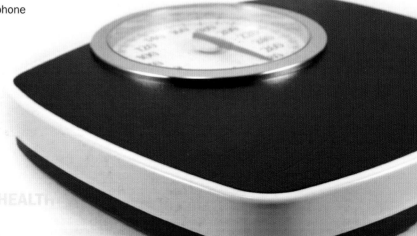

medical checks

have a ... Dental check-up

Gum disease and tooth decay not only hurt your smile and your breath but can also lead to the type of low-level inflammation that increases your risk of a host of health conditions, including heart disease. Your dentist will tell you how often you need to go for check-ups.

have an ... Eye test

See your optometrist for an eye exam at least once every two years. Tests are free for certain groups, such as school students and anyone aged 60 or over.

have a ... Blood pressure check and cholesterol test

Your GP will monitor these as necessary. If you're over 40 and you've never had them checked, ask to be tested, especially if you have a family history of heart disease, high blood pressure or high cholesterol.

have a ... Cervical screening test

All women between 25 and 64 will be invited for a cervical screening test every three to five years to check for early abnormalities that can be treated to prevent cancer developing.

have a ... Mammogram

Women aged 50–70 are invited for a screening mammogram every three years to look for signs of breast cancer at an early stage, when treatment is most successful. Once you're over 70 you won't automatically be invited for screening, but you can ask for further mammograms. Research has shown that breast-screening programmes significantly reduce cancer mortality.

have a ... Prostate-specific antigen (PSA) test

Not everyone agrees on the need for PSA testing, so talk to your doctor. If you have a high risk of prostate cancer (men with one or more first-degree relatives [father, brother] diagnosed before the age of 65), talk to your doctor about whether screening is a good idea for you.

have a ... Bowel cancer screening test

An NHS programme offers screening for bowel cancer and polyps every two years for all aged 60–69. People over 70 can request a screening kit. Screening uses a faecal occult blood (FOB) test, which detects minute amounts of blood in stools. You can also buy a kit to use at home and send off for analysis (see page 383). Regular bowel cancer screening has been shown to reduce the risk of dying from bowel cancer.

7 symptoms never to ignore

1 Sudden 'worst-I've-ever-had-in-my-life' headache. Could signify an aneurysm, or bleeding in the brain. Get to A&E immediately.

2 Black, tarry stools or blood with a bowel movement. Could indicate internal bleeding. Call your doctor.

3 Slurred speech, weakness or paralysis (particularly on one side of your body), numbness, confusion. Could be a stroke. Get to A&E.

4 Vaginal bleeding after menopause. Could be a sign of uterine cancer. Call for a doctor's appointment.

5 Sudden weight gain or loss with no change in eating habits. Could indicate liver or thyroid disease, diabetes or cancer. Call your doctor.

6 Sudden flashes of light. Could indicate that your retina is becoming detached. Have someone drive you to A&E immediately.

7 Never-before-experienced pain in your chest, throat, jaw, shoulder, arm or abdomen. It could be a heart attack. Get to A&E immediately.

Resources

BBC Health & Fitness
www.bbc.co.uk/health/healthy_living/fitness
BBC website offering information on health and fitness.

British Association for Behavioural and Cognitive Therapies
BABCP, Victoria Buildings, 9–13 Silver Street, Bury BL9 0EU email: babcp@babcp.com
tel: 0161 797 4484 www.babcp.com
Charity and leading UK organisation for cognitive behavioural therapy, including help to find an accredited therapist.

British Heart Foundation
14 Fitzhardinge Street, London W1H 6DH
tel: 020 7935 0185, 0845* 070 80 70 (Heart HelpLine) www.bhf.org.uk
Charity supporting research in, and promoting prevention, care and support for, heart disease.

British Nutrition Foundation
High Holborn House, 52–54 High Holborn, London WC1V 6RQ email: postbox@nutrition.org.uk
tel: 020 7404 6504 www.nutrition.org.uk
Charity promoting scientifically based nutritional knowledge and advice, and providing healthy eating information to the public.

British Pain Society
Third Floor, Churchill House, 35 Red Lion Square, London WC1R 4SG email: info@britishpainsociety.org
tel: 020 7269 7840 www.britishpainsociety.org/patient_home.htm
Information for people with chronic pain, including a list of UK-based patient organisations and information about local pain clinics.

Diabetes UK
Macleod House, 10 Parkway, London NW1 7AA
email: info@diabetes.org.uk tel: 0845* 120 2960 (Careline), 020 7424 1000 (office)
www.diabetes.org.uk
Charity devoted to the care and treatment of people with diabetes. Funds research and provides practical support and information.

Food Standards Agency
Aviation House, 125 Kingsway, London WC2B 6NH
tel: 020 7276 8829 (helpline), 0845* 606 0667 (publications) www.food.gov.uk, www.eatwell.gov.uk, www.salt.gov.uk
Independent agency providing advice to the public and the Government on food safety, nutrition and diet.

Hearing Concern LINK
19 Hartfield Road, Eastbourne, East Sussex BN21 2AR email: info@hearingconcernlink.org
tel: 01323 638230 www.hearingconcernlink.org
Charity providing support, advice and information to deaf and hard of hearing people.

Help the Aged
207–21 Pentonville Road, London N1 9UZ
email: info@helptheaged.org.uk
tel: 020 7278 1114 www.helptheaged.org.uk
Charity offering a wide range of advice on getting the most out of your later years.

International Glaucoma Association
Woodcote House, 15 Highpoint Business Village, Henwood, Ashford, Kent TN24 8DH
email: info@iga.org.uk tel: 01233 648 170 (SightLine) www.glaucoma-association.com
Independent charitable organisation offering patient information about glaucoma.

Keep Fit Association
1 Grove House, Foundry Lane, Horsham, West Sussex RH13 5PL email: kfa@keepfit.org.uk
tel: 01403 266000 www.keepfit.org.uk
National governing body offering local classes aimed at all ages to improve stamina, strength and suppleness, movement skills, balance, agility, co-ordination and posture.

Macular Disease Society
PO Box 1870, Andover SP10 9AD
email: info@maculardisease.org
tel: 01264 350 551, 0845* 241 2041 (helpline)
www.maculardisease.org
A self-help society, with a nationwide network of local support groups, providing information and practical support for people with central vision impairment.

Mindfulness-Based Cognitive Therapy (MBCT)
Wellcome Building, University of Oxford,
Department of Psychiatry, Warneford Hospital,
Oxford OX3 7JX www.mbct.co.uk

Information about MBCT for depression, with links
to classes, books and CDs.

**National Independent Bowel Cancer
Screening Programme**
Point Of Care Testing Ltd, Unit 5, Arbroath
Business Centre, Arbroath, Angus DD11 1RS
email: info@pocl.co.uk tel: 0845* 603 5709
www.pocl.co.uk

Private testing for bowel cancer (carried out by post).

NHS
www.nhs.uk

Information on health conditions and treatment
options within the NHS, including a facility to
compare hospitals.

NHS Direct
tel: 0845* 4647 (24 hours, 365 days a year)
www.nhsdirect.nhs.uk

Immediate health advice, information and access
to NHS resources.

NHS Smokefree
tel: 0800 022 4332 (free helpline seven days a
week, 7am to 11pm) www.gosmokefree.nhs.uk

Free stop-smoking help, resources, nicotine
replacement products, local support groups
and more.

Over50
www.over50.gov.uk

Government website including information on
health and well-being for the over-50s.

Patient UK
www.patient.co.uk

Website offering authoritative information on all
aspects of health and disease.

Relate
tel: 0300 100 1234 (to find your local branch)
www.relate.org.uk

Charity providing relationship advice, counselling,
sex therapy, workshops, mediation, consultations
and support.

Royal National Institute for Deaf People (RNID)
19–23 Featherstone Street, London EC1Y 8SL
tel: 020 7296 8000, 0808 808 0123 (Free
information line) www.rnid.org.uk

The UK's largest charity for deaf and hard of
hearing people.

Royal National Institute of Blind People (RNIB)
105 Judd Street, London WC1H 9NE
tel: 020 7388 1266, 0845* 766 9999 (helpline)
www.rnib.org.uk

Charity offering help and support for blind and
visually impaired people.

Seasonal Affective Disorder Association
PO Box 989, Steyning BN44 3HG www.sada.org.uk

Support organisation for people with Seasonal
Affective Disorder ('winter depression').

Light box suppliers:

Goldstaff Ltd, Hexgreave Hall, Farnsfield,
Newark NG22 8LS tel: 0800 1388 567
(freephone) www.britebox.co.uk

Lumie, 3 The Links, Trafalgar Way, Bar Hill,
Cambridge CB23 8UD email: info@lumie.com
tel: 01954 780 500 www.lumie.com

The S.A.D. Lightbox Company, Lane End Business
Park, Lane End, High Wycombe HP14 3BY
email: customerservice@sad.uk.com
tel: 01494 883328 www.sad.uk.com

Walking the Way to Health
Natural England, John Dower House, Crescent
Place, Cheltenham GL50 3RA
email: whiinfo@naturalengland.org.uk
tel: 01242 533337 www.whi.org.uk

A joint initiative between Natural England and the
British Heart Foundation promoting and setting
the standards for organised health walks.

Weight Concern
Brook House, 2–16 Torrington Place, London
WC1E 7HN email: enquiries@weightconcern.org.uk
tel: 020 7679 6636 www.weightconcern.com

Charity addressing the health needs of overweight
people, promoting self-help programmes and support
groups, and developing new treatments for obesity.

*Calls cost more than the standard rates.

Index

A

abdominal exercises 211, 216
abdominal fat 23, 24, 88, 115, 180, 182, 318, 329
ACE inhibitors 309
acetaldehyde 334
acetylcholine 308
acupressure 61, 287
acupuncture 278, 310, 338
acyclovir (Zovirax) 300
addiction
    alcohol 67
    painkillers and sedatives 60–61
    smoking 63
adrenaline 258, 280
advanced-care directive 376
aerobic exercise 26, 41, 178, 181, 184, 197, 282, 291, 366
aerobic fitness 104, 347, 369
aerobics, water 287, 348
ageing 14–35
    changes in attitudes towards 11, 12, 13
    classic signs of 115
    diet and 118–19
    happiness and 17
    mental decline 178, 341
    myths about 15–17
    positive view of 244, 245
    role models 245
    self-perception about 29
    studies 14–15
    successful ageing, components of 12, 13, 20–35, 102–3, 238, 239
    through the decades 18–19
    toxic thinking about 244, 245
age-related macular degeneration (AMD) 354, 355, 357
air pollution 58
alcohol
    addiction 67
    alcohol-related damage 43, 53, 66
    benefits of 53, 66, 320, 344, 362

binge-drinking 53
    and cancer 334
    excessive consumption 45, 46, 53, 66–67, 252, 334
    healthy limits 128, 321, 334, 365
    see also wine
alcoholic hepatitis 66
aldosterone 258
allergic rhinitis 303
allergies 303
almonds 117, 128, 137, 139, 147, 161, 362, 367
alpha blockers 309
alpha cells 364
alpha-hydroxy acids (AHAs) 298
alpha-linolenic acid 139
aluminium 280, 307
Alzheimer's disease
    brain changes 34
    diet and 124, 136, 148
    exercise and 26, 27, 179
    protection against 31, 136, 148, 179, 342, 344
    risk of 23, 25, 32, 71, 115, 246, 252, 273, 342, 364
amaranth 135
amino acids 61, 114, 284
anaemia 285
anger 31, 44, 45, 47, 88, 241, 260, 291
angina 325, 327
antacids 280, 307, 325
anterior cruciate ligament 57
anthocyanins 338, 367
anti-arrhythmia drugs 267
antibiotics 116, 170, 361
anticholinergics 280, 309
anti-clotting drugs 296
anticoagulant medications 171
anticonvulsants 339
antidepressants 90, 116, 267, 280, 339, 340
Antidote to Ageing fitness routine 200, 201, 214–25
antihistamines 61, 276, 280, 300, 311
anti-inflammatory gels and creams 287, 348
anti-malaria drugs 361

antioxidants 21, 25, 77, 120, 121, 123, 127, 168, 272, 285, 298, 320, 330, 357
    protective 25, 49, 51, 55, 58, 63, 165, 337, 338, 344
    superfoods for 121, 128–9
    top 20 of 129
anti-snoring strips 304
antiviral medication 271, 300
anxiety 26, 32, 70, 104
aortic aneurysm 324, 381
appetite 178
apples 123, 124, 129, 154, 161, 165, 320, 333
apricots 325, 362
arm exercises 205, 229
arm strength 104
arnica 287
art 257
arteries
    clogged 31, 47, 293, 294, 295, 317
    hardening of 252, 293
    plaque 26, 78–79, 117, 126, 294, 295, 317, 319, 322, 325, 341
arthritis 57, 80, 102, 136, 267, 287, 315, 335, 346–9
    exercise for 26, 181, 187, 349
    prevention 346–7
    reducing pain from 61, 338, 347–8
    rheumatoid 171, 253
    strength training and 347, 349
    supplements for 348
    see also osteoarthritis
artificial sweeteners 71
artificial tears 356
asparagus 338
aspirin 280, 286, 296, 323, 339, 361
    for blood clots 323, 325, 327
asthma 56, 62, 120, 136, 171
    asthma drugs 309
    exercise-induced 162
atherosclerosis 25, 31, 42, 117, 180, 293, 320
Ativan (lorazepam) 278
atrial fibrillation (AF) 327
aubergines 126

avocados 117, 254, 321, 325, 338
Axid (nizatidine) 281

B

back, exercises for 202, 203, 204, 205, 207, 208, 214, 215, 216, 217, 220, 226, 227, 228
back pain 57, 61, 315, 335, 373
  lower back pain 181, 199, 286, 291
  reducing 289, 291–2, 338, 339
bacon 151, 163, 164, 367
bad breath 274, 276
badminton 194, 264
baked beans 163
balance 23, 61, 101, 264–7
  dynamic 193
  foot lifts (exercise) 265
  improving 27, 187, 193–4, 197, 264–6
  knee lifts (exercise) 265
  static 193
  testing 194, 264
bananas 124, 307, 325
barley 132, 135, 321, 322
Barret's oesophagus 278
baths 289, 298, 307
beans 121, 122, 131, 147, 322, 365
  canned 163, 321
bed rest, effect on bones and muscles 174–5
beef 136, 149, 151, 164
beef liver 347
beetroot 126
belching 277
bending 291
benign prostatic hyperplasia (BPH) 308, 311
  see also prostate, enlarged
benzodiazepines 278
berries 165, 344
beta-agonists 280
beta-carotene 55, 168, 357, 358
beta cells 320, 363, 364
betacyanin 126
beta-glucan 117, 322

beta-sitosterol 117, 139
biceps, exercises for 215, 226, 229
bile acids 317
biofeedback 279–80, 310, 337
biscuits 164
black beans 122
blackcurrants 123, 344
black-eyed peas 122
bladder 308, 309
bladder cancer 62, 334
bladder training 310
bleeding
  in the brain 381
  vaginal 381
blessings, counting 242
blindess 81
blinking 356
blood cells
  red 40, 41
  regeneration 40, 41
  white 120
blood clots 26, 117, 316, 318, 319, 322, 323, 324
  aspirin and 323, 325, 327
blood clotting 25, 120, 171
blood glucose see blood sugar
blood pressure
  checks 49, 81, 381
  diastolic 70, 324, 325, 326
  drugs for 90, 325
  high 16, 25, 28, 29, 60, 62, 66, 69, 70, 81, 88, 115, 246, 286, 318, 324–6, 328, 329, 341–2
  lowering 43, 63, 77, 114, 128, 181, 296, 324–5
  systolic 70, 246, 324, 325, 326
blood pressure monitor, home 326
blood sugar 21, 29, 66, 131, 296, 363
  fasting levels 329
  fluctuations in 71, 72, 121
  high 47, 81, 88, 136, 167, 328, 361, 365
  stabilisation 113, 342, 367
body clock 301, 302

body fat
  abdominal fat 23, 88, 115, 180, 182, 318, 329
  visceral 23, 318
body mass index (BMI) 23, 25, 342, 371, 377
bone density 350, 351, 352, 353
bone density, loss of 23, 42, 56, 70, 74, 180
bone mineral content (BMC) 174–5
bone resorption 350, 353
bones
  brittle 142, 169
  fractures 23, 56, 57, 142, 170, 193, 264
  growth of 57
  health 177
  strength 19, 26, 42
  see also osteoporosis
boron 169
Boswellia serrata 348
bowel cancer 130, 334, 381
bowel movements 130, 280
bowling 185, 193, 249
brain
  bleeding in 381
  blood flow 344
  damage 43
  development 17
  hippocampus 17, 179, 341, 343
  regeneration of 42
  rewiring 108–9
  shrinking 17
  stimulation 34–35, 178, 244
  see also memory; mental decline; thinking; thinking skills
brain cells 41, 42, 340, 341, 343, 344
brain-derived neurotrophic factor (BDNF) 35, 42, 178, 343
Brazil nuts 147
bread
  white 131
  whole-grain 107, 108, 113, 131, 133, 161, 328
  wholemeal 130, 131

breakfast 45, 47, 72, 104
  skipping 72, 157, 284
breakfast cereals 134, 154,
    163, 170
  fortified 169, 347
  whole-grain 108, 132, 134
  wholemeal 131
breast cancer
  diet and 112, 126, 130,
    139, 140, 333
  protection against 21, 26,
    112, 126, 130, 139, 140,
    171, 333
  risk of 25, 66, 80, 93, 169,
    332, 334
  surgery 378
breasts
  breast awareness 380
  mammograms 380
breathing
  control of 58
  deep 89, 299, 369
  relaxation breathing 285, 349
breath, shortness of 49, 52,
    195, 371
broad beans 122
broccoli 112, 126, 129, 147, 149,
    161, 165, 329, 333, 344
bronchitis 62, 368
brussels sprouts 112, 126,
    149, 333
bulgur wheat 132, 135, 321
burgers 153
butter 166
B vitamins 114, 116, 148,
    254, 279, 283, 329

C

cabbage 112, 126, 129, 329,
    333
caffeine 61, 70, 93, 250, 284,
    303, 311, 320
  in cola 75
  diuretic 311
  osteoporosis and 351–2
  tinnitus and 362
cakes 338
calcium 56, 74, 114, 116,
    126, 280, 289, 326, 332,
    350, 351, 353

calcium carbonate 170, 351
calcium channel blockers 280,
    309
calcium citrate 170, 351
calcium gluconate 170
calcium lactate 170
calcium phosphate 170
calcium-rich foods 142–7
calcium supplements 116,
    143, 169–70, 265, 307
calories
  burning 177
  restriction 24, 25, 114–15,
    152–7
calorie supplements 371
calves, exercises for 207, 209,
    220, 221
cancer 16, 19, 23, 25, 330–4
  age and 330
  anti-cancer diet 111, 165, 332–3
  bladder 62, 334
  bowel 130, 334, 381
  breast 21, 25, 26, 66, 80,
    93, 112, 126, 130, 139,
    140, 169, 171, 332, 333,
    334, 378
  cervical 54
  childhood 56
  colon 26, 80, 93, 114, 126,
    139, 142, 169, 171, 334
  colorectal 332, 333
  gall bladder 332
  intestinal 21
  laryngeal 66, 333
  liver 66, 332, 334
  lung 49, 58, 62, 64, 77,
    112, 126, 165, 168, 331,
    332, 333, 334
  mouth 62, 64, 123
  myths 331
  oesophageal 53, 62, 66,
    278, 332, 334
  oral 64, 333
  ovarian 112, 128, 169, 333,
    334
  pancreatic 62, 80, 332, 334
  preventive measures 332–4
  prostate 21, 25, 26, 66, 80,
    112, 116, 126, 139, 165,
    169, 171, 332, 333, 334

rectal 334
risk of death from 331
skin 46, 50, 51, 82, 83,
    330, 357
stomach 112, 330, 332, 334
throat 62, 66
triggers and causes 330
uterine 334, 381
canoeing 185
cappuccino 144, 166
capsaicin cream 287
carbohydrates 136
  refined 21, 25, 71, 152,
    164
  simple 338
card games 249
cardiovascular disease 30, 32,
    93, 316, 325, 327
  see also angina;
    atherosclerosis; heart
    attacks; heart disease;
    strokes
cardiovascular fitness 175,
    177, 186
cardioversion 327
carotenoids 120, 121, 123
carpets and rugs 266, 267
carrots 121, 125, 161, 323,
    362
cartilage 287, 346, 348
cashews 137, 161, 367
cataracts 19, 267, 354, 357,
    358
  surgery 355
catechins 332
cauliflower 129, 329, 333
cavities 273, 274, 275
celecoxib (Celebrex) 286
cell regeneration 40, 41, 42,
    43
centenarians 13
central nervous system 178
cereal bars 161
cereals see breakfast cereals
cerebral cortex 41
cervical cancer 54
cervical smear tests 54, 55,
    381
chamomile oil 298, 299
change, gradual 107–9

cheese 144–5, 163
  cream cheeses 323
  low-fat 142, 144
  low-sodium 163
  processed 163
  yoghurt cheese 146
cherries 338, 367
chest, exercises for 203, 204,
    214, 216, 217, 229
chestnuts 147
chest pain 49, 52, 58, 195, 381
chewing gum 275, 276
chicken 79, 148, 149, 150,
    153, 161, 165, 367
chickenpox virus 297
chickpeas 122, 365
childhood, cancer in 56
childhood illnesses and
    accidents 46, 56–57
chiropractic 338
chloride 169
chlorogenic acid 126
chlorophenamine 300
chocolate 120–1, 128, 165,
    306, 338, 344
cholesterol 25, 317, 319–21
  checks 49, 381
  HDL ('good') cholesterol 62,
    66, 73, 79, 117, 175, 176,
    317, 318, 329, 341, 352
  HDL ('good') cholesterol,
    raising 136, 138, 295,
    296, 320–1, 323
  LDL ('bad') cholesterol 26,
    77, 78, 117, 131, 138,
    175, 176, 294, 295, 317,
    318, 341, 352
  LDL ('bad') cholesterol,
    lowering 131, 296, 319,
    322, 323
  very low density (vLDL) 177
chondrocytes 346, 347
chondroitin sulphate 287
chromium 169
chromosomes 258
chronic fatigue syndrome 282,
    285
chronic inflammation 86, 91,
    113, 252, 315, 327,
    342, 368

chronic obstructive pulmonary
    disease (COPD) 45, 58, 62,
    335, 368–71
  natural remedies 369, 371
  prevention 368–9
chronic pain 81, 88, 103, 188,
    315, 335–9
Chronic Systemic Inflammation
    Syndrome 368
Churchill, Winston 32
cigar smoking 64
cimetidine (Tagamet) 280, 281
cinnamon 320
circadian rhythms 302, 305
circulation problems 293–5
cirrhosis 66
citrus fruits 123, 128, 329, 362
  see also individual fruits
clams 355
cleaning 261, 298
clementines 123, 128, 357
clubs and groups 249, 337
clutter control 259, 302
coaching 185
cocoa 75, 128, 142, 144,
    149, 344
coconut oil 164
codeine 303, 339
cod-liver oil 116, 171
coenzyme Q10 285, 323
coffee 46, 47, 70, 132, 166,
    284, 306, 311
cognition, exercise and 178,
    329
cognitive behaviour therapy 89,
    260, 306, 337
cognitive reserve 34
cognitive skills 42
colas 74, 75, 306
cold compresses 288
colds and flu 32, 103, 111,
    182, 195, 252, 263, 268,
    268–72
  flu vaccine 84, 180, 270, 272
  prevention of 268–71
  treatment 271–2
coleslaw 333
collagen 19, 297
college and university courses
    249

colon cancer 26, 80, 93, 114,
    126, 139, 142, 169, 171,
    334
colorectal cancer 332, 333
computers 90
concentration problems 57
concussions 57
condiments 162
confusion 61, 76, 341, 381
constipation 21, 76, 113, 169,
    277, 279–80
contact dermatitis 297
continuous positive airway
    pressure (CPAP) 278
control, lack of 44, 45, 47
COPD (chronic obstructive
    pulmonary disease) 45, 58,
    62, 335, 368–71
copper 169, 358
cornea, burns on 357
corneal degeneration 357
corn oil 136
coronary artery disease 335
  see also heart disease
corticosteroids 170, 339
cortisol 30, 84, 258, 343
coughing, persistent 49, 52,
    58, 81
coughing up blood 58
couscous 135
crackers 133, 142, 164
cranberry juice 124, 281
C-reactive protein (CRP) 88,
    318, 327–8, 368
creativity 16
credit cards 68
Cretan diet 110, 111
  see also Mediterranean diet
crisps 163
cucumbers 161
cumin 163
cupric oxide 358
cycling 184, 287
cytokines 252, 253, 371

D

dairy products
  fat-free 294
  lactose intolerance 142
  see also cheese; milk; yoghurt

dance 185, 193, 194, 264
DDT (dichlorodiphenyl-trichloroethane) 137
Dead Sea salts 289
death, risk of 27, 176, 264, 316
debt 46, 68
decaffeinated drinks 70
decongestants 276, 311
deep breathing 89, 299, 369
dehydration 76, 265, 279, 289, 306, 341
delayed-onset muscle soreness (DOMS) 288
dementia 34, 35, 324, 364
  exercise and 178, 179
  protection against 342, 344, 345
  vascular 341, 342, 344, 345
  see also Alzheimer's disease
dental health 45–46, 81, 102, 273–6
  check-ups 381
  see also gum disease; teeth
dentine 273
dentists 276
depression 16, 28, 30, 32, 57, 66, 84, 104, 136, 171, 341
  causes 252
  chronic pain and 339
  constipation and 280
  dementia and 343
  endogenous depression 252
  exercise and 108, 182, 187
  falls and 267
  fatigue and 283
  management 91, 239, 252–5
  screening test 283
  self-testing 255
  stress and 33, 34, 253
  symptoms 252, 283, 343
  vulnerability to 252
desserts 155, 166, 167
Devil's Claw 348
DHA (docosahexaeonoic acid) 117, 136, 137, 171, 322, 344
diabetes 16, 21, 29, 90, 240, 243, 288, 306, 315, 363–7, 373

complications 296, 335, 358, 364
diet and 113, 121, 136, 363, 365
drugs for 116
exercise and 26, 184, 187, 199, 366
hearing loss 361
neuropathy and 335, 339, 340
obesity and 363
prevention 364–7
risk of 23, 25, 32, 33, 46, 59, 86, 115, 167, 252, 328, 367
strength training and 364, 366
type 1 41, 363
type 2 (adult-onset) 41, 59, 66, 69, 70, 74, 187, 320, 342, 363, 364, 367
diabetic foods and drinks 635
diabetic retinopathy 358
diarrhoea 113, 169
diazepam (Valium) 278
diclofenac 60
diet 24–25, 110–16
  anti-cancer diet 165
  anti-inflammatory 337–8
  bad food habits 160
  and brain function 344
  calorie restriction 24, 25, 114–15, 152–7
  and cancer protection 111, 165, 332–3
  eating patterns 21, 157, 159, 284, 320
  enjoying food 115, 158–9
  fibre see fibre
  gradual changes 108
  grounded fork rule 157
  harmful foods 162–6
  healthy 110–16
  Japanese 24, 110, 111, 114, 115, 120, 152, 157, 158
  older people, nutritional shortfalls and 115
  poor 45
  quiz 118–19
  rosacea and 299
  seasonal 159

second-helpings rule 157
spicy 299
3 hour rule 157
vegetarian 80, 110
dietary fibre see fibre
dieting 152–3
  fad diets 73
  older people 22
  yo-yo 45, 47, 73
digestion 277
  problems 277–81
digoxin 267
dinner parties 249
dinnerware 157
disability, ageing and 176, 282
diuretics 76, 116, 267, 276, 280, 311
diverticulitis 19, 113, 277, 309
dizziness 61, 76, 81, 265
DNA 24, 120, 332, 333, 334
docosahexaenoic acid (DHA) 117, 136, 137, 171, 322, 344
doctors
  evaluation of 375
  getting the most from 372, 373–5
  importance of seeing 81
DOMS (delayed-onset muscle soreness) 288
doorway thresholds 266
dopamine 108, 109, 178, 280, 339
doughnuts 338
driving 46, 355
dry eyes 356
dry mouth 276
dumbbells 187, 190, 192
dyspnoea 371

E

earplugs 304, 360–1
ear protectors, custom-fitted 304
ears
  hair cells 359, 362
  see also hearing problems
earwax 360, 361
Easy Does It fitness routine 200, 201, 202–12

eczema 136, 297
eggs 161, 347, 355
eicosapentaenoic acid (EPA)
    117, 136, 137, 171, 322
eighties, signs of ageing in 19
elastin 297
electrical sockets and switches
    266
electrolytes 289
emotional eating 160
empathy 241–2
emphysema 45, 62, 368
enamel, tooth 274
endorphins 32, 85, 92, 160, 338
endurance exercise 184, 186,
    197
energy 21, 26
energy bars 72
environmental toxins 46, 103
Epsom salts 289
erectile dysfunction 182
erythromycin 361
evening primrose oil 298–9
exercise 174–237
    activities of daily living 27, 59,
        91, 184, 185, 193, 196, 197
    antidote to ageing 26–27,
        41, 175, 176, 188
    Antidote to Ageing fitness
        routine 200, 201, 214–25
    antidote to pain 336
    balance and 27, 187,
        193–4, 197, 264–6
    benefits 174–8, 182–3
    bodily regeneration and 40,
        41, 42, 174, 175
    cancer prevention and 334
    clothing and shoes 91
    cold prevention and 268
    constipation and 280
    for creaky joints 15
    delayed-onset muscle
        soreness (DOMS) 288
    dementia and 178, 179
    diabetes and 26, 184, 187,
        199, 329, 366
    Easy Does It routine 200,
        201, 202–12
    endurance activities 184, 186
    fatigue and 282

fitness pyramid 197
fitness routines 200–37
flexibility 27, 101, 191, 193,
    197, 349
goals 188, 199
high-impact exercise 57
lack of 91, 174–5
low-impact activities 287
for mental sharpness 371
motivation and social support
    for 198–9
natural ways 185
overexertion 288
painful 109
plan 91, 188
prescribing 107
recovery time 190
for sleep problems 301, 305
Spread Stopper routine 200,
    201, 226–37
starting an exercise
    programme 188
weight-bearing 56
when not to 195
see also strength training;
    weight training; and
    individual activities
exercise balls 181, 192
exercise classes 181, 198, 265
exercise gear 188, 192
exfoliation 298
eyedrops 358
eyes
    dry 356
    intraocular pressure 355
    lens 41, 354
    tests 81, 355, 381
    see also vision problems

F

falls 23, 264
    balance training 193–4, 199
    reasons for 267
    reducing risk of 181, 199, 266
family 30–31
family medical history 375
famotidine (Pepcid) 281
fast food 25, 45, 47, 78–79,
    136, 162, 165
fat cells 182

fatigue 282–5
fats 136–7, 164–6
    animal 148
    bad 164–6
    hydrogenated 163, 164, 165
    monounsaturated 117, 321,
        365
    omega-3 fatty acids 61, 80,
        103, 113, 116, 117, 136,
        137, 140, 165, 166, 171,
        253, 286, 298, 317, 321,
        328, 356, 357, 371
    omega-6 fatty acids 113,
        136, 140, 165, 254, 357
    saturated 21, 25, 65, 115,
        134, 144, 162, 163, 294,
        317, 319, 320, 365
    trans fats 21, 25, 43, 65,
        78–79, 162, 163, 164–5,
        166, 294, 317, 319
feet
    arches 292, 348
    cold and numb 293
fertility 19
fibre 19, 49, 77, 104, 113,
    117, 121, 130, 134, 135,
    154, 161, 328, 353
    constipation prevention 130,
        133, 279
    insoluble 131
    recommended servings 130,
        279
    soluble 131, 322
    supplements 322
fibrinogen 246
fibromyalgia 335, 338
fifties, signs of ageing in 19
figs 147, 155
financial advisers 31
fish 80, 103, 136, 137, 138,
    321, 344
    canned 138, 163
    frozen 138
    oily 113, 115, 137, 138,
        165, 253, 338, 344, 347,
        357, 365
    smoked 162
fish-oil capsules 171, 286, 299,
    321, 322, 344, 356, 371
fitness pyramid 197

fitness routines 200–37
  Antidote to Ageing 200, 201, 214–25
  Easy Does It 200, 201, 202–12
  Spread Stopper 200, 201, 226–37
fitness test 179
fizzy drinks 74–75, 79, 103, 167, 274–5, 278, 321, 338
flavonoids 21, 120
flavonols 165, 344
flaxseeds 139, 253, 326, 338, 357, 361
flexibility 27, 101, 191, 193, 197, 349
flooring 266, 267
floor wax 266
flossing 274, 327
flour 133, 168
flu see colds and flu
fluoride 274
fluoride gel treatments 274
folate 126, 254, 295, 329
folic acid 77, 116, 329, 344, 361–2
food diary 198
food poisoning 277
football 194, 264
forgetfulness see memory, problems
forties, signs of ageing in 19
fractures 23, 56, 170
  childhood 57
  hip 142, 193, 264, 351
free radicals 19, 24, 25, 26, 112, 115, 120, 319, 330, 332, 334, 337, 353
fridge makeover 173
friendships 30, 41, 43, 86–87, 91, 247–9, 260–1
fruit juices 124, 132, 167, 307, 344
  processed 321
fruits
  canned 123
  chopped 154
  'convenience' 173
  dried 128
  eating more 123–4

frozen 123, 173
  health benefits 24, 25, 43, 49, 63, 76, 104, 112, 120, 121, 131, 165, 295, 321
  seasonal 173
  snacks 161
  two-colour rule 127
functional decline 364
functional reserve 46

G

gall-bladder cancer 332
gallstones 66, 328
game 80
gardening 195, 199, 261
gardens, visiting 254
garlic 129, 326, 333
garlic salts 164
garlic supplements 269
gastric cancer 162
gastrointestinal (GI) bleeding 60, 61, 286, 296, 323, 339
gastrointestinal problems 93
gastro-oesophageal reflux disease (GORD) 277, 278, 303
genetics 15–16
gentamicin 361
geosmin 126
geranium essential oil 298
ginkgo biloba 295
ginseng 285
glaucoma 32, 267, 354, 355, 358
glucagon 364
glucosamine 287
glucosamine sulphate 348
glucose 104, 163, 183
glucosinolates 126
glutathione 281
glutes, exercises for 208, 218, 219, 220, 221, 230, 231, 232
glycaemic index 131, 365
glycogen 364
glycolic acid 298
golf 184, 193, 249, 287
gout 120, 338
grapefruits 123, 129, 319–20
grape juice 120, 124, 167

grapeseed oil 137, 140
gravity 278
greens, leafy 136, 142, 147, 347, 355, 357
green tea 83, 110, 366
groin, exercises for 209
groundnut oil 140
guacamole 254
guided imagery relaxation 371
gum disease 46, 81, 273, 275–6, 327, 353
  bleeding 274, 275
  receding 273

H

haemochromatosis 169
haemorrhoids 113, 120
hair 19
hair cells 40
halibut 361, 367
ham 162, 164
hamstrings, exercises for 206, 208, 221, 232
handbags 291–2
hands
  age spots 19
  exercises for 205
  washing 104, 271
hand sanitiser 269, 379
hand washing 104, 271
happiness 33, 102, 239
  ageing and 17, 238
  health and 269
haricot beans 122
hats 357
hazelnuts 137, 147
HCAs (heterocyclic amines) 80
HDL cholesterol 62, 66, 73, 79, 117, 175, 176, 317, 318, 329, 341, 352
  raising 136, 138, 295, 296, 320–1, 323
headaches 57, 60, 61, 103, 381
head injuries 57, 331, 341, 345
headphones 360, 362
head protection 57
health-care records 376–7
healthcare system, getting the most from 372–81
healthy life quiz 96–105

hearing 19
  protection of 359–62
hearing aids 359
hearing problems 315, 359–62
hearing tests 360, 380
heart
  cells 41
  exercise and 42
  heart health 322–3
  maximum pumping ability 175
  muscle 41, 42
heart arrhythmias 136
heart attacks 21, 25, 32, 66,
    114, 132
  risk of 26, 27, 43, 60, 62, 76,
    79, 88, 92, 246, 286, 293,
    316–17, 324–5, 327–8
  symptoms 381
heartbeat, irregular 117,
    195, 327
  see also heart arrhythmias
heartburn 277–8
heart disease
  alcohol and 53
  aspirin and 296
  depression and 252
  diabetes and 364
  diet and 43, 80, 113
  endurance activities and 199
  pollution and 58
  protection from 32, 66, 108,
    128, 139, 162, 184, 187,
    199, 317
  red meat and 80
  risk of 16, 21, 23, 28, 29,
    30, 31, 32, 33, 43, 46,
    64, 69, 71, 80, 84, 86,
    92, 115, 164, 167, 246,
    311, 318, 324–5, 327–9
  smoking and 49, 62
  strength training and 187
  unhappy relationships and 84
heart failure 60, 311, 324
heart rate 185, 258
  resting 175
heart rate monitors 192
heating pads 287, 288–9, 290
Helibacter pylori 277, 280,
    281, 300
hemp oil 113

herbal tea 306
herbs 306
hernias 195, 278
herpes 55
herring 137, 165
heterocyclic amines 149
hiatus hernia 278
high blood pressure 16, 25, 28,
    29, 60, 62, 66, 69, 70, 81,
    88, 115, 246, 286, 318,
    324–6, 328, 329, 341–2
high-density lipoprotein (HDL)
    cholesterol see HDL
    cholesterol
high-fibre cereals 128, 165, 326
hiking 264
hip fractures 142, 193, 264,
    351
hippocampus 17, 179, 341,
    343
hip protectors 266
hips, exercises for 219, 221,
    231, 233
histamine 281
HIV status 55
hobbies and interests 28, 29,
    87, 89, 101–2, 197
holidays 13, 46, 47, 92
homocysteine 131, 148, 295,
    318, 329
honey 125
hormones
human growth hormone (HGH)
    178, 183, 302
  sleep 123
  stress 32, 33, 47, 84, 86,
    88, 103, 109, 256, 260
horseback riding 185
hospitals 269
  errors 378
  hospital stays 378–9
  hygiene 379
hot dogs 367
hotel rooms 269
hot flushes 179
hula (exercise) 265
human growth hormone (HGH)
    178, 183, 302
human papilloma virus (HPV)
    54, 55

tests for 54
vaccine for 55
humidifiers 298, 356
hunger 65, 160
  emotional 65, 160
hydration 104, 279
hydrocarbons 52
hypertension see high blood
    pressure
hypnosis 300
hypoglycaemia 365
hyssop essential oil 298
hysterectomies, total 55

I

ibuprofen 60, 61, 286, 296,
    323, 326, 339
ibuprofen gel 287, 348
ice 280
  for muscle pain 288, 290
  for shingles 300
ice cream 71, 166
iced tea 75, 108
immune system 26, 28, 81,
    180
  boosting 272
  overactive 252, 315
  psychological states, link with
    269
  suppressing 180
immunisations 377
immunity 116, 180
impotence 16
  see also erectile dysfunction
incontinence 306, 307
  reduction of 308–10
  urinary 308–11
indigestion 81, 90
inflammation 46, 78–79, 103,
    117, 182, 183, 258
  anti-inflammatory diet 337–8
  chronic 86, 91, 113, 252,
    315, 327, 342, 368
  depression and 252–3
  diet and 25, 136
  heart 88
  skin 297, 299
inflammatory markers 368
influenza see colds and flu
injections 363

insomnia 21, 61, 70, 90, 101, 301, 303, 305, 306
insulin 167, 180, 183, 334, 363
insulin-producing cells 41
 receptors 364
 secretion 366
insulin resistance 23, 71, 77, 78, 90, 108, 114, 142, 175, 182, 258, 318, 328, 363–4
 see also metabolic syndrome
insulin sensitivity 366
intense pulse light (IPL) 300
interleukin-6 30
intermittent claudication 293
internet
 older internet users 248
 researching medical conditions 374
 social connections 87, 248
intestinal cancer 21
inulin 322
iodine 169
iron 113, 126, 149, 168–9, 280
iron supplements 170, 285
irritable bowel syndrome 113
ischaemic strokes 327
isothiocyanates 126

J,K

jasmine 305
jasmine tea 128
jaw pain 381
jogging 175
joint pain 57, 188, 195, 286–92
 relief from 286–7
joints
 creaky 15
 flexibility exercises 191
 inflammation 349
 lubrication 287
 swollen or painful 195, 349
junk food 21, 25, 43, 47, 65, 78–79
kale 126, 147, 165, 347
Kegel exercises 309
kettlebells 181
kickboxing 181
kicking 181
kidney beans 121, 122, 365

kidney diseases and failure 60, 81, 324, 328
kidneys 114, 171, 279
kidney stones 279
kitchen scissors 294
kiwi fruit 123, 129
knees
 arthritis 15, 348
 injuries 57
 joints 348
 pain 61, 287

L

lactose intolerance 142
larder makeover 172–3
laryngeal cancer 66, 333
laughter 32–33, 241, 260
lavender essential oil 289, 299, 305
laxatives 76, 116, 279
LDL cholesterol 26, 77, 78, 117, 131, 138, 175, 176, 294, 295, 317, 318, 341, 352
 lowering 131, 296, 319, 322, 323
 oxidised 295
learning style 342
legs
 cramps 307
 exercises for 206–7, 208–9, 232, 234
 weakness 267
legumes *see* beans
lemons 123, 128, 129
lentils 365
lethargy 81
 see also fatigue
lettuce 127
leucine 114
libido 16
life expectancy 10, 11, 111
life satisfaction 47
lifestyle history 375
lifting 291
ligaments 57, 191
light box 305
lighting 266
lignans 140
linoleic acid 139

linseed (flaxseed) oil 113, 140, 356
lipofuscin 19
liquorice 280
listening to your body 262–3, 289
liver 41, 364
liver cancer 66, 332, 334
liver damage 66, 323, 328
loneliness 30, 41, 47, 246
longevity 11, 12–13, 87, 152
 see also ageing
long health 11–12
lorazepam (Ativan) 278
loud noise 360, 361, 362
Lucentis (ranibizumab) 355
lunch 157
lung cancer 49, 58, 62, 64, 77, 112, 126, 165, 168, 331, 332, 333, 334
lung disease 58, 368–71
 bronchitis 62, 368
 emphysema 45, 62, 368
 see also chronic obstructive pulmonary disease (COPD)
lung health 49, 58
lungs 43
 damage 58, 62
lupus 282
lutein 120, 126, 355, 357
lycopene 51, 83, 117, 121, 334

M

macadamia nuts 137
mackerel 137, 165, 344, 347
macular degeneration 25, 171, 267
 age-related 354, 355, 357
magnesium 113, 114, 116, 126, 132, 142, 143, 169, 289, 353, 361, 366–7
magnesium supplements 265, 307
make-up 299
mammograms 380
mandarins 129
manganese 126, 132, 169
mangetout 129
mangoes 123, 124, 362
maple syrup 134

margarine 294, 319
  cholesterol-lowering 323
marijuana 46, 52
marinades 150
marriage, happiness in 84, 85
massage 289
mattresses 291
meat
  cured 369
  free-range 136
  lean 148–51, 319, 355
  processed 80, 164, 367
  red 149, 338, 367
  smoked 162
  see also individual types of
medical records 376–7
medications
  constipation and 280
  dry mouth and 276
  falls and 265, 267
  fatigue and 283
  fear of dependency 339
  and hearing loss 361
  incontinence and 309, 311
  management 378
  memory problems and 341
  new prescriptions 375, 378
  polypharmacy 283
  prescribing errors 375
  prostate enlargement and 311
  reviews of 265
  side effects 339, 375, 377
  and sleep problems 303
meditation 21, 89, 103, 181,
    258, 272, 336–7
Mediterranean diet 110, 111,
    368–9
melanomas 50, 51, 83
melatonin 21, 93, 307, 331
melons 325
memory 91
  ageing and 14–15, 340
  exercise and 178
  problems 52, 57, 102, 171,
    340–5
  stimulation 340–5
  stress, impact of 14, 15, 33
  tests 14–15
memory loss 66, 114, 142,
    152, 341

Ménière's disease 362
menopause 19, 23, 179
mental decline
  age-related 178, 341
  contributory factors 345
  protection against 340–5
  see also dementia
mercury 137, 270
metabolic syndrome 108, 182,
    328–9, 368
  see also insulin resistance
metabolism 19, 22, 72, 177,
    187
methylation 16
methylcellulose 322
methylmercury 137
micronutrients 315
migraines 61
milk 128, 134, 144, 166
  low-fat 326, 366
  skimmed 108, 134, 142,
    144, 169, 170
  soya 142, 147, 366
millet 135
mind-body connection 28, 41,
    238
mindfulness 109, 260
Mindfulness-based Cognitive
    Therapy (MBCT) 260
mitochondria 26
mobile phones 326, 331
moisturisers 298
moles 83
molybdenum 169, 380
money management 68
monounsaturated fats 140,
    149, 166
mood swings 57, 71
morphine 303, 339
mouth cancer 62, 64, 123
mouth, dry 276
mouthwash 274, 275
mozzarella 145
muffins 279
multiple sclerosis 169, 252, 335
multi-tasking 261
multivitamins 116, 167, 168–9
muscle cramps 289
muscle pain 188, 195, 286, 373
  relief 288–9

muscles
  aching 272, 293
  building 23
  cells 148, 366
  delayed-onset muscle
    soreness (DOMS) 288
  density 22
  loss of 22–23
  mass 73, 114, 175
  relaxation 33, 337
  weakness 180, 187
muscle strength 27, 177, 181,
    186–7, 189–91, 282
  exercise and 27, 42, 182–3,
    282, 286
music 257, 260, 306, 307,
    360, 362
mussels 355
myrrh essential oil 298

N

naproxen 280
naps 283, 302
narcotic pain relievers 309, 339
neck, exercises for 204
neck pain 302, 338
neck pillows 302
neckties 358
neighbours 31, 87, 249
nerve cells 41
neurobics 34, 35, 345
neurons 35
neuropathy 335, 339, 340
neurotransmitters 178
neurotrophins 35
niacin 113, 114, 132, 148,
    149, 168, 321, 323
nickel 169
nicotine 325
  see also smoking
nicotine fading 63
night shift 93
nizatidine (Axid) 281
nociception 335–6
nonsteroidal anti-inflammatory
    drugs (NSAIDs) 60, 61, 280,
    281, 286, 296, 326, 339
noodles 367
noradrenaline 258, 339
Nordic walking 190

nosebleeds 120
numbness 381
nursing homes, visiting 250
nutritional deficiencies 115, 116
nutritionists 373
nuts 128, 131, 136, 137,
    139, 142, 147, 161, 165

O

oatmeal 117, 131, 134, 322,
    355, 366
  in baths 298
oats 134, 319
obesity 59, 88, 183
  abdominal 23, 24, 88, 115,
    180, 182, 318, 329
  arthritis and 346–7
  cancer and 334
  diabetes and 363
  incontinence and 310
oesophageal cancer 53, 62,
    66, 278, 332, 334
oestrogen 309, 333, 334
oil mister 140
oils, healthy 140
Okinawan diet 110, 111, 114,
    115, 120, 152, 157, 158
Okinawan philosophy 239
old, defined 11
olive oil 113, 136, 137, 140,
    166, 321, 332, 338, 365
  extra-virgin 140
olives 163
omega-3 fatty acids 61, 80,
    103, 113, 116, 117, 136,
    137, 140, 165, 166, 171,
    253, 286, 298, 317, 321,
    328, 356, 357, 371
omega-6 fatty acids 113, 136,
    140, 165, 254, 357
omeprazole (Zanprol) 280
onions 129, 165, 333
onion salts 164
opioids 280, 339
optic nerves, damaged 354, 358
optimism 32–33, 89, 102, 283
oral cancer 64, 333
oral contraceptives 54
orange juice 124, 147, 167,
    295, 361–2

oranges 123, 128, 129, 357
oregano 163
orthopaedic lifts 57
oseltamivir (Tamiflu) 271
osteoarthritis 15, 287, 338,
    339, 346, 348
osteoblasts 350
osteoclasts 350
osteophytes 346
osteoporosis 15, 56, 315,
    350–3
  exercise and 184, 187, 199,
    351, 352
  prevention 142, 169, 184,
    199, 350–3
ovarian cancer 112, 128, 169,
    333, 334
overeating 157, 160
  see also obesity
overflow incontinence 308, 309
oxidation 24, 26, 281, 332, 367
oxygen 25, 40
oysters 355

P

PAD (peripheral arterial
    disease) 293–6, 325
PAH (polycyclic aromatic
    hydrocarbons) 80
pain 263
  acute 335
  anti-inflammatory diet 337–8
  chronic 81, 88, 103, 188,
    315, 335–9
  management 336–9
  rating 337
  and sleep problems 303
painkillers 45, 116, 276, 303,
    348
  addiction 60–61
  long-term use 60–61, 326
  opiod-based 339
pak choi 129, 147
palm oil 164
pancreas 363
pancreatic cancer 62, 80, 332,
    334
pancreatitis 66
panic, avoiding 242
papaya 362

paracetamol 286, 287, 339
paralysis 381
Parkinson's disease 25, 70,
    252, 308, 335
Parmesan 145, 163
parsley 347
pasta 113, 172
PCBs (polychlorinated
    biphenyls) 137
peanut butter 114, 137, 139,
    161
peanuts 139, 154, 321
pearl barley 135
pears 319–20
pecans 128, 137, 161, 320–1
pectin 319–20
pedometers 192
pelvic-floor muscle exercises
    309, 310
pelvic tilt exercise 210
Pepcid (famotidine) 281
peppermint essential oil 298
peppers 127, 161, 329, 357,
    362
periodontitis 273, 276
peripheral arterial disease
    (PAD) 293–6, 325
persimmons 129
pessimism 32
pets 30, 31
  cats 31
  dander 303, 305
  dogs 31, 247
  and falls 266
  sleeping with 305
pharmacists 373
phosphoric acid 74
phosphorus 113, 132, 149
photokeratitis 357
physical therapists 188
physiotherapists 373
phytochemicals 112, 120, 121,
    123, 127, 133
phytonutrients 123
phytosterols 139, 140, 323
pickles 163
Pilates 181, 193, 199
pilchards 142
pillows 302, 365
pineapple 121

pinto beans 121, 122
pistachios 128, 161, 261, 362
pizza 144, 145, 163
plant sterols 323
plaque, arterial 26, 78–79, 117, 126, 294, 295, 317, 319, 322, 325, 341
plaque, dental 273, 274, 276
play, sense of 241
plums 123, 129
pneumonia 182, 252
  vaccine 180
polio 56
pollen 303
pollution 331, 369, 371
polycarbophil 322
polycyclic aromatic hydrocarbons (PAH) 80
polypharmacy 283
polyphenols 344
polysomnography 304
popcorn 135
pork 149, 151
porridge 131, 134, 319, 355
portion control 73, 80
'portion distortion' 154
post-herpetic neuralgia 297
posture 190
potassium 114, 117, 142, 289, 325, 353
potato fries 79
poultry see chicken; turkey
PPI (proton pump inhibitor) 61, 280
practice nurses 373
pranayama yoga 285
prawns 138
prayer 159, 257
presbyopia 19, 354
probiotic bacteria 143
processed foods 43, 59, 112, 136, 162, 163, 172, 325
processed meats 80, 164, 367
progressive relaxation 89, 306–7
prostate cancer 21, 25, 26, 66, 80, 112, 116, 126, 139, 165, 169, 171, 332, 333, 334
prostate, enlarged 19, 306, 308, 309, 311

prostate-specific antigen (PSA) test 381
protein 113, 114, 161
  daily requirement 149, 284
  lean 114, 148–51
proton pump inhibitor (PPI) 61, 280
prunes 128, 353
psoriasis 88, 136
psychological health 177, 240
psychotropic medications 280
psyllium seeds 279, 322
pterygium 357
pulse, checking 327
pumpkin seed oil 137, 140
pumpkin seeds 113, 147, 361
pyjamas 303, 305

Q, R

quadriceps 347
  exercises 206, 221, 347
quercetin 333
quinoa 135, 321
racquet sports 287
raisins 128, 165
ranibizumad (Lucentis) 355
ranitidne (Zantac) 281
rapeseed oil 140, 165, 365
raspberries 333
rate of perceived exertion (RPE) 186
Raynaud's syndrome 288
reading, bedroom 303
reading glasses 19, 266
rear, exercises for 207
Recommended Daily Amount (RDA) (nutrients) 168
rectal cancer 334
red beans 121, 122
red meat 149, 338, 367
regeneration of the body 40–43
relationships 30–31, 103, 254, 261
  internet connections 87, 248
  unhappy 45, 84–85, 253
  see also family; friendships; marriage; neighbours
relaxation 21, 103, 343, 349
  guided imagery 371

muscular 337
  progressive 89, 306–7
relaxation breathing 285, 349
Relenza (zanamivir) 271
religion 256, 257, 282–3
resilience 239, 240–3
  building 241–3
  coherence, strong sense of 240
  spirituality and 256
  stress and 240
resistance training 23, 27, 320
resolvins 113
restless legs syndrome 305
resveratrol 165, 344
retinal detachment 381
retinol 168
rheumatoid arthritis 171, 253
rhubarb 147
riboflavin 113, 126, 143, 149, 168
rice
  brown 108, 113, 132, 135, 321, 361
  white 132
  wild 135
  rice bran 323
romantic partners 30–31
  see also relationships
rosacea 32, 297, 299–300
rosemary 125
rose oil 299
RPE (rate of perceived exertion) 186
rubber gloves 298
rubdowns 289

S

SAD (seasonal affective disorder) 254
salad dressings 162, 164, 319
salads 79, 125, 127, 154
  fruit 166
  as snacks 155
salicylic acid 137
saliva flow 273, 275, 276
salmon 114, 117, 136, 137, 138, 142, 165, 169, 344, 347, 357

salt 134, 162–4, 365
   garlic salts 164
   onion salts 164
   sea salt 164
salt substitutes 325
SAMe (S-Adenosyl methionine)
   348
sardines 137, 142, 344, 347
saturated fats 21, 25, 65,
   115, 134, 144, 162, 163,
   294, 317, 319, 320, 365
sauerkraut 333
sausages 162
saw palmetto 311
schizophrenia 52
sciatic nerve 292
screening
   medical checks 381
   self-checks 380
seasonal affective disorder
   (SAD) 254
seasonal eating 159
seaweed 110
second-hand smoke 43, 45,
   49, 52, 368
sedatives 60–61
sedentary lifestyle 91, 101,
   338–9, 358
seeds 113, 137, 139, 147
selenium 132, 149
self-esteem 91
   exercise and 179–80
self-tanning products 83
semen 334
serotonin 178, 253, 339
sertraline 182
sesame oil 140
sesame seeds 147
Seventh Day Adventists, diet of
   110–11
seventies, signs of ageing in 19
sex hormones 317
sex and sexuality
   in later life 16–17, 54, 55, 182
   prostate cancer and 334
sexually transmitted diseases
   (STDs) 17, 54, 55
sexual partners, multiple 46,
   54–55
shellfish 355

shift working 93
shingles 182, 297, 300, 335
shoes
   low/high heels 292
   vibrating 265
   walking 265
shoulders
   exercises for 202, 204, 214,
      215, 216, 217, 226, 227,
      229
   pain 381
Siberian ginseng 285
silicon 169
singing 185
sinuses 90, 272
sitting disease see sedentary
   lifestyle
sitting positions 291
sixties, signs of ageing in 19
skin
   ageing 19, 297
   renewal 297
skin cancer 46, 50, 51, 82,
   83, 330, 357
skin cells, regeneration of 40, 41
skin problems 297–300
   contact dermatitis 297
   dry and itchy skin 297–8
   rosacea 32, 297, 299–300
shingles 182, 297, 300, 335
sleep 26, 92, 281, 367
   cycles 302
   naps 283, 302
   patterns 21, 301–2, 343
   problems 30, 57, 90, 93,
      301–7
   sleep hygiene strategies 61,
      90, 93, 302–3, 305–7
   sleeping too much 101
sleep apnoea 90, 278, 304, 305
sleep hormones 123
sleeping pills 45, 47, 61, 306,
   341
sleep specialists 278
slow-cooker 319
slurred speech 381
smell 116, 319
smoking 43, 44–45, 47, 49,
   62–63
   addiction 63

blood pressure and 325
cancer and 331, 334
cigars 64
hearing loss and 362
heart disease and 43
incontinence and 310
lung disease and 45, 58, 368
marijuana 46, 52
mental function and 345
nicotine-replacement therapy
   63
oral health and 276
osteoporosis and 351
PAD and 294
quitting 49, 53, 63, 294,
   320, 325, 334
second-hand smoke 43, 45,
   49, 52, 368
skin cancer and 51
vision problems and 358
smoothies 72, 146
snacks 59, 65
   bedtime 307
   healthy 65, 128, 137, 142,
      154, 155, 161, 294–5, 329
   persistent snacking 65
   television and 59
sneezing, etiquette of 269
snoring 90, 304, 305, 361
   remedies for 304
soap, dry skin and 297–8
soba noodles 367
social connections 30–31,
   42–43, 44, 86–87, 103,
   239, 246–51, 344–5
   committing to 250
   internet and 87, 248
   mealtimes and 158, 159
   mutual assistance 239
   spirituality and 256
   weeding out 250
   see also relationships
socks 305
sodium 21, 76, 114, 162–4, 325
   excess 325, 362
   Ménières's disease and 362
   see also salt
soft drinks 45, 47, 59, 74–75,
   167, 306
   see also fizzy drinks

sorbets 166
sores 293
sorghum 135
soup 154
soya bean oil 136
soya beans 122, 142, 323, 325–6, 338, 367
soya milk 142, 147, 366
soy sauce 164
spices 163
spinach 50, 121, 126, 147, 295, 325, 329, 347, 357, 367
spinal disc movement 291
spiritual advisers 257
spirituality 239, 256–7
sports
  companion sports 249
  risky 375
  see also individual activities
sports creams 272
sports injuries 57
sports teams 185
Spread Stopper fitness routine 200, 201, 226–37
squash 323
stair-climbing 98, 196, 197, 199
stairways 266
stanols 323
statin drugs 116, 285, 296, 319, 320, 321
STDs (sexually transmitted diseases) 17, 54, 55
stearic acid 149
steroids 56, 303
stock cubes 164
stomach cancer 112, 330, 332, 334
stomach ulcers 60, 61, 84, 277, 280–1, 296
stools 61, 380, 381
storecupboard makeover 172–3
strawberries 123, 129, 357, 362
strength 104
strengths, personal 242
strength training 91, 186–7, 189–91, 193, 197, 199
  Antidote to Ageing programme 214–15, 218–19, 222–3

for arthritis 347, 349
Easy Does It programme 202–3, 206–7, 210–11
gardening as 195
recovery time 190
Spread Stopper programme 226–7, 230–1, 234–5
streptomycin 361
stress 88–89
  bad/good 34–35
  and brain shrinkage 17
  change and 109
  chronic 88, 258, 291
  detrimental effects 33, 44, 47, 244
  exercise, benefits of 160, 180, 181
  financial 31, 46, 68
  management 21, 28, 29, 88–89, 91, 92, 104, 239, 240, 260–1
  and memory problems 14, 15
  resistance to 258, 260–1
  stress-eating 158, 160
  stress resiliency 32, 240
  workaholism and 69
stress hormones 32, 33, 47, 84, 86, 88, 103, 109, 256, 260
stress incontinence 308, 309, 310
stretching 191, 193, 264, 287, 289
  for arthritis 349
  for back pain 291
  exercises 204–5, 208, 208–9, 212–13, 216–17, 220–1, 224–5, 228–9, 232–3, 236–7, 291
  gardening as 195
  and muscle pain 288
strokes 25, 29, 114, 136, 162, 167, 171, 240, 322
  aspirin and 296
  depression and 252
  ischaemic 327
  PAD and 293
  risk of 46, 62, 71, 115, 246, 252, 293, 316, 317, 318, 324–5, 327–9, 345

smoking and 49
symptoms 381
vascular impairment 344
substance P 287
sugar 21, 134, 162, 166–7, 321
  brown 134
  cravings 71, 114, 167
  refined 163, 167
  sugary foods 71
sugar-free gum 275, 276
sugar rush 284
sulphoraphane 126
sunburn 46, 50, 82–83, 331
sun damage 50–51, 82–83, 297, 357
sunflower oil 136
sunflower seeds 139, 147
sunglasses 356, 357
sunlight 54, 269, 271, 289, 347
  eye protection 356, 357
sun protection factor (SPF) 82–83
sun-protection water shirt 83
sunscreens 50, 51, 82–83
sun-sensitising drugs 357
superfoods 121, 128–9, 131, 137
superoxide dismutase 26
supplements 167–71
  for arthritis 348
  calcium 116, 143, 169–70, 265, 307
  calorie supplements 371
  fibre 322
  fish oil 171, 286, 299, 321, 322, 344, 356, 371
  garlic 269
  iron 170, 285
  magnesium 265, 307
  multivitamins 116, 167, 168–9
  vision-protecting 357–8
  vitamin D 116, 167, 169, 265, 289
surgeons 378
sweetcorn 355
sweeteners, artificial 71
sweet potatoes 323, 325, 362

swimming 184, 287, 291, 347–8
Swiss chard 347, 357, 361
symptoms
  common 263
  emergency 381
  ignoring 81, 262
systemic lupus erythematosus (SLE) 56

T

tabbouleh 135
table tennis 185
Tagamet (cimetidine) 280, 281
tahini 147
tai chi chuan 181, 182, 191, 193, 194, 199, 264, 305, 367
Tamiflu (oseltamivir) 271
tangerines 128, 357
tanning beds 82
tannins 128, 165
taste 116
taygay philosophy of life 239
tea 21, 128, 132, 155, 159, 306, 326, 332
  black 366
  chamomile 306
  green 83, 110, 366
  herbal 306
  jasmine 128
  oolong 366
teeth
  brushing 274, 275, 327
  colour changes 276
  flossing 274, 327
  plaque 273, 274, 276
  tooth decay 273
  tooth loss 273, 353
  whitening treatments 276
  see also gum disease
telephones 266
television 47, 59, 108, 245, 345
telomerase 258
telomeres 258
tendons 27, 191
tennis 185, 249, 264, 287
testicles 380
tetracycline 170, 361

TFF2 protein 281
thiamin 113, 168
thighs, exercises for 209, 218, 219, 230, 231, 233
thinking
  fuzzy 115
  negative 32
  positive 32, 33, 89, 102, 198
thinking skills 340, 341, 342
thirties, signs of ageing in 19
throat cancer 62, 66
throat pain 381
thymus gland 120
thyroid disorders 341
thyroid hormones 170
thyroid, underactive 252
tin 169
tinnitus 362
tiny bladder syndrome 306
tiredness 282
  see also fatigue
tofu 110, 147, 338
tomatoes 51, 83, 117, 129, 154, 161, 329
tomato juice 117, 127
tomato sauce 121, 334
tongues, cleaning 274
tongue-scrapers 274
toothbrushes, electric 274
Townshend, Pete 11
toxins 137, 170, 330, 337, 369
tranquillisers 116
trans fats 21, 25, 43, 65, 78–79, 162, 163, 164–5, 166, 294, 317, 319
treadmills 287
triceps, exercises for 203, 227, 228
triglycerides 78, 138, 171, 317, 318, 320, 321, 323, 328, 329
tryptophan 61
tumours see cancer
tuna 137, 149
turkey 148, 149, 150, 161, 164
turmeric 281
turnips 129, 347, 362
twenties, signs of ageing in 19

U,V

ulcers 60, 61, 280–1
  duodenal 60
  stomach 60, 61, 84, 277, 280–1, 296
ultraviolet (UV) rays 82, 357
unhappiness 47
unhealthy habits and choices
  current 45–46, 47
  of the past 39, 44, 46, 48
  repairing 48–93
urethra 308, 309, 311
urge incontinence 308, 309, 310
urinary problems 279, 308–11
urination schedule 310
urine 132, 279, 380
  paint card test 279
uterine cancer 334, 381
UVA rays 51
UVB rays 51
UV (ultraviolet) rays 82, 357
vaginal bleeding 381
vaginal cones 310
Valium (diazepam) 278
vanadium 169
vancomycin 361
vascular dementia 341, 342, 344, 345
vasopressin 258
vegetable juices 77, 125–6, 344
vegetable oil 254
vegetables
  canned 163
  cruciferous 149, 333
  eating more of 77, 125–7
  frozen 125
  green 112, 113
  health benefits 24, 25, 43, 45, 47, 49, 50, 55, 63, 77, 101, 112, 120, 121, 131, 165, 295
  leafy green 136, 142, 147, 347, 355, 357
  raw 77, 125
  seasonal 173
  snacks 161
  two-colour rule 127

vegetable soup 154
vegetarians 80, 110
vending machines 161
venison 80
visceral fat 23, 318
vision problems 19, 267, 315, 354, 354–8, 355, 357, 358
  cataracts 19, 267, 354, 355, 357, 358
  diabetic retinopathy 358
  falls and 267
  glaucoma 32, 267, 354, 355, 358
  macular degeneration 25, 171, 267, 354, 355, 357
  protection against 355, 357–8
  retinal detachment 381
  vision-protecting supplements 357–8
vitamin A 120, 125, 126, 168, 298, 362
vitamin B_1 see thiamin
vitamin B_2 see riboflavin
vitamin B_3 see niacin
vitamin B_6 126, 132, 143, 148, 149, 168, 329
vitamin B_{12} 143, 149, 168, 254, 329
vitamin C 24, 117, 126, 168, 269, 281, 295, 298, 344, 353, 357, 358, 362, 367
vitamin D 51, 56, 83, 115, 142, 168, 269, 271, 317, 330, 332, 338, 347, 351
  deficiency 115, 269, 289
  supplements 116, 167, 169, 265, 289
vitamin E 117, 132, 140, 168, 298, 344, 358, 362, 367
vitamin K 126, 347, 351
volleyball 287
volunteering 13, 87, 249, 250

W

waist size 23, 377
walking 108, 183, 184, 185, 194, 265, 272, 321
  for back pain 291
  barefoot 348
  for circulation problems 294
  dog walking 185
  fatigue and 282
  for lowering blood pressure 326
  mood, positive effects on 254
  Nordic walking 190
  pace 183, 199, 245
  PAD and 294
  'walkable' neighbourhoods 253
  weight loss and 199
wallets 292
walnut oil 140
walnuts 113, 114, 128, 137, 139, 161, 294–5, 307, 320–1, 328, 338
warfarin 171, 286, 322, 323, 327, 351
water
  drinking sufficient 21, 76, 133, 265, 276, 284
  excessive intake 76
  health benefits 132, 334
  incontinence and 306
  instead of sugary drinks 74, 155, 161
  sparkling 132
water aerobics 287, 348
weight
  checks 380
  healthy 342, 371
  older people 19, 22–23
  swings 22
  see also dieting
weight loss
  for arthritis 346–7
  benefits of 108, 278, 286, 321, 334
  exercise and 182, 199
  for incontinence 310
  for joint pain 286
  in old age 22–23
  overemphasis on 152–3
  unexplained 58, 377, 381
  walking and 199
weight training 23, 26, 176, 187, 351
  lower-body training 190
  posture 190
  repetitions 189
  sets 189
wet heat 287
wheat germ 323, 355, 362
white beans 122
white noise 362
white noise machines 304
whole-grain bread 107, 108, 113, 131, 133, 161, 328
whole-grain cereals 108, 132, 134
whole-grain pasta 113
whole grains 113, 130–5, 321, 344, 355, 366
wild rice 135
wine 306
  red 128, 344
  white 165
  see also alcohol
workaholics 46, 69
working after retirement 249
worry 88, 102
worry time, scheduling 305–6
wound healing 116, 120
wrinkles 19, 43, 49, 50, 62, 77, 82, 297, 369
wrists, exercises for 205

X, Y, Z

xylitol 275, 276
yeast infections 120
yoga 89, 165, 191, 193, 199, 261, 264, 285, 291
yoghurt 142–3, 146, 167, 323, 329, 355
  fat-free 142, 146
  frozen 146
  live-culture 281
zanamivir (Relenza) 271
Zanprol (omeprazole) 280
Zantac (ranitidine) 281
zeaxanthin 120, 355, 357
zinc 113, 114, 116, 148, 149, 169, 355, 367
zinc lozenges 271, 353
zinc oxide 358
Zovirax (acyclovir) 300

The Body Repair and Maintenance Manual is published by The Reader's Digest Association Limited, 11 Westferry Circus, Canary Wharf, London E14 4HE
Copyright © 2009 Reader's Digest Association Limited
Copyright © 2009 Reader's Digest Association Far East Limited
Philippines Copyright © 2009 Reader's Digest Association Far East Limited
Copyright © 2009 Reader's Digest (Australia) Pty Limited
Copyright © 2009 Reader's Digest India Pvt Limited
Copyright © 2009 Reader's Digest Asia Pvt Limited

The Body Repair and Maintenance Manual is adapted from *Long Life Prescription*, published by The Reader's Digest Association, Inc., USA, in 2008.

We are committed both to the quality of our products and the service we provide to our customers. We value your comments, so please do contact us on **08705 113366** or via our website at **www.readersdigest.co.uk**

If you have any comments or suggestions about the content of our books, email us at **gbeditorial@readersdigest.co.uk**

Origination Colour Systems Limited, London
Printing and binding in China

Reader's Digest Project Team
Writers Sarí Harrar, Debra Gordon
Consultant Sheena Meredith MB BS
Nutritionist Fiona Hunter BSc Hons (Nutrition), Dip. Dietetics
Project Editor John Andrews
Art Editors Jane McKenna, Simon Webb
Editor Ali Moore
Researcher Angelika Romacker
Picture Researcher Rosie Taylor
Proofreader Barry Gage
Indexer Marie Lorimer

Reader's Digest General Books
Editorial Director Julian Browne
Art Director Anne-Marie Bulat
Head of Book Development Sarah Bloxham
Managing Editor Nina Hathway
Picture Resource Manager Sarah Stewart-Richardson
Pre-press Account Manager Dean Russell
Product Production Manager Claudette Bramble
Production Controller Katherine Tibbals

Picture credits

L = left, R = right, T = top, C = centre, B = bottom

Front cover Getty Images Ltd/Tony Anderson/Taxi **Back cover** Corbis/© Benelux/zefa **Spine** Punchstock/DigitalVision **1** ShutterStock, Inc/Johanna Goodyear **2** iStockphoto.com/Andresr **19** ShutterStock, Inc/Martina Ebel **26** ShutterStock, Inc/Lisa F. Young **29** ShutterStock, Inc/Xalanx **30** ShutterStock, Inc/Monkey Business Images **32** ShutterStock, Inc **46** iStockphoto.com/Christine Balderas **48 C** ShutterStock, Inc/ nazira_g **R** ShutterStock, Inc/Dana Bartekoske **50** ShutterStock, Inc/Dana Bartekoske **52** ShutterStock, Inc/Marc Dietrich **53** iStockphoto.com/Alex Bramwell **62** iStockphoto.com/NickyBlade **63** ShutterStock, Inc/Jasenka Luköa **67** ShutterStock, Inc/Tomasz Trojanowski **70** ShutterStock, Inc/Maksymilian Skolik **72** ShutterStock, Inc/Westbury **75** ShutterStock, Inc/Scott Karcich **76** ShutterStock, Inc/Cloki **78** ShutterStock, Inc/Mariusz Szachowski **82** ShutterStock, Inc/Michal Bednarek **86** ShutterStock, Inc/Monkey Business Images **89** ShutterStock, Inc/nazira_g **106** Alamy Images/Kirsty-Anne Glubish/Design Pics Inc **110 L** ShutterStock, Inc/Sasa Petkovic **R** iStockphoto.com/Floortje **113** ShutterStock, Inc/Monkey Business Images **117** iStockphoto.com/Klaudia Steiner **118 L** ShutterStock, Inc/Artemis Gordon **R** ShutterStock, Inc/Juriah Mosin **121** ShutterStock, Inc/Kai Hecker **124** ShutterStock, Inc/Monkey Business Images **126-7** ShutterStock, Inc/Bernd Jurgens **129 T** ShutterStock, Inc/Mashe **B** ShutterStock, Inc/Iakov Kalinin **132** ShutterStock, Inc/Valeriy Velikov **138** ShutterStock, Inc/Paul Turner **141** iStockphoto.com/Che McPherson **143** ShutterStock, Inc/Olga Lyubkina **145** Punchstock/Ciaran Griffin/Stockbyte **147** ShutterStock, Inc/Freddy Eliasson **153** ShutterStock, Inc/Apollofoto **159** ShutterStock, Inc/Mike Flippo **165** iStockphoto.com/Jason Reekie **166** ShutterStock, Inc/Ultimathule **171** iStockphoto.com/Malgorzata Korpas **184** ShutterStock, Inc/Eric Gevaert **185** ShutterStock, Inc/chasmer **186** ShutterStock, Inc/Tom Grill **191** ShutterStock, Inc/Glenda M. Powers **199** ShutterStock, Inc/Miodrag Gajic **200 L** ShutterStock, Inc/Val Thoermer **R** ShutterStock, Inc/Yuri Arcurs **241** iStockphoto.com/Michael Kemter **244** ShutterStock, Inc/James Steidl **246** ShutterStock, Inc/Andresr **251** ShutterStock, Inc/Monkey Business Images **261** ShutterStock, Inc/Galina Barskaya **262 L** ShutterStock, Inc/Junial Enterprises **C** ShutterStock, Inc/Jason Stitt **267** ShutterStock, Inc/Yurok **268** ShutterStock, Inc/Tamasz Trojanowski **270** ShutterStock, Inc/Tatiana Popova **275** iStockphoto.com/Roman Kob Zarev **279** ShutterStock, Inc/Lai Seet Ying **281** Punchstock/Jutta Klee/fStop **284** ShutterStock, Inc/Peter Blottman **288** ShutterStock, Inc/Martin Novak **290** ShutterStock, Inc/Marc Dietrich **292** ShutterStock, Inc/Alexsandra Nadeina **296** ShutterStock, Inc/iofoto **299** ShutterStock, Inc/IKO **300** ShutterStock, Inc/Yuri Arcurs **304** ShutterStock, Inc/Monkey Business Images **307** ShutterStock, Inc/Diego Cervo **311** ShutterStock, Inc/Levent Aydin **314 L** ShutterStock, Inc/Monkey Business Images **C** iStockphoto.com/Joan Vicent Canto Roig **316** ShutterStock, Inc/Monkey Business Images **318** iStockphoto.com/Ljupco **322** ShutterStock, Inc/Noel Powell, Schaumburg **323** ShutterStock, Inc/Khomulo Anna **328** iStockphoto.com/Andrew Manley **330** ShutterStock, Inc/Monkey Business Images **333** ShutterStock, Inc/LockstockBob **335** ShutterStock, Inc/Monkey Business Images **340** ShutterStock, Inc/Tatiana Popova **349** ShutterStock, Inc/Losevsky Pavel **353** iStockphoto.com/Joe Potato **354** ShutterStock, Inc/Alex James Bramwell **356** ShutterStock, Inc/Elena Elisseeva **361** ShutterStock, Inc/Kulish Viktoriia **362** ShutterStock, Inc/Edwin Verin **366** ShutterStock, Inc/Monkey Business Images **380** iStockphoto.com/Chris Hutchison

Photography by Jill Wachter is © Jill Wachter

Additional photography courtesy of Jupiter Images, Reader's Digest Publications and Getty Images

Concept code: US4792/G
Book code: 400-418 UP0000-1
ISBN: 978 0 276 44501 9
Oracle Code: 250013208S.00.24